Community-Based Health Care

Other Books by Management Sciences for Health

Beyond the Clinic Walls: Case Studies in Community-Based Distribution
James A. Wolff et al.

Ensuring Equal Access to Health Services: User Fee Systems and the Poor
William Newbrander, David Collins, and Lucy Gilson

*Extending Access to Health Care through Public-Private Partnerships:
The PROSALUD Experience*
Carlos J. Cuéllar, William Newbrander, and Gail Price

*The Family Planning Manager's Handbook: Basic Skills and Tools for
Managing Family Planning Programs*
ed. James A. Wolff, Linda J. Suttenfield, and Susanna C. Binzen

*Health Care in Muslim Asia: Development and Disorder in Wartime
Afghanistan*
ed. Ronald W. O'Connor

*Lessons from FPMD: Decentralizing the Management of Health and Family
Planning Programs*
Riitta-Liisa Kolehmainen-Aitken and William Newbrander

Lessons from MSH: Strategic Planning: Reflections on Process and Practice
Sylvia Vriesendorp

*Management Strategies for Improving Health and Family Planning Services:
A Compendium of* The Manager *Series, Vols. V–IX*
ed. Janice Miller, Claire Bahamon, Laura Lorenz, and Kim Atkinson

*Managing Drug Supply: The Selection, Procurement, Distribution, and Use
of Pharmaceuticals,* with the World Health Organization, 2nd edition

MOST—Management and Organizational Sustainability Tool

Myths and Realities about the Decentralization of Health Systems
ed. Riitta-Liisa Kolehmainen-Aitken

Private Health Sector Growth in Asia: Issues and Implications
ed. William Newbrander (Chichester, England: John Wiley & Sons)

Community-Based Health Care

Lessons from Bangladesh to Boston

edited by Jon Rohde and John Wyon

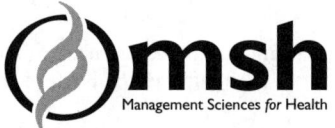

in collaboration with the Harvard School of Public Health

Management Sciences for Health Tel.: 617.524.7799
165 Allandale Rd. Fax: 617.524.2825
Boston, MA 02130-3400 Web site: www.msh.org/publications
  Orders: bookstore@msh.org
ISBN 978-0-913723-83-8

Interior design and composition: Jenna Dixon
Proofreader: Beth Richards
Indexer: Pierce Butler

Library of Congress Cataloging-in-Publication Data
Community-based health care : lessons from Bangladesh to Boston / edited by
  Jon Rohde and John Wyon.
       p.   cm.
    Includes bibliographical references and index.
    ISBN 978-0-913723-83-8 (softcover : alk. paper)
      1. Community health services—Cross-cultural studies. 2. Public health—Cross-
    cultural studies. 3. Medical care—Cross-cultural studies. I. Rohde, Jon E. II. Wyon,
    J. B. (John Benjamin), 1918-
    RA425.C737   2002
    362.1'2—dc21   2001059080

Printed in the United States of America on acid-free paper by Thomson-Shore
with vegetable-oil based ink.

♾The paper used in this publication meets the minimum requirements of the American
National Standard for Information Sciences—Permanence of Paper for Printed
Library Materials, ANSI Z39.48-1984.

10 9 8 7 6 5 4 3 2 1   08 07 06 05 04 03 02

Contents

Foreword

The importance of this book drawn from the Symposium on Community-Based Health Care: Lessons from Bangladesh to Boston, and of the meeting itself, is to lay to rest the notion that we have little to learn from societies very different from our own, that our systems and experience are so narrowly constrained by our culture and economic status as to be irrelevant to those in very different material circumstances or with different histories.

What these lessons teach us is that Boston *should* understand Bangladesh, *not solely for intellectual purposes,* nor so that it can assist Bangladesh, but to better understand itself and its own programs, and to see models and ideas that will have relevance for Boston's work. Policymakers in the wealthy nations can learn much about community education for behavior change, about outreach to disempowered and marginalized populations, about the use of community workers and ancillary personnel, and about relating health and other sectors in a great variety of settings.

These lessons show us that Bangladesh has something to learn from Boston that it can *use,* not merely a fantasy system of care beyond the reach of all but the richest societies. Program directors in the developing world can learn much about community empowerment and control, about the use of data and evaluation, and about management and information systems. Both the symposium itself in November 2000 and this compilation and analysis demonstrate the utility of learning from each other, even when the lesson learned is "Don't do what we did!"

We have much to learn from one another, and what we learn is not always what we have started out to study. Often an examination of teaching and communication materials leads to an understanding of cultural diversity and sensitivity and its utility in improving health by making services more appropriate as well as more accessible. Often a look at using paraprofessional and community workers as a cost-saving device leads to an understanding of the improved outcomes produced by peer educators and leaders. Similarly, a study of data can lead us to better understand and identify proxies when hard data are not available; and frequently a search for explanations and causes leads to better understanding of the relationship between health and economic status, or education, or environment, or housing, or violence.

We have too often assumed that models of health care, delivery systems, financing, and community-based approaches could only be studied—or used—in similar situations, in peer societies, with similar material means and economic or political systems. What we have learned, and what the symposium furthers, is that very dissimilar societies, with very different constraints, can benefit from understanding how others work and what can be used in organizing societies to improve health.

In Boston, arguably the medical center of the United States, health status in poor neighborhoods was improved more by adopting the community health center model of South Africa than by the presence of a multitude of world-class research institutions. The infant mortality initiatives of Costa Rica, the system of community health workers in Jamaica, and the outreach to young fathers in Kenya have all informed and shaped programs in Boston's neighborhoods. As Commissioner of Health and Hospitals in Boston 10 years ago, I looked as much to communities in the southern hemisphere for ideas and models as I did to those in other big American cities. Healthy Boston, like the healthy communities movement worldwide, benefits from this sharing of information, ideas, and approaches. Lessons Without Borders, a project of the US Agency for International Development, adapted this approach and examined the programs it funded or designed in the developing world. It returned those to the United States that would improve both inner city and remote rural health.

At the same time, we found that our colleagues from those countries from whom we had borrowed ideas or programs were equally interested in the transformation that occurred to them in our society and often regarded them as improvements or evolutions of the original model, and adopted our adaptations.

This process of sharing, shaping, and redesigning occurs only where there is openness of spirit as well as of mind. But increasingly, both

occur. These lessons also broaden our understanding of the determinants of health and the barriers to care. When we examine other societies who have resources we do not, or barriers we have overcome, and
still see health and access disparities, we have greater understanding
and purpose.

From Boston to Bangladesh, from Haiti to Hamburg, there is much
to learn, much to excite us about the possibilities of communities' role
in their own health; when we look through a window, we often see our
own reflection.

—*Judith Kurland*
Regional Director, US Department
of Health and Human Services

Preface

The gathering of health ministers from around the world at Alma-Ata, Kazakhstan, in 1978 was arguably the most influential meeting of its kind in the history of public health. The Declaration of Alma-Ata remains one of the most influential yet debated documents in the field of health, with its call for meaningful involvement of communities in the design and control of affordable health services. Can it work for the billions of poor today? Or is it simply an ideal?

The symposium on which this book is based was held in November 2000, sponsored by the Harvard School of Public Health, Management Sciences for Health, and the Rockefeller Foundation. The meeting was an opportunity both for those who were involved in the Alma-Ata conference and for those who have been practitioners of its recommendations to share experiences, debate the principles, and attempt once again to interpret the lessons of primary health care (PHC) in an effort to reach "health for all." The symposium, and the book that emerged from it, reached back to the antecedents of PHC in the mid-19th century, considered the technological advances following World War II, and looked to see how experiences since Alma-Ata have influenced health and health services in countries as poor as Bangladesh and as rich as the United States.

Can it work? Surely yes! Many projects have amply proven this: Jamkhed in India has reduced infant mortality from 160 to 18 or less, endemic malnutrition has virtually disappeared, and fertility has fallen to under 3 children per family in a poor rural area with a population of 200,000. (See the bibliography for sources on this and other projects.) The Narangwal Project in the Punjab proved the success of the Bhore Commission model of family planning and essential care provided by health auxiliaries in rural villages. Piaxtla in Mexico demonstrated the power of an activated community to provide care for itself. Sidney Kark, before he was driven by apartheid from his home country of South Africa, demonstrated the power of social medicine by treating families in a community context and addressing the cultural-behavioral determinants of health. This book presents examples from Bangladesh, Bolivia, Germany, Haiti, Nepal, Peru, Tibet, the United States, and Vietnam. All of these had a common factor: visionary leaders to drive the process. While all involved the community in some way, it was the vision and energy of dedicated leaders that made the projects work. Indeed, often the results did not outlast the presence of the founding leader. Alma-Ata was silent on this crucial element.

Can community-based PHC reach large populations? Again yes! But with caveats. Barefoot Doctors, a national extension of the Ting Hsien model of John Grant and Jimmy Yen of the 1930s, surely reached most of China in a sustainable fashion. Top-down in policy and organization, it was grounded and paid for by each work group, each community. Accountability was entirely local. Yet this remarkably effective, equitable, and affordable system folded with the collapse of the centrally directed economic system, which left communities prey to the uncertainties of the marketplace. A fee-for-service system replaced work points, and with it both preventive medicine and equity were largely lost. One wonders whether market forces can support an equitable health system.

Indonesia has pioneered a system of village initiatives to make health for all affordable. The Dana Sehat scheme, initiated in Solo with small monthly payments by each family into a common pool to pay for medicines, had shared benefits that helped the poorest gain some access to care. But significant health payments exceeded the savings and bankrupted many village schemes. Indonesia's *posyandus* (village health posts) are run entirely by volunteer women who work only one or two days a month, a sustainable level of effort in a community where service is recognized by public approval. These posts started only to weigh children monthly and for mothers to share advice on child rearing. Later they added oral rehydration packets for the most common illness, diarrheal disease, and periodic vitamin A supplements. Then the Indonesian Family Planning Program saw these posts as an easy and reliable way to resupply contraceptive pills. Still later, health outreach workers added immunization services to improve coverage of infants. More recently, some posts have added treatment of minor ailments, and a few are monitoring chronic ailments like arthritis and hypertension in older patients. There are now some 250,000 posts in 65,000 villages, all run by volunteers. The services are of very mixed quality and limited in scope, but the phased approach, embedded in the village tradition of a monthly women's meeting called *arisan,* made this a viable and sustainable large-scale activity reaching most of the country.

These experiences led James Grant of UNICEF to champion GOBI (growth promotion, oral rehydration, breastfeeding, and immunization)—a few things for everyone, needed by rich and poor alike. No doubt the idea was very top-down, but UNICEF chose just a few interventions aimed to be relevant to all children in all nations that would support and strengthen health systems of any design. All too often GOBI became target driven and not built into any system, so it was not sustained. Where it was embraced by a health system, it has lasted and contributed substantially to declining infant and childhood deaths. Where carried out in campaigns, its benefits rapidly faded.

Is community-based PHC affordable? Who pays for it and for how long? As the world swings to the tune of the market economy, we have seen many programs wither and die. Social-sector budgets are early targets of the International Monetary Fund—communities are asked to pick up the tab for health services, and equity is lost. The governments of Sri Lanka and Costa Rica made the unusual decision to give priority to village-based health posts manned by midwives, even at the expense of hospitals. Both those countries have seen their rewards in sustained reduction in mortality and fertility, although their high levels of female education have probably contributed as least as much to this result as the health care system.

A more usual response is seen in Bangladesh, where the government has provided a few essential services and encouraged NGOs to work with communities through a large array of approaches to provide responsive health and development initiatives. BRAC has covered this country of 110 million people with house-to-house demonstrations of oral rehydration therapy and achieved a high rate of TB cure with trained community workers paid largely through sale of a few inexpensive drugs. BRAC's annual budget is US$132 million, of which 74% is generated within Bangladesh from BRAC's own activities and programs. NGOs immunized the country and distribute vitamin A twice annually. This book explores some of those approaches and finds the results impressive (see chapters 4 and 5). Meanwhile, the government has concentrated on family planning, modifying its approach with a strong element of continuous operational field research, achieving the most dramatic fall in fertility of any poor nation. Affordability may mean learning what you can pay for and staying within those limits, leaving the communities to set their own priorities with their own resources. In Bangladesh, many have found it necessary to *exclude* those who can best afford to pay, as they tend to take over the system, be it health, credit, or education. This inverts the standard wisdom of cross-subsidy often applied to social insurance schemes.

Is community-based PHC sustainable? Here the record falters. Often projects do not outlast their founding leaders. Overambitious expansion in both population served and range of services can exceed financial resources and management capacity. Especially vulnerable is the voice of the community, which these studies show to be critical to success. Chapters describe issues of financing (chapter 10); choice and adaptation of technologies (chapter 7); and various levels of community involvement and tradeoffs between scale and comprehensiveness (chapter 6). While large government systems run by tax revenues have the scale, they rarely have the responsiveness to or ownership by the people they serve and are thereby less effective, even in health outcomes.

No discussion of PHC can be considered comprehensive today in the absence of strategies to deal with the HIV epidemic. Some 45 million infections worldwide are estimated to date, with 25 million deaths, and in many countries the curve continues to rise. In contrast to many infections, HIV is often shrouded in secrecy, shame, and recrimination, the victims blamed for their fate. Yet this epidemic underscores the failure of the very fundamentals of PHC, for it can *only* be prevented, not cured, and *only* through knowledge, social action, and culturally sensitive measures taken by the people themselves. While the power of science has found means to ameliorate and defer the devastating clinical effects of this infection, social inequities between nations deny the majority of sufferers the respite these advances could offer. The inequities exposed by this epidemic challenge the very principles of global public health. The symposium regrettably did not grapple with this important issue.

The second part of this collection discusses recent experiences in the United States and Germany, uncovering a remarkable parallel with poorer countries. We are reminded that the antecedents of the community health center movement in this country lay in South Africa, India, and postwar Europe. The principles developed and applied at Many Farms (Arizona), Columbia Point (Boston), Lexington (Kentucky), and more recently Watts (Los Angeles) and Roxbury (Boston) emphasize social determinants of health, teamwork, and a strong role for the community. Linking such grounded programs with academic centers, to ensure that graduates have a pragmatic appreciation for social issues and the ability and inclination to work with community representatives, is an ongoing challenge. John Knowles pointed out years ago that 80 percent of the advance in life expectancy since World War II has been due to social factors and behavioral change; medical technology plays a steadily decreasing role. Yet when budget cuts come, it is the social services, the poverty reduction strategies, the home visits, and health education that go first.

Whether we are considering rural Nepal or the Mayo Clinic, good health information plays a central role in enabling planners to design appropriate interventions as well as to share with communities an understanding of the epidemiology. From an initial situation analysis to design of service mix and choice of technologies to research on better approaches to health care, to monitoring and reporting on progress, a robust health information system is a critical part of reaching health for all. It is also a critical tool in motivating communities, donors, and governments to provide needed funds. Nothing speaks like the facts, whether in Bangladesh or Boston!

The following questions may help the reader explore the diverse lessons of this book:

- What is the role of the community in this approach? How is it involved?
- Who should choose the priorities for implementation and how?
- What is the role of measurement in planning? Implementation?
- What is the mix of technologies chosen? And the modifications to suit cultures?

- Is it sustainable? How? How cost-effective is it compared to other approaches?
- What is the role of charismatic leadership? Can the approach outlast the leader?
- What political considerations contributed to the success or difficulties faced by the community-based PHC program?
- How does one avoid being taken over by vested interests and the rich?
- What is the role of women and how does this approach empower or liberate them?
- Is there evidence to support the belief that female education is an important determinant of health, perhaps even more than health care?
- How important are health technology and specific antidisease programs, in contrast to health behavior and healthy lifestyles?
- What is the relationship between community-based health services run by the community and government health services?
- What is the optimal mix of professional capacity and ratios of different levels of workers in a large-scale community program?
- How does one address the fundamental problem of poverty as a prime determinant of health among the poor?
- What should a health program do about nutrition and food?
- What are the distinct roles of international, national, and local voluntary and professional agencies?
- What are the crucial roles of universities in poor and in rich countries?

The discussions at the symposium often addressed these questions, which will be raised again in the conclusion.

—Jon Rohde

Acknowledgments

This book is based on a symposium held on November 11 and 12, 2000, at the Harvard School of Public Health in Boston. More than 100 people experienced in primary health care, in poor and wealthy countries, met to explore developments since 1978, the year of the meeting of health ministers at Alma-Ata. This symposium was designed to exemplify the main stages of this evolution up to the year 2000, derive their common principles for application elsewhere, and encourage the creation of approaches and methods to improve the health of communities of people.

The symposium had its roots in the Working Group on Community-Based Primary Health Care, a committee of the International Health Section of the American Public Health Association. Many of the contributors have participated in this working group. As the group was planning an event to celebrate the new millennium at APHA's annual meeting in Boston, they learned that the Alumni Council of the Harvard School of Public Health was developing a symposium to showcase models of community-based health care, with a focus on the United States. Its purpose was not only to establish principles for community-based health services but also to produce materials for physicians and others preparing to work as public health and preventive medicine specialists. With the support of Dean Barry Bloom of the Harvard School of Public Health, these two groups, led by Drs. John Wyon and Joan Altekruse (president of the HSPH Alumni Council), joined forces to plan the symposium. The symposium thus expanded to focus on community-based health care in both international and domestic settings.

The planning committee also drew upon Professor John O. Field, retired from Tufts University; Dr. Eliot Putnam, Jr., the former Director of the National Council on International Health (now the Global Health Council); and Ms. Gail Price, the current president of the HSPH Alumni Council and a Senior Program Associate at Management Sciences for Health. MSH is a nonprofit organization, with headquarters in Boston, that has worked in more than 100 countries to improve health systems and services. Dr. Ron O'Connor, MSH's Chief Executive Officer, championed this book, and Ms. Catherine Crone-Coburn, MSH's President, provided support for its development.

The HSPH's Office of Alumni Programs provided extensive assistance for the symposium. The Assistant Dean for Students and Alumni, Dr. Robin Worth, and the staff of that office, principally Ms. Catherine Fratiani, organized the event. We are deeply indebted to HSPH for managing and hosting the symposium. Participants from universities, hospitals, and public and private health institutions in a dozen countries attended. Many MSH staff members participated in the symposium, which MSH also supported.

Dr. Jon Rohde, Senior Advisor to MSH's EQUITY Project in South Africa, was a key participant in the symposium and served as the lead technical editor of this book. Jon Rohde, with assistance from his colleague Dr. Barbara Timmons at MSH, assembled and edited the chapters in this book. Ms. Ceallaigh Reddy copyedited many of the chapters. John Wyon was active in reviewing them, suggesting improvements, and following up; some were entirely rewritten. Five new chapters were written especially for this book.

Ms. Judith Kurland composed an inspiring foreword, while Drs. Hugh Fulmer and Anthony Adams contributed the introduction to Part II. Dr. Robert Northrup of Project Hope assisted Dr. Joseph Valadez with the revision of his chapter. Mr. John Pollock of MSH reviewed several chapters and made helpful suggestions. Dr. Paul Farmer of Partners in Health and Brigham and Women's Hospital provided some background materials on HIV/ AIDS. We are grateful to all these people for giving generous amounts of their time so that this book could become more than the proceedings of a conference.

We extend special appreciation to the Rockefeller Foundation for partial funding of the symposium and this book and to the James M. and Cathleen D. Stone Foundation for its contribution to the publication costs.

PART I

EXPERIENCES IN DEVELOPING COUNTRIES

Introduction to Part I:
A Brief History of Community-Based
Primary Health Care

John Wyon and Jon Rohde

In 1865, Prussia's Chancellor Bismarck, concerned about the quality of recruits entering his army, created the first system of primary health care for a whole nation, providing access to a doctor for all poor families. In 1911, the British parliament, led by Lloyd George and Winston Churchill, passed a National Health Insurance Bill to give every family earning less than 500 pounds a year access to a doctor of their choice. The 1911 law was extended in 1948 to all living in the British Isles. By now, most relatively wealthy countries have similar arrangements for medical care, yet many people around the world are still left out. This book presents experiences in poor and wealthy countries, seeking lessons relevant in both settings.

Where did the concept of community-based primary health care originate? Many historians of health would say from the efforts of John Grant working in China at Peking Union Medical College for the Rockefeller Foundation in the 1920s and '30s. Leaving the compounds of the most modern hospital and medical school in that vast country, Grant established health services based on locally recruited lay workers in rural Ting Hsien county. His effort to reach an entire defined population with major attention to preventive measures to preserve and promote health and only modest efforts to treat disease initiated the

20th-century model of PHC. He teamed up with Jimmy Yen, who carried the literacy movement into rural China, believing that human welfare and progress depended on the ability to read and write. Grant's emphasis on preventive measures and the use of locally recruited and trained paraprofessionals was extended by Dr. John L. Hydrick to the Dutch East Indies and later, by Grant, to India. His work was eventually embraced throughout China in the Barefoot Doctors movement of the 1960s that followed the Cultural Revolution and brought improved health to a population nearing one billion people.

In the early days of the Japanese invasion of China, Grant moved to India, where his efforts, still aimed at serving entire communities, evolved into the concept of a "health center" with both medical care provided by doctors and nurses and preventive measures led by lay outreach workers. This population-based approach became the center of the plan for India's national health system. As the secretary of the Bhore Commission, Grant guided independent India's plan for an organized health care system, which extended from a few villages with small midwife centers, through comprehensive primary health centers to district hospitals and higher levels of referral, a model which has been pursued for the past 50 years and imitated in most developing countries throughout the world. The emphasis on prevention and promotion of health, the use of low-level workers, and the definition of an entire population for which the health services are responsible were common features of Grant's models. These principles of population-based PHC still hold good today.

During the early 1940s, Sidney Kark in South Africa, following the report of the Gluckman Commission that identified striking disparities in health among different ethnic and racial groups, established a rural health center as a learning and teaching environment for the provision of comprehensive health promotion and care in Pholela, Natal. Kark, his wife, Emily, and their colleagues focused more on the social aspects of health, recognizing distinct determinants of health and health behavior in the different communities around Durban and in rural Natal. Home visits and community meetings enabled the workers to better understand the cultural context of nutrition, reproduction, hygiene, and social interaction and poverty, which were clearly shown to be the major determinants of health and disease in this population.

Kark called his approach community-oriented primary care (COPC). Drs. Mervyn Susser and Zena Stein, students of Kark, carried the model to the slums of Johannesburg, where they developed the Alexander Community Health Model as perhaps the first large population-based health care system in urban slums. The strong recognition of social, economic, and cultural factors in determining health and the need to address these factors to improve it landed Kark and his colleagues into trouble with the apartheid government, which labeled such concerns "communist" and therefore subversive. By 1960, Kark and others had fled, carrying their lessons to the United States, Israel, and other more receptive environments. The concern about the social determinants of health became an integral part of PHC projects in many nations.

After World War II, increased attention was paid to the technologies of health that could be applied to diseases of entire populations. Epidemiologists had long recognized the role of vectors in the spread of important diseases such as yellow fever and malaria. Although vector control had successfully reduced these scourges in the Western hemisphere, making such engineering accomplishments as the Panama Canal possible, the application of vaccines, insecticides, and new medicines made the prospect of the control of infectious diseases a powerful possibility. In some cases, such as yellow fever, widespread immunization and vector control were largely successful in reducing the burden of illness in large previously infected populations. But an even more ambitious and well-planned global effort to eradicate malaria was confounded by the complexity of the disease epidemiology and of the human environments in which it was found, as well as by the emergence of resistant organisms and vectors, leaving malaria a major scourge even today. Technological approaches can have complex social ramifications.

The widespread application of the oldest vaccine, smallpox, using good epidemiologic surveillance with containment measures, led to the eradication of this disease in the mid-1970s. This triumph continues to lure health planners to the attractiveness of technical interventions, properly applied with good epidemiology, to the needs of world populations. This global success, at a total cost only 5–10 times the annual costs of protecting rich nations from smallpox, fueled enthusiasm for technical solutions to worldwide health problems that offered ultimate eradication or at least control. James Grant, son of John Grant and Executive Director of UNICEF, saw immunization as the "Trojan horse," the intervention that could bring modern health services to every family and, for the first time, offer the prospect of "health for all." His demonstration of global mobilization behind a common health goal led not only to the polio eradication effort, but also to the concept that progressively more comprehensive services could reach into every home, rich or poor. But while Grant envisioned equity in health by incremental inclusion of well-designed, technically sound universal efforts, his detractors found this approach disempowering, dependency producing, devoid of community input. Limited health for all, James Grant's idea of doing a few essential things that could reach everyone, was seen as a threat to comprehensive health under local control. How does one choose between a few health measures for all and all health measures for a few? This is a central dilemma of PHC.

Meanwhile, the relative success of public health measures in the early decades of the century resulted in burgeoning populations and recognition in the second half of the century that human fertility was itself a major threat to health. John Wyon, one of the organizers of the symposium on community-based health care on which this book is based, showed that there was a broad receptivity to birth control, even in the poor agricultural communities in India where he worked. With the development of oral contraceptives and other modern means of birth control, including surgical sterilization procedures, family planning campaigns were launched on a scale and with an approach comparable to those used to control infectious diseases. These family planning methods had limited success when offered simply as technical interventions, however. The experience of the past 50 years has demonstrated the complexity of social and cultural, as well as physiologic, factors in influencing human fertility and epidemic diseases. Public health —that is, the health of the public—can rarely be manipulated by technology alone.

Research has played an important role not only in developing appropriate technologies that can be applied in the field, but also in the study of populations and increasingly the application of social sciences to enable health programs to engage with the very communities they wish to help. Technology turns out to be the simplest part of applied public health. The earlier lessons of Grant and Kark have been found to be essential to the success of even the targeted so-called vertical programs. Thus, in the latter third of the century, notable efforts were made to combine both the social population-based preventive thrusts of the earlier pioneers with the newer technologies becoming available as a result of research in the area of vaccines, effective drugs, and contraceptives.

A further key contribution was the demonstration by John Gordon of the importance of community-based epidemiology to the understanding of disease and health determinants in a population. He had demonstrated the value of house-to-house surveillance in documenting an epidemic of scarlet fever in a defined community in Romania in the 1930s, delineating the spread and consequences of the disease. To measure the impact of new birth control technologies on health and fertility in a rural population, he designed the Khanna Study in rural India based on similar household surveillance. Over several years, John Wyon, who led a staff of 30 interviewers, recorded monthly data on each family, revealing not only determinants of fertility previously unappreciated, such as lactational amenorrhea and gender preference, but also the high rates of tetanus, diarrhea, and pneumonia as causes of early childhood death, and resulting high fertility. Surprisingly, over 50 percent of couples of reproductive age used contraceptives at some time during the five years of observation.

In the early 1960s, when US and Pakistani public health investigators opened the Cholera Research Laboratory in East Pakistan (today Bangladesh), they established a field study area in Matlab, a rural riverine district, to study the protective effect of cholera vaccines. A household census of over 100,000 people was conducted on principles developed at Khanna and updated fortnightly to monitor the impact of various health interventions, eventually demonstrating the ineffectiveness of cholera vaccine to control epidemics, as well as defining a wide range of demographic and health parameters. The census continues to be updated every two weeks. This population has grown to 200,000 and is today the most thoroughly studied rural population of its size in the world, the central field laboratory of the International Centre for Diarrheal Disease Research, Bangladesh (ICDDR,B) and its Centre for

Health and Population Research. This field-based study area, with its support hospital and laboratories, has been central to many of the advances made in public health over the past 40 years and features prominently in the story of improved health and declining fertility in Bangladesh, which is described in chapters 4 and 5.

Following the Khanna Study, Carl Taylor demonstrated the affordability of using auxiliary nurses to provide community-based services in Narangwal in the Punjab, lessons which were extended to Companyganj in Bangladesh by Colin McCord and colleagues at the outset of that country's independence in 1972. The larger community-based health systems established by the Aroles of Jamkhed in central India (see chapter 3) and Zafrullah Chowdhury at Gonoshasthaya Kendra near Dhaka demonstrated the importance of doctors gaining people's acceptance through first providing quality medical care for the sick, in both these cases in a simple but effective rural hospital setting. Once the confidence of the community had been gained, the doctors extended preventive and promotive services into the villages, eventually addressing the underlying social and crucial economic determinants of health, which became the central focus of these programs. While the community was surely the prime concern of these dedicated and imaginative doctors, they responded initially to the community's wish to have effective curative care by introducing preventive measures in the fields of nutrition, immunization, and *only later* family planning. They extended activities in both of these large population areas (roughly 250,000 population each) slowly and in consultation with the community by training community members to increasingly provide for the most common problems. Activities progressed from curative medical services, through social and economic interventions, and then preventive health services.

The Indian government, recognizing the importance of the Jamkhed approach, undertook a massive program in the late 1970s, the village health volunteer (VHW) scheme, which eventually recruited and trained more than half a million community workers throughout India. Unfortunately, this initiative was an expensive failure. Although it attempted to extend health services into the community through the use of locally trained volunteers, it made no accommodation for their ongoing training, supervision, motivation, and direct linkage with a caring and responsive health care system such as that provided by the Aroles in Jamkhed. The government scheme lacked concerned and committed leaders. The assumption that the communities would see the PHC system of the government as caring and responsive was rarely fulfilled, and the community health workers were often left without guidance, motivation, or support. The token payment of 50 rupees (then about US$5) per month became a crushing economic burden when more than 500,000 VHWs became involved and began to ask for wage increases and other benefits. The unsupported volunteers came to see government salaries as the logical fruit of their efforts rather than recognition of service to their neighbors.

A further reason for the failure was the lack of appreciation for all the nonmedical elements of the Jamkhed approach: water supply, improved market access, agricultural inputs, land reclamation, and animal rearing. Had the vision of the community development blocks, the integrated approach to rural development that India initiated in the 1950s across the entire nation, been linked to the community health effort of the VHWs, the synergy of health and economic improvement might well have made the effort a success.

While the conference of 110 national ministers of health at Alma-Ata in 1978 encouraged community ownership, "going to scale" or meeting the health needs of large populations became the challenge of the late 20th century. Programs constantly sought to balance the need to involve the community in both determining and providing the conditions for improved health with the desire to apply available and affordable technologies to vast populations over large areas. The malaria eradication effort had addressed this complexity through a highly standardized approach, recruiting its own staff, including not only field workers but also management. This vertical structure enabled the service to function independently and extend activities from its national headquarters to the most peripheral village. When malaria eradication turned out to be unsustainable, this failure fueled some unwarranted pejorative characterizations of vertical programs.

Similarly, family planning programs, notably in India and Indonesia, and initially in Bangladesh, recruited their own workers, who were accountable through a system independent of the regular Ministry of Health for their performance and through which they received their salaries, supplies, training, and supervision. In Indonesia, the system reached into all 65,000 villages with family planning field workers. It was then enlarged at the community level through the *posyandu* (village health post) system. This system too depended on support and encouragement from above, but it thrived as an extension of a well-supported vertical family planning program. It was jeopardized throughout the country with the political disruption surrounding the overthrow of President Suharto. The rehabilitation of this community-based volunteer system is a large undertaking presently challenging the Indonesian Ministry of Health. Sustainability of PHC, both in financing and in leadership, has proved a recurring challenge in all PHC models, whether vertical or community based.

Surely the largest effort at provision of community health services was the Barefoot Doctors program of China, a successful effort to apply a mixture of modern medicine, traditional health practices, and promotive health behaviors, designed from above but sustained by local economic self-reliance. While this system, along with the major public health campaigns directed from the central ministry in China, accounted for tremendous improvements in the health and longevity of the Chinese people, it collapsed precipitously with the privatization of health services and the economy in the 1980s. While medical care services are still widely available in China, the preventive and promotive aspects for which the Barefoot Doctors were recognized worldwide have yet to reach previous levels in the new privatized China.

Bangladesh was a latecomer to PHC, with a weak government-operated, top-down system of health services under the Pakistani government from 1947 until independence in 1971. The experiences of many motivated young Bangladeshi health professionals working among the 10 million refugees who fled to India during the War of Liberation, as well as the experiences of many who stayed behind to contribute to the liberation by addressing the most pressing health, social, and economic needs of the population, helped shape the new Bangladesh. Those who returned in 1972 found an ailing country in great poverty with virtually no functioning health care.

Bangladesh, the "international basket case" of Henry Kissinger some 25 years ago, has made more progress in the past 30 years than any other poor country. The rapid fall in mortality, the control of the most common diseases, the fall in fertility through use of modern contraceptives, in the context of imaginative social and economic development, based on strong research foundations, including efforts to address widespread malnutrition and environmentally conditioned illness, are documented in chapters 2, 4, and 5. These approaches provided the starting point for the discussions at the symposium. They illustrate the concepts of Nobel laureate Amartya Sen, himself a Bengali, in which development is aimed at maximizing the freedoms of the poor: freedom from ill health, from early death, from illiteracy, and from dependency.

This anthology explores the diversity of experiences from Bangladesh and other poor countries in an attempt to unravel the complexity of what works under what conditions and how it can be sustained. The diversity of experiences, mix of approaches, choice of technologies, and indeed the promotion of various ideologies have contributed to the wealth of lessons available. There was not one model forced by government but rather a proliferation of efforts by nongovernmental groups of all kinds, most with a firm base in the community. Experiences range from the national house-to-house education effort by BRAC (chapter 4), teaching every woman how to prepare oral rehydration solution to treat diarrhea, the most common killer of children, to the efforts by the ICDDR,B to entice the villages of Chakaria to take full control of their health through planning and providing health services as they see fit in their own villages (chapter 5). These examples are followed by experiences from as far abroad as Haiti (chapter 7), where the experience of the Hôpital Albert Schweitzer has for over 40 years provided a defined population with a high quality of health care. This care has produced a measurably improved life expectancy and quality of life for those fortunate enough to live in the hospital's catchment area. The story of Andean Rural Health Care (chapter 8) provides experience with the interface of government, NGO, and community, and the tensions that emerge when control is vested in the community. Chapter 9 on Nepal reflects on how information systems can drive performance and involve community members in seeking higher levels of participation in their own health.

With the emergence of the HIV epidemic in the 1980s, the challenge to PHC has become profound. Even the wealthy nations discovered the necessity of engaging the people themselves in a full understanding of the determinants and consequences of this infection. The most difficult challenge in public health is changing behaviors, and those underlying HIV infection are the most difficult of all. During the last decade of the 20th century, as tens of millions became infected with this deadly virus, over 90% of these living in poor countries, some communities learned to deal with the devastating threat of AIDS through education, local action, and compassion. The story of community action in Boston (chapter 14) could be repeated from communities across the United States, Uganda, Thailand, and numerous other countries, showing the power of community action in the face of ineffective private and government health services.

The failure of health care systems to stem the AIDS epidemic has left communities to fend for themselves. Success has often grown upwards from grassroots efforts, through which various approaches are providing care for those suffering from AIDS as well as decreasing new infections. Global public health has no greater challenge than its response to this unprecedented epidemic. The only solution in view at the outset of the 21st century is a sound, community-based PHC approach. Only the application of the principles enunciated in the symposium on a universal scale will stem this terrible epidemic. This publication is a small contribution to that end.

1 Origins, Evolution, and Prospects for Primary Health Care in a Changing World

John H. Bryant

One of the authors of the Alma-Ata declaration describes the wavering of major agencies in guiding the world from the principles that led to the optimism of "health for all" to today's increasing attention on private services and medical care. Can the new attention to medical care from the World Bank and WHO along with marketplace economics really place knowledge and technology in the hands of all people to make health for all possible? Equity then becomes the critical issue to establish a floor below which no one should fall. Community-based primary health care still offers the best strategy.

—*Jon Rohde*

This chapter focuses on the place of primary health care (PHC)—past, present, and future—in the larger health system context in which it functions, keeping in mind its global reach. Those who might benefit often live in desperate circumstances. How do global deliberations and declarations affect their lives?

The broadest issues of PHC—the health system, the global context, and equity of access to services—include:

- the origins and evolution of PHC, beginning with the Alma-Ata meeting, including a lively example of PHC at work;
- new concepts and components of health system development: WHO's new Framework for Measuring Health System Performance, the Surveillance for Equity and the Equity Gauge, and Benchmarks of Fairness for health care reform;
- how these evolving and emerging concepts and methods fit into or shape our understanding of health system development.

THE ORIGINS AND EVOLUTION OF PRIMARY HEALTH CARE

PHC was first defined at the meeting in Alma-Ata, Kazakhstan, in 1978:

PHC is essential health care based on practical, scientifically sound, and socially acceptable methods and technology, made universally accessible to individuals and families in the community through their full participation, and at a cost the community and the country can afford to maintain at every stage of their development in the spirit of self-reliance and self-determination.

In 1998, 20 years after Alma-Ata, a meeting in Almaty (same city, different name) brought together a number of the original participants. The consensus statement of the participants reaffirmed their belief in:

> the values of equity, participation, and intersectoral development which are expressed in the 1978 Declaration of Alma-Ata. They are as valid today as they were twenty years ago. We also believe that the understanding and implementation of PHC needs to be revitalized in view of the changes taking place on the threshold of the 21st century. The challenge will be to operationalize the values of Alma-Ata by developing, on the one hand, sustainable health systems for managing PHC and by establishing, on the other hand, complementary systems for governance that will ensure equity and intersectoral response to health needs of people, thereby, effectively uniting PHC and health for all (Primary Health Care 21, 1998).

Dr. Gro Harlem Brundtland, Director General of WHO, supported the meeting in Almaty with the following statement: "PHC remains a key strategy in implementing the policy of HFA. We will continue to work with our partners in UNICEF as well as new partners including the World Bank, UNDP and UNFPA in ensuring that the PHC movement continues and builds on the lessons learned and the gains achieved and the leadership and commitment of the many who have tirelessly worked to make PHC a reality."

The meeting concluded that the insights of 1978 into health problems and societal responses were strikingly accurate, and the proposed solutions have proven to be highly appropriate. These insights included:

- Human values (such as equity, fairness, and gender sensitivity) play a critical role in the pursuit of health for all and PHC;
- Accurate information about problems and the effectiveness of responses to them is essential;
- Community participation is important for improving the health and well-being of communities;

- Weaknesses in health systems research and research capacities must be addressed.

Not surprisingly, however, some problems of the time were less apparent and came more fully to light as the struggles to pursue health for all and PHC continued. Examples of these problems are:

- the limitations of governmental capacity to carry out comprehensive approaches to health care;
- the need for health services to be integrated with other sectors, with PHC as the centerpiece of health development;
- the social and cultural parameters of identifying and addressing health problems in particular societies;
- the challenge of incorporating PHC into health systems, which requires health care reform in virtually every nation, whatever its level of development.

There were yet other problems in the health sector that were unpredictable. Some examples are:

- emerging and re-emerging diseases, such as HIV/AIDS;
- dramatic advances in market orientation and information technologies that have led to the globalization of interactions across the world, benefiting some immensely, but aggravating inequities for others;
- armed conflicts at local levels and widespread civil disorder emerging as threats to peace and human well-being;
- in increasingly pluralistic societies, the call for PHC to embrace the major components of different lifestyles and environments, for example, through programs in schools and workplaces.

EMERGING AND EVOLVING EXAMPLES OF HEALTH SYSTEM DEVELOPMENT

As Dr. Jo Asvall (previously Regional Director for WHO/Europe) noted, the Alma-Ata concept of PHC in Europe is very much "alive and kicking," steadily growing in comprehension and depth, solidifying its position as the most sensible way forward for the 51 member states of our region as they enter the 21st century. It has also been successfully applied in countries as diverse as Haiti and Kenya.

PHC and the Hôpital Albert Schweitzer in Haiti

The Hôpital Albert Schweitzer (HAS) was founded by Larimer and Gwen Mellon 50 years ago in rural Haiti, inspired by Albert Schweitzer and his philosophy of reverence for life. In the early years, the hospital responded to those who came seeking care, but it later expanded its vision and mission to include the health and well-being of all of the 285,000 people in the Artibonite Valley, most of them living in poverty. The hospital is committed to equity-oriented health and development, with three interactive programs: hospital, community health, and community development.

The health and development programs are largely funded from gifts and grants from outside Haiti, with communities sharing the costs in ways that do not dissuade them from seeking care. The entire program costs $16 per capita per year, with hospital services at $10, community health at $5, and community development at $1. Twelve percent of the costs are recovered through patient fees.

It is useful to see the impact of HAS programs over the years—health status and service indicators are considerably better in the HAS service area than in rural Haiti more generally (Table 1).

The HAS recently undertook an evaluation and visioning exercise to ensure that equity and quality of care were being pursued. Working

TABLE I
Health Status and Health Care Indicators

	HAS Service Area	Rural Haiti
Infant mortality rate	51.6	88.9
< 5 mortality rate	68.2	144.3
Total fertility rate	4.8	5.9
Immunizations	78%	26%

with the government of Haiti and other partners, the hospital developed a monitoring and evaluation system for health status and other health-related indicators. One of the findings related to the physical structure of the valley. About three-fourths of the population lives on the plains of the valley, which is generally flat and reasonably fertile, and has roads. The remainder of the population lives on the mountainside, which is extremely rugged, and where, with few exceptions, the only transport is by foot or donkey. The evaluation process revealed that those living on the mountainside are seriously disadvantaged relative to those on the plains (Table 2).

It is interesting that HAS and its community partners have decided that, while all of the indicators noted in Table 2 need to be addressed, priority will be given to education to reduce illiteracy. Based on the widely accepted understanding that education is a fundamental requirement for health, this decision is consistent with the principle of justice that calls for protecting the opportunity to be healthy (Daniels 2002).

The experience of HAS is an example of PHC that has matured over the years to a health care system that reaches virtually everyone, poor though they may be, with care according to need, as called for by the commitment to equity. And there is an openness to new ideas and to discovering oversights (such as the differences between the mountains and the plains), and the place of a principle of justice in shaping decisions for rationing health services. Additionally, the need to scale up throughout the country is constantly recognized. The Director of HAS, Dr. Henry Perry, has also shown how complementary approaches to

TABLE 2

Health and Education Indicators in the Artibonite Valley

	Mountains	Plains
< 5 mortality rate	90	50
Malnutrition	48%	23%
Illiteracy	65%	33%
Total fertility rate	6	3.6
> 2 hours to care	80%	20%

PHC have produced great progress in health for all in Bangladesh (Perry 2000).

WHO's Framework for Assessing the Performance of Health Systems

WHO's Framework for Assessing Health System Performance is a fresh conceptualization of health, described in the *Bulletin of the World Health Organization* (Murray and Frenk 2000) and elaborated in WHO's *World Health Report 2000.* It has generated considerable debate on its methodology for international comparisons of health attainment. It also represents an encompassing perspective of the function of health systems at the national level.

World Health Report 2000 provides a conceptual description of the framework, including the statistical base for national indices and detailed descriptions of health system realities. It also presents the defining goals of the health system, including:

- improving health of the population, both the average level and the distribution of health;
- enhancing the responsiveness of the health system to the expectations of the population;
- fairness in financing and financial risk protection for households.

Pursuing these goals gives rise to three critical concepts:

- quality: the level of goal attainment for health and responsiveness;
- equity: fair distribution of health, responsiveness, and financial burdens;
- efficiency: achievement of the socially desired mix of the goals compared to available resources.

Stewardship is a key factor in defining strategic directions for the entire health system. It focuses on the changing role of the state in health system development and includes the notion of good governance and policymaking that serves the public interest.

At a meeting of the APHA in 1999, Julio Frenk, one of the authors (along with Chris Murray) of the WHO framework, made the following comments: "We hope this Framework will help in reaching to the future with a constructive perspective. We see the commitment to health for all as persisting and permanent, and we see our understanding of PHC undergoing positive changes as we advance our capabilities for assessing system performance."

In short, WHO's framework provides a fresh conceptualization of how health services need to be organized and managed to achieve equity, quality, and efficiency. I agree with Julio Frenk in seeing a place for PHC in the framework. However, I am willing to be a bit provocative by insisting that, for the framework to achieve its goals of health attainment with a fair distribution of health improvements, increased responsiveness to the expectations of the population (again with fair distribution), and stewardship that defines strategic directions for the entire health system, effective approaches to PHC must be included. The capacity of PHC to reach out to entire populations with basic services and participatory interactions is foundational for the WHO framework. Having said that, I also see the framework as providing a place for PHC in a variety of health systems across all levels of socioeconomic development.

Surveillance for Equity and the Equity Gauge

Surveillance for Equity, championed by Carl Taylor for many years, brings special insights to this field (Taylor 1992). Seeing equity as the distribution of benefits according to demonstrable need, Taylor goes further by insisting that equity is not only morally right, but that it can also help make PHC more effective and efficient. Thus, Surveillance for Equity is a management tool that fits synergistically with a moral imperative. From a practical perspective, sustainable PHC depends on continuing dialogue between health workers and community leaders, supported by health information that includes a concern for equity.

Equity, so often mentioned but so seldom measured and monitored, is now the subject of extensive development of such measures. The South African Equity Gauge Project, under the leadership of the Health Systems Trust in Durban, is developing indicators for equity.

They observe that equity has a number of different meanings, and the Equity Gauge is based on the following broad meaning: Equity means "fair shares" and "fair opportunities" in the distribution of and access to resources and services (Ntuli, Khosa, and McCoy 1999).

The clusters of Equity Gauge indicators include the following:

- private versus public sector;
- health status;
- health financing in the public sector;
- access (distribution of personnel in the public sector and distribution of services);
- quality of care;
- race inequalities in South Africa;
- rural-urban inequity.

These indicators are being tested through the participation of an Equity Gauge Network. Some 100 researchers in 14 countries, supported by the Rockefeller and Henry J. Kaiser foundations, are working in collaboration. We see here important advances in the pursuit of equity. Because inequities are often relative to the context in which they are being studied, the approach of the Equity Gauge invites further exploration of indicators in various social, cultural, political, and economic settings. Certainly these indicators invite interaction with the other health system components under discussion.

Benchmarks of Fairness for Health Care Reform

Norman Daniels, philosopher at Tufts University in Medford, Massachusetts, has long been concerned with interactions of justice and health. His writings have included *Just Health Care* (Daniels 1985) and *Am I My Parents' Keeper?* (Daniels 1988). In 1996, working with the Clinton Task Force on Health Care Reform, he and colleagues published *Benchmarks of Fairness for Health Care Reform* (Daniels, Light, and Kaplan 1996).

While health care reform in the US has remained somewhat stagnant, the benchmarks attracted the interest of a number of us who are interested in justice and health in developing countries. Over the past three years, a cluster of colleagues from Asia, Africa, and Latin America has been working toward adapting the benchmarks to the realities and needs for reform in those countries, using the benchmarks as a new tool for health care reform (Daniels et al. 2000).

The benchmarks are seen as promoting change related to fairness at the local and national levels through policy change. Fairness is viewed as a multifaceted concept, broader than equity and including:

- equity in health outcomes, access to all forms of care, and financing;
- efficiency in management and allocation (inefficiency can be costly to efforts to promote equity);
- accountability, in order for the public to have influence over health care.

There are nine benchmarks:

- intersectoral public health
- financial barriers to equitable access
- nonfinancial barriers to access
- comprehensiveness of benefits and tiering
- equitable financing
- efficacy, efficiency, and quality of health care
- administrative efficiency
- democratic accountability and empowerment
- patient and provider autonomy

The intent is not to provide a blueprint of health care reform calling for insistent action following a fixed pattern. Rather, the benchmarks are a tool for facilitating deliberation and reflection on reform options. The following brief examples illustrate some of the emphases of four of the benchmarks:

- intersectoral public health
  - basic education and health literacy
  - improvements in social determinants of health
- nonfinancial barriers to access

- □ reduction in geographical maldistribution
- □ reduction in gender and cultural discrimination
- ■ efficacy, efficiency, and quality of health care
  - □ focus on PHC with community participation
  - □ implementation of evidence-based practice
- ■ democratic accountability and empowerment
  - □ explicit procedures for resource allocation with transparency
  - □ strengthening civil society and advocacy groups

Reflecting for a moment on some of the most serious aspects of poverty and despair, we should note that the benchmarks reach well beyond the health sector as such, calling for assessment of fairness across sectors and with respect to social determinants of health.

The benchmarks make it possible to score reform options in terms of their fairness. We developed a scale of −5 to +5 to judge reform options according to the fairness of their assessed intent or impacts. The scoring can be applied to the national, district, and local levels.

Two examples of applications of the benchmarks follow. First, in Thailand and Pakistan, the results of workshops on the benchmarks were presented to policymakers, who then invited follow-on field projects using the benchmarks to facilitate consideration of health system change. Those follow-on projects are underway.

Second, in Kenya, graduate students studying health policy and management applied the benchmarks to health sector reform actions promoted by the Ministry of Health. After analyzing and scoring the reform options, they engaged health system personnel and policymakers in dialogue about the benchmarks. There was both agreement and disagreement over interpretations of the intention of the reforms, and lively debate about scoring the extent of fairness of the reforms at local, district, and national levels. This process was constructive for all parties: policymakers, health system managers, students, and faculty.

INTERACTIONS OF HEALTH SYSTEM COMPONENTS

We have examined four sets of ideas and processes that are components of health system development:

- Primary Health Care
- WHO Framework for Assessing Health System Performance
- Surveillance for Equity and the Equity Gauge
- Benchmarks of Fairness for Health Care Reform

An overarching observation is that none of these four stands alone, functioning in isolation, in the context of addressing the health needs of populations. Each is defined to a considerable degree by the context in which it functions. They are interdependent. Each needs a health system context. Each brings essential strengths to that health system context. These are not necessarily the only four candidates for such system roles, but they are exemplary of such system components.

Figure 1 shows that the WHO framework can provide an encompassing structure for addressing the health and development needs of populations at a national level. For it to do so with the measures it pro-

FIGURE I

Potential Interactions among Health System Components

■ **Framework for Assessing Health System Performance**
Health attainment and distribution of services
Responsiveness and distribution
Fairness in financing
Stewardship
Quality, equity, efficiency

■ **Primary Health Care**
Population-based
Community participation
Integration with rest of the
   health system
Intersectoral integration
Information-based

■ **Benchmarks of Fairness**
Intersectoral public health
Nonfinancial barriers to access
Efficacy, efficiency, and quality
   of health care
Democratic accountability and
empowerment

■ **Surveillance for Equity**
■ **The Equity Gauge**
Ensuring fair distribution of and access to
resources and services

poses for assessing health system performance calls for including other components.

The four components are interactive, and there is an interdependence between the framework and the three health system components. Without PHC, the Equity Gauge, and the Benchmarks of Fairness, the task of stewardship under the framework would be difficult indeed. PHC is an essential component without which the other components would have great difficulty achieving their intentions. For example, in relation to the framework, PHC can achieve total coverage of populations, including their participation, as would be required by the goals of health attainment as well as responsiveness to expectations.

Surveillance for Equity and the Equity Gauge provide mechanisms for ensuring equity in the fair distribution of health services, responsiveness, and financial burdens, which are central to the framework. These approaches to equity also complement the intentions of PHC and the benchmarks.

The Benchmarks of Fairness are intended to promote change in the interest of fairness across the system, and from bottom to top. They provide a tool for considering reform options that can be applied in a wide variety of circumstances: developed and developing countries; national, district, and local settings; and public and private sectors. The benchmarks clearly complement the other components.

CONCLUDING OBSERVATIONS

This chapter has examined the components of health care systems and their potential interactions. Let us consider what history has shown. The world converged at Alma-Ata to take action in the interest of human well-being. We emerged with a set of ideas—health for all and PHC—based on fundamental human values and on the most practical perspective of the time with respect to advancing community health care.

The ideas were not perfect, but they broke new ground, reached out to all nations, and advanced critical dimensions of health care. Complexities emerged that were unforeseen: changing roles of governments, lack of support of higher levels of health systems, increasingly complex and costly health care, and inequities that accompany privatization. There were also some very positive examples of PHC: the

Aroles' work in India, BRAC in Bangladesh, and Hôpital Albert Schweitzer in Haiti.

Now, the world has moved onward, benefiting from the lessons of Alma-Ata, and recognizing important problems of health and development that call for new dimensions of understanding and action. The four health system components discussed in this chapter are not a final answer. But there is no final answer—there will only be steps toward improved answers, and the health system components represent such steps.

Given the complexity of health-related factors in our world that must be addressed, and given the complexity of health systems and related responses, we are continually building structures and processes for ensuring health and well-being. Seeking constructive interactions of the components that lie before us is an example of that never-ending process.

The key question remains: Can the health and well-being of all the people be enhanced by an international determination to achieve a convergence of the best current knowledge to shape health system development?

While there are many uncertainties, we believe it is reasonable at least to address this question and bring these four components together into some form of synergy and interdependence. Step by step, an integrated system can emerge as a real possibility. If this is such a possibility—at this time in our history of global health that is tinged with such inadequacy and uncertainty—is this not a time to take some definitive steps of inquiry and exploration toward a more fully integrated system?

Is It Time for Another Alma-Ata?

Would it be helpful to have another Alma-Ata conference? The striking thing about Alma-Ata was that it brought the nations of the world together to focus on health problems that were not being adequately addressed, and to do so through the development and application of new concepts of health care buttressed by the moral values of equity and justice. It was also clear that while Alma-Ata did not have final answers to the health problems of the world, it provided important steps toward coping with current as well as emerging problems. We now have long lists of pressing problems. Is there among them a set of challenges comparable to those that called forth the international response of Alma-Ata? Three examples of gross health system inadequacies illustrate the extreme scope of change necessary and the need to develop a strategy to effect this change.

First, the field of public health has always been pulled in two directions: towards a broad focus on the underlying social and economic causes of death and disease, and, in contrast, towards a narrow focus on medical technology and the needs of individuals. Currently, public health movements, including epidemiology, in most countries are heading down the narrow, disease-focused route; only serious and concerted effort will divert public health to a broader perspective. Clearly what is needed is a combination of concerns—for disease entities and for broader population well-being. Public health is described as being at a crossroads (Beaglehole and Bonita 1997).

Second, the problem of HIV/AIDS reaches beyond all other problems of our time in terms of human suffering and difficulty of effective and affordable management. This is surely so in Africa, and with seriously increasing burdens in Asia. There is no doubting the importance of grappling with the complexities of the disease itself. At the same time, there must be actions to ameliorate the devastating impacts of this disease on the larger society—the massive loss of productive lives of young adults, the burden on the remaining elderly, and the helplessness of AIDS' orphans, who will number 35 million by the year 2010. Concerns for equity are largely submerged by the scope of tragedies. Mutually supportive actions at the community level are often the only responses that touch households and afflicted families.

Third, limited resources have led the governments of many developing countries to limit their involvement in the provision of health care. In doing so, they have often fallen short of ensuring that other arrangements (such as through privatization and nongovernmental organizations) meet the basic health needs of populations. This failure reveals deep-seated flaws in economic and social system management as well as a diminished expression of moral responsibility for the well-being of the people.

We have also described two sets of challenges. The first is that of bringing about a constructive convergence of the four contemporary components of health system development: community-based PHC, WHO's Framework for Assessing Health System Performance, Surveillance for Equity and the Equity Gauge, and the Benchmarks of Fairness for Health Care Reform. The second is the challenge of corrective actions to address the three problem areas described above.

It is clear that serious consideration of this range of actions would require coherent international deliberation with readiness for far-reaching policy change. This process could readily build on the insights and commitments of Alma-Ata—community-based PHC and health for all remain cornerstones for further action. But, of course, they are only a beginning. Constructing the process for bringing together the ideas, resources, and commitments for addressing these issues represents dramatically new terrain. The rewards in terms of human well-being could be immense.

Is it time for another Alma-Ata? Why not?

REFERENCES

Beaglehole, Robert, and Ruth Bonita. 1997. *Public Health at the Crossroads.* Cambridge: Cambridge University Press.

Daniels, Norman. 1985. *Just Health Care.* Cambridge: Cambridge University Press.

————. 1988. *Am I My Parents' Keeper? An Essay on Justice between the Young and the Old.* New York: Oxford University Press.

————. 2002. "Justice, Health and Health Care. An Essay." Tufts University. Forthcoming.

Daniels, Norman, Donald W. Light, and Ronald Kaplan. 1996. *Benchmarks of Fairness for Health Care Reform.* New York: Oxford University Press.

Daniels, Norman, et al. 2000. "Benchmarks of Fairness for Health Care Reform: A Policy Tool for Developing Countries." *Bulletin of the World Health Organization* 78: 740–50.

Murray, Christopher J. L., and Julio Frenk. 2000. "A Framework for Assessing the Performance of Health Systems." *Bulletin of the World Health Organization* 78: 717–31.

Ntuli, Antoinette, Solani Khosa, and David McCoy. 1999. *The Equity Gauge.* Durban, South Africa: Health Systems Trust.

Perry, Henry B. 2000. *Health for All in Bangladesh: Lessons in Primary Health Care for the 21st Century.* Dhaka: University Press.

"Primary Health Care 21, Everybody's Business." 1998. An International Meeting to Celebrate 20 Years after Alma-Ata. Almaty, Kazakhstan, November 27–28, 1998. Organized by WHO, Geneva, and the WHO Regional Office for Europe, Copenhagen.

Taylor, Carl E. 1992. "Surveillance for Equity in Primary Health Care: Policy Implications for International Experience." *International Journal of Epidemiology* 21: 1043–49.

World Health Organization. *World Health Report 2000.* Geneva: World Health Organization.

2   Primary Health Care in Bangladesh: Challenges, Approaches, and Results

Henry B. Perry

The post-independence proliferation of small NGOs in Bangladesh is doing much to meet the varying health needs of communities. Meanwhile, large programs such as BRAC (formerly the Bangladesh Rural Advancement Committee), CARE, and the government Ministry of Health address the most pressing problems of population growth, common infectious diseases, and environmental health, yielding good results on a population-wide basis. This is an optimistic chapter that looks at the progress in primary health care in the world's poorest large country.

—Jon Rohde

T here is perhaps no country in the world that has made more progress in achieving health for all with fewer resources during the past three decades than has Bangladesh. Hence, it is appropriate that this chapter focus on the challenges that Bangladesh faced at the time it obtained nationhood in 1971, to review the approaches that were taken to address these challenges, to point out some of the remarkable results that have been achieved, and to consider a few of the underlying factors that made these achievements possible.

BANGLADESH IN 1971

Bangladesh is located on a large river delta. Annual flooding from the Padma, Jamuna, and Meghna rivers, which drain the Himalayas, produces very rich farmland. At the time of independence in 1971, Bangladesh had just over 70 million people (Bangladesh Bureau of Statistics 1984), and it was one of the most rural countries in the world, with less than 5% of the population living in urban areas (Bangladesh Bureau of Statistics 1998).

The gross national product in 1971 was US$80 per capita (Haq and Haq 1998). (See Figure 1 for a comparison of the GNP in Bangladesh and Pakistan between 1973 and 1999.) Seventy-six percent of the adult population was illiterate, comprising 91% of women and 53% of men (Haq and Haq 1998). Women were not allowed to travel more than a short distance from their homes because of social customs.

The infant mortality rate was 150 deaths per 1,000 live births (Figure 2), and one-quarter of live-born infants died before reaching the age of five years (Haq and Haq 1998). The life expectancy at birth was

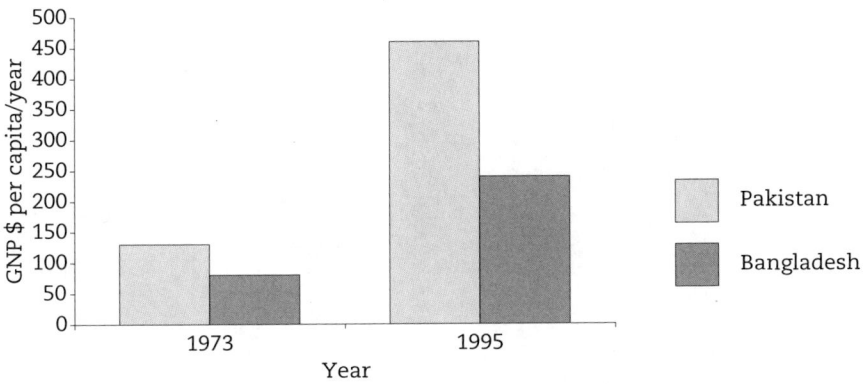

FIGURE I

Comparison of GNP per Capita
in Bangladesh and Pakistan, 1973–99

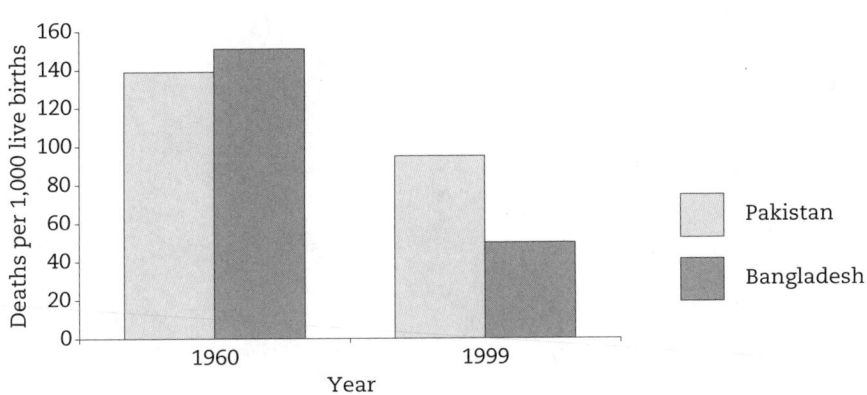

FIGURE 2

Comparison of Infant Mortality Rates
in Bangladesh and Pakistan, 1960–99

only 40 years (Haq and Haq 1998). The total fertility rate was 6.2 births per woman (Haq and Haq 1998, Figure 3). Fewer than 2% of children were fully immunized (Figure 4) and fewer than 2% of newborns were protected against neonatal tetanus through maternal immunization (World Health Organization 1995, Expanded Programme on Immunization 1998). Fewer than 5% of women of reproductive age were

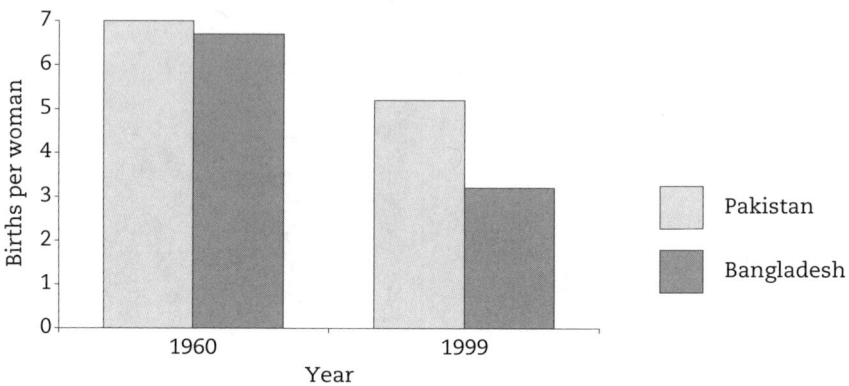

Comparison of Total Fertility Rates
in Bangladesh and Pakistan, 1960–99

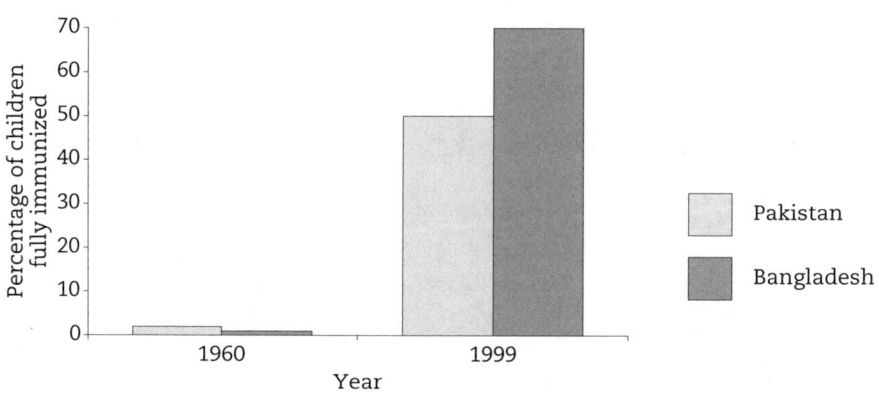

FIGURE 4
Comparison of Childhood Immunization Coverage
in Bangladesh and Pakistan, 1960–99

using a modern method of contraception (Mitra et al. 1997, Figure 5).
Childhood malnutrition, cholera, and smallpox were rampant, as were
neonatal tetanus and measles. Thirty thousand children were going
blind in both eyes each year because of vitamin A deficiency, often pre-
cipitated by measles (Keiss 1999).

In spite of pervasive ill health, by 1971, the population had begun to

FIGURE 5

Comparison of Contraceptive Prevalence Rates in Bangladesh and Pakistan, 1960–99

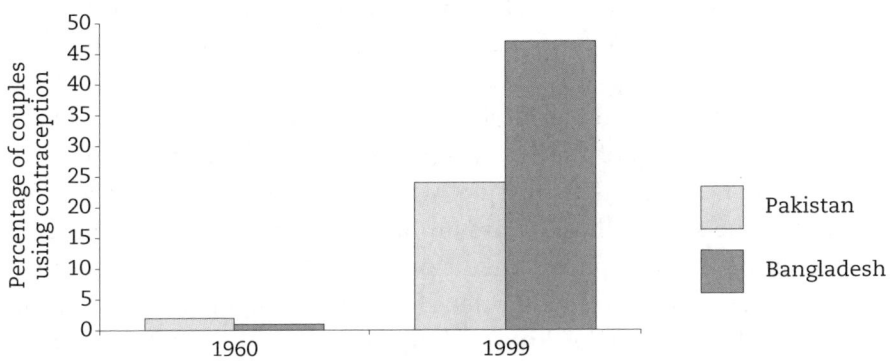

FIGURE 6

Comparison of Annual Growth Rates of the Population in Bangladesh and Pakistan, 1960–99

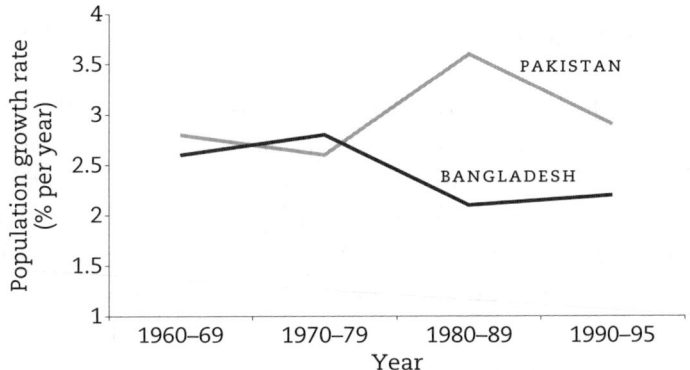

grow rapidly because of a rapidly falling crude mortality rate and only a minor fall in the crude birth rate (Figure 6). The annual growth rate was 2.8% (Haq and Haq 1998).

Much of the country's infrastructure, including many health facilities, had been destroyed in its war of independence with West Pakistan —a war during which up to three million Bangladeshis died. The physician-to-population ratio was 1:65,000 (Cash 2000). Health care providers with training in modern methods of medicine and public health were virtually nonexistent outside of urban areas.

Thus, the new country of Bangladesh in 1971 faced a daunting set of challenges in socioeconomic development, including health and family planning. Henry Kissinger, United States Secretary of State at that time, referred to Bangladesh as an "international basket case." No doubt, the needs of the people of Bangladesh were among those that N. R. E. Fendall was thinking of when he wrote his famous statement about the state of health care around the world: "If I were asked to compose an epitaph on medicine throughout the 20th century it would read: 'Brilliant in its scientific discoveries, superb in its technological breakthroughs, but woefully inept in its application to those most in need'" (Fendall 1972).

The leaders of the independence movement in Bangladesh, along with their 70 million Bangladeshi supporters, fervently believed that, with political freedom, abject poverty would be eliminated and health care would become available to those most in need.

APPROACHES TAKEN

Bangladesh's initial progress in socioeconomic development was difficult, partly because of the large numbers of very poor people throughout the country. The new government gave high priority to slowing the rate of population growth. In 1975, the government proclaimed population growth to be its most important development problem (Haider et al. 1995), and international donors also gave priority to this problem. A bifurcated Ministry of Health was established with a semi-independent family planning "wing," which received most of the country's international donor assistance for family planning. In 1976, the Government of Bangladesh established the ambitious goal of reaching near-replacement fertility (that is, a total fertility rate of 2.6) by 1985 (Government of Bangladesh 1976).

In 1982, Bangladesh adopted its first national drug policy, largely due to the leadership of Dr. Zafrullah Chowdhury (Chowdhury 1996). This policy promoted the use of essential drugs and restricted the use of drugs with no scientifically proven efficacy. This bold and far-reaching policy provoked, and still provokes, criticism from the Bangladesh Medical Association and from the international pharmaceutical community (Chowdhury 1996).

In 1988, a four-member committee (including Dr. Chowdhury) established by the government proposed a national health policy calling for the decentralization of the Ministry of Health's activities, integration of the two "wings" of the Ministry, and limitation of the widespread private practice of physicians in government hospitals and in government medical colleges. This proposal provoked a storm of protest from the Bangladesh Medical Association; in fact, the proposed policy and the opposition to it, led by physicians, was the beginning of the downfall of the government then in power, which was planning to adopt the proposed policy (Chowdhury 1996).

The lack of a strong government infrastructure and service delivery system throughout the country and the slowness in developing this system after independence left a void that was increasingly filled by what has become one of the most dynamic NGO sectors in the world. Organizations such as the Bangladesh Rural Advancement Committee (BRAC) and Gonoshasthaya Kendra (which Dr. Zafrullah Chowdhury founded) began to grow and received world-class technical assistance and international financial support.

Beginning in 1971 and continuing over the next three decades, Bangladesh was able to build an extensive government infrastructure of rural health facilities, train and deploy 44,500 government field workers in health and family planning, establish 108,000 government EPI outreach sites and 34,000 satellite clinics, and increase the number of physicians per population tenfold, from 1:65,000 to 10:65,000 (Perry 2000).

In addition, more than 4,000 NGOs began to work in the health, population, and nutrition sector (Perry 2000). An environment developed in which the government came to view NGOs as partners that are vital to the achievement of health and development goals for the country, and the government encouraged their work in many ways. Two of the most important NGOs in Bangladesh are BRAC and the Grameen Bank.

BRAC has become the largest nonsectarian national private agency in the world (see chapter 4). It has 25,000 full-time employees, 34,000 part-time teachers, and 25,000 nonsalaried community health workers, called *shasthya shebikas*. BRAC carries out multisectoral development activities in 50,000 of the country's 86,000 villages, and its programs serve more than 38 million people (Perry 2000).

The Grameen Bank of Bangladesh, world-famous for originating the microcredit programs of poverty alleviation for women that are now in place around the world, has more than 11,000 employees and a network of more than two million borrowers in 34,000 villages. The Grameen Bank is now beginning a national system of community-based health services. One of the main reasons for this major undertaking is that illness as well as the cost of medical care are major reasons for loan default, and often families pay for treatments that have no actual benefit (Perry 2000).

In support of this growing health partnership between government and NGOs, a unique institution was founded in 1962: the Cholera Research Laboratory. The large number of cholera cases in East Pakistan made it an ideal site for research into this devastating epidemic disease. Because of the interests of the United States and its allies in preventing cholera among its troops should they be called into duty in areas where cholera is endemic, the US Department of Defense supported a biomedical research lab for cholera in Dhaka with a field research station in a rural area called Matlab, where field trials to test new cholera vaccines could be carried out.

To assess the effectiveness of new vaccines against cholera, a method had to be developed to compare mortality rates from diarrhea among people who had received the vaccine and among similar people who had not. The pioneering community epidemiological research carried out in India just prior to that time by two Harvard School of Public Health faculty members—Dr. John Gordon, then Professor of Epidemiology, and Dr. John Wyon, then a project field director working in India under Dr. Gordon—was adapted for the cholera vaccine trials in Matlab.

The research of Wyon and Gordon, summarized in their classic volume entitled *The Khanna Study* (Wyon and Gordon 1971), was based on prospective visitation of all homes in the population under study and the recording of vital events (that is, births, deaths, and migrations) that had taken place since the previous visit. This method was adopted for the cholera vaccine assessment, and all homes in a population of 200,000 people were visited every two weeks to record vital events. One-half of the population was in an intervention area where new cholera vaccines could be administered and the other half was in a control area—similar in all respects except that no cholera vaccine would be administered there. These studies demonstrated the ineffectiveness of the vaccines then widely in use.

In 1975, the Cholera Lab expanded its activities in Matlab, which became a field research site for testing innovative approaches for family planning and soon thereafter for child health. These inquiries had strong community-based components studied by Bangladeshi researchers with academic researchers from other countries. The family planning approaches developed in Matlab served as the prototype for Bangladesh's renowned family planning program (Perry 2000). Because of the proven effectiveness in Matlab of community health workers visiting the homes of every woman of reproductive age every two weeks to promote family planning and to distribute birth control pills and condoms, a national family planning program was gradually established in which community-based family planning workers called Family Welfare Assistants visited the homes of women of reproductive age. With the introduction of injectable contraceptives, which rapidly became the most popular method, the frequency of visits was reduced to a manageable two months. Later, NGOs throughout Bangladesh adopted this approach, so that by the late 1990s, over 30,000 community-based family planning workers were carrying out more than 50 million home visits per year to promote and provide family planning services. These workers took on a few other important simple activities as well, such as routine immunizations and participation in polio and vitamin A-deficiency eradication campaigns (Perry 2000). The scaling-up of this community-based family planning program took place gradually and with careful monitoring and evaluation of the process.

The Cholera Lab (as it was called initially) achieved international renown for its development of oral rehydration therapy (ORT) for diarrhea and for documenting its effectiveness through field trials in the late 1960s and early 1970s. Many consider this one of the most significant scientific achievements of the 20th century. The development of ORT and the extensive practical experience with its use at the

Cholera Lab (now the International Centre for Diarrhoeal Disease Research, Bangladesh, ICDDR,B) made it possible for BRAC to develop and implement the BRAC National Oral Rehydration Therapy Project between 1979 and 1990. Through this project, ORT workers visited every home in the country to teach mothers how to prepare home-based ORT (Chowdhury and Cash 1996). The project's activities were "taken to scale" gradually. A strong monitoring and evaluation program made it possible to identify weaknesses that could be corrected before scaling up to the next level. Eventually, women in 13 million households were taught how to make and use ORT.

Progress in improving immunization coverage stalled until the mid-1980s, when the Government of Bangladesh made a commitment to establish the Expanded Programme on Immunization (EPI) and actively sought the participation and collaboration of NGOs such as BRAC and CARE in its immunization efforts (Huq 1991). Much of the later progress of EPI in Bangladesh was built on the lessons from the smallpox eradication program in Bangladesh during the 1960s and early 1970s, with strong elements of the Matlab home visitor program.

RESULTS ACHIEVED

Bangladesh's achievements over the past three decades using the approaches described above are admired around the world. I will point to only a few.

The infant mortality rate has fallen by two-thirds, from 150 to around 50 deaths per 1,000 live births (Figure 2), and the total fertility rate has fallen by half, from just over six to just over three births per woman (Figure 3). This is the most rapid fall in fertility ever observed in a country where social, economic, and institutional circumstances have been so unfavorable (Perry 2000).

The percentage of children who are fully immunized increased from less than 2% to 70% (Figure 4), and the percentage of newborns protected through maternal immunization increased from less than 2% to 86% (World Health Organization 1995, Expanded Programme on Immunization 1998). The percentage of children receiving high-dose vitamin A capsules at the time of biannual campaigns increased from less than 2% to 80% (Keiss 1998).

The percentage of women of reproductive age using a modern method of contraception increased from 5% to 47%, and the rate of increase still shows no signs of slowing (Figure 5). The national EPI has prevented an estimated 1.2 million deaths from neonatal tetanus, pertussis, measles, and polio (Khan and Yoder 1998). The number of children going blind as a result of vitamin A deficiency has declined from 30,000 per year to 6,000, and the lives of an estimated 25,000 children are being saved each year through the mortality reduction effects of high-dose vitamin A supplementation (Keiss 1998). The total number of active cases of leprosy has fallen from 136,000 to 30,000, and virtually all newly detected cases are receiving multidrug therapy (Lobo 1997, 1998).

At the time of the completion of the BRAC National Oral Rehydration Therapy Project in 1990, 90% of all 12.5 million mothers of young children knew about and could prepare oral rehydration salts (Chowdhury and Cash 1996). More recent studies have documented that the ORT use rate for cases of childhood diarrhea is over 50% and, in cases of severe diarrhea, it is 80% (Chowdhury et al. 1997b).

These achievements have all taken place with a minimal amount of financial resources. In 1996–97, only US$8.63 per capita was spent on primary health care services and US$1.97 was spent on hospital services (Health Economics Unit and Data International 1998).

Some of the results of the BRAC community health care program, made possible through the work of shasthya shebikas, merit special attention. These include the following:

- In a pilot area of "only" 4.8 million inhabitants, shasthya shebikas, with the help of a strong training and supervisory program, were able to reduce the rate of tuberculosis to half that of comparison areas. This was made possible through an aggressive case-detection strategy and through a home-based, directly observed treatment program in which 85% of patients completed their full course of therapy (Chowdhury et al. 1997a).
- In a project area of approximately 10 million persons, shasthya shebikas were trained to implement the World Health Organization protocol for diagnosis and treatment of pneumonia. Of

60,222 cases of acute respiratory infection detected by shasthya shebikas, 18,609 cases of uncomplicated pneumonia were treated, and 181 cases of severe pneumonia were identified and referred. The cure rate for the cases of uncomplicated pneumonia treated with antibiotics by shasthya shebikas was 98% (BRAC 1998, Haque 1999).

Comparisons of Bangladesh's progress with that of Pakistan have generated particular interest because of the fact that they are both South Asian countries and they have a common political and religious heritage. Although the gross national product (GNP) per capita increased substantially less in Bangladesh than in Pakistan between 1973 and 1999 (Figure 1), the decline in infant mortality has been much more pronounced in Bangladesh (Figure 2). Improvements in childhood immunization coverage rates have been much greater in Bangladesh than in Pakistan (Figure 4). The decline in the total fertility rate has also been much greater (Figure 3). The increase in the contraceptive prevalence rate has also been much greater (Figure 5), and the annual growth rate of the population has become substantially less (Figure 6).

Pakistan has a notably higher level of military spending than Bangladesh. Pakistan spends four times more, as a percentage of GNP, for military purposes than Bangladesh does. For every rupee spent in Pakistan on education and health, 1.25 rupees are spent for military purposes, while in Bangladesh, only 0.41 taka are spent for military purposes for each taka spent on education and health (Figure 7).

ACCOUNTING FOR BANGLADESH'S PROGRESS

Accounting for Bangladesh's progress is not simple. Nevertheless, a number of factors taken together appear to provide a reasonable explanation:

- There has emerged a strong partnership among the Government of Bangladesh, NGOs, and communities for the provision of basic primary health care services. The government has actively pursued partnerships with NGOs, and both govern-

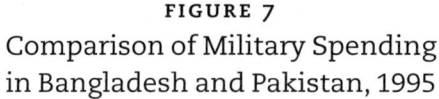

FIGURE 7

Comparison of Military Spending
in Bangladesh and Pakistan, 1995

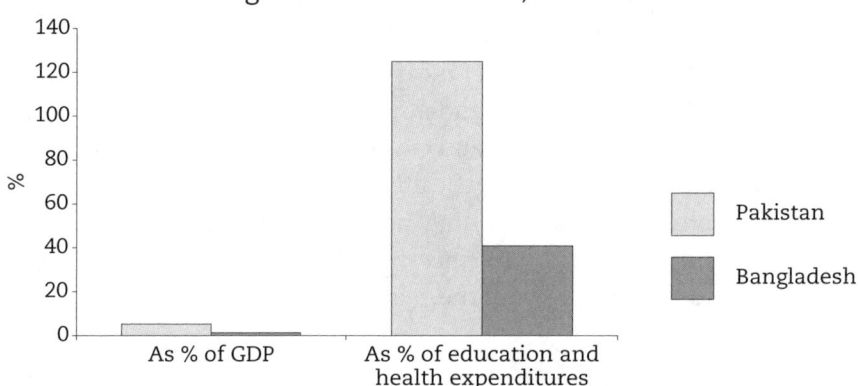

ment and NGO health services have worked actively with communities to carry out their programs.

- There is a tradition in Bangladesh of high-quality field and operations research that has guided changes in government and NGO programs. This tradition has also made it possible to scale up several programs nationally, a feat that has failed in many other countries. BRAC and ICDDR,B have played important roles in these activities.

- The government has been open to international donor support for its own health and family planning programs, and it has encouraged international donor support for NGO programs as well. The international donor community has responded generously. There has been a healthy balance of expatriate and Bangladeshi technical expertise.

- There has emerged a tradition of strong outreach services down to the household level, particularly for basic health and family planning services. The tradition of home visitation in delivery of basic health and family planning services is one that, in my opinion, deserves much more recognition as a reason for Bangladesh's progress than it has received. Home visitation has been an essential ingredient in Bangladesh's success in reducing childhood mortality and in reducing fertility—

both essential steps in achieving health for all. This tradition of home visitation partly owes its intellectual roots to John Gordon and John Wyon, who demonstrated the viability of this approach as a demographic and epidemiological tool with which to prospectively measure rates of mortality and fertility, and effects of health and family planning interventions within a population (Wyon and Gordon 1971).

- High-impact primary health care services, namely immunizations and family planning, have been emphasized.
- Multisectoral approaches have helped Bangladesh to move more quickly toward the goal of health for all.

CONCLUSION

Enormous progress at modest cost can be made in reaching health for all when community-based approaches designed to reach the entire population are led by government–NGO partnerships and if strong political and professional leadership is present. A "friendly" policy environment promotes success. That is, when the government supports collaboration with the NGO sector and with communities and when the government is open to new ideas based on solid field research, the probability of success will be greater.

The historian Arnold Toynbee remarked, "The 20th century will be chiefly remembered in future centuries not as an age of political conflicts or technical inventions, but as an age in which human society dared to think of the welfare of the whole human race as a practical objective" (quoted in UNICEF 1995). Perhaps no other extremely poor country of the developing world has made more progress in such a short time in improving the welfare of its people. This remarkable achievement is a tribute to the hard-working and deeply motivated people of Bangladesh. This remarkable achievement is also a tribute to the international donor and public health community, which has worked hand in hand with the Bangladeshi people.

REFERENCES AND RESOURCES

Bangladesh Bureau of Statistics. 1984. *Bangladesh Population Census: 1981.* Volume 1.

————. 1998. *1997 Statistical Yearbook of Bangladesh.* Dhaka: Ministry of Planning.

————. 1999. Data supplied by Hamidul Hoque Bhuiyan.

BRAC. 1998. *Annual Report of the Reproductive Health and Disease Control Project, 1997.* Dhaka: BRAC.

Cash, Richard. 2000. Personal communication.

Chowdhury, A. Mushtaque R., and Richard A. Cash. 1996. *A Simple Solution: Teaching Millions to Treat Diarrhoea at Home.* Dhaka: University Press.

Chowdhury, A. Mushtaque R., et al. 1997a. "Community Health Workers Can Control Tuberculosis: The BRAC Experience in Bangladesh." *The Lancet* 350: 169–72.

Chowdhury, A. Mushtaque R., et al. 1997b. "The Status of ORT: How Widely Is It Used?" *Health Policy and Planning* 12: 58–66.

Chowdhury, Zafrullah. 1996. *The Politics of Essential Drugs. The Makings of a Successful Strategy: Lessons from Bangladesh.* Dhaka: University Press.

Expanded Programme on Immunization. 1998. *Findings of the National Coverage Survey.* Dhaka: Expanded Programme on Immunization, Directorate General of Health Services, Government of the People's Republic of Bangladesh.

Fendall, N. R. E. 1972. "Auxiliaries and Primary Medical Care." *Bulletin of the New York Academy of Medicine* 48: 1291–1300.

Government of the People's Republic of Bangladesh. 1976. *Bangladesh National Population Policy: An Outline.* Dhaka: Population Control and Family Planning Directorate, Ministry of Health and Family Welfare.

Haider, Syed J., Kim Streatfield, and Md. Azizul Karim. 1995. *Comprehensive Guidebook to the Bangladesh Family Planning-MCH Program.* Dhaka: Research Evaluation Associates for Development; The Population Council; Ministry of Health and Family Welfare.

Haq, Mahbub ul, and Khadija Haq. 1998. *Human Development in South Asia, 1998.* Dhaka: University Press.

Haque, Raisul (BRAC). 1999. Personal communication.

Health Economics Unit and Data International. 1998. *Bangladesh National Health Accounts 1996/97.* Dhaka: Ministry of Health and Family Welfare and Data International, Ltd.

Huq, Mujibul, ed. 1991. *Near Miracle in Bangladesh*. Dhaka: University Press.

Keiss, Lynnda. 1999. Personal communication. Dhaka: Helen Keller International.

Khan, M. Mahmud, and Richard A. Yoder. 1998. "Expanded Report on Immunization in Bangladesh: Cost, Effectiveness, and Financing Estimates." Technical Report No. 24. Partnerships for Health Reform. Bethesda, MD: Abt and Associates.

Lobo, Derek. 1997. "National MOHFW Tuberculosis and Leprosy Programmes." Unpublished documents.

————. 1998. Personal communication. Dhaka: World Health Organization.

Mitra, S., et al. 1997. *Bangladesh Demographic and Health Survey 1996–1997*. Dhaka: National Institute of Population Research and Training; Mitra and Associates; Calverton, MD: Macro International Inc.

National Institute of Population Research and Training (NIPORT), Mitra and Associates, and ORC-Macro International. 2000. "Bangladesh Demographic and Health Survey 1999–2000: Preliminary Report." Dhaka: NIPORT and Mitra and Associates; Calverton, MD: ORC-Macro International.

Perry, Henry B. 2000. *Health for All in Bangladesh: Lessons in Primary Health Care for the 21st Century*. Dhaka: University Press.

Rashid, Haroun Er. 1991. *Geography of Bangladesh*. Dhaka: University Press.

UNICEF. 1995. *The State of the World's Children, 1995*. New York: UNICEF.

World Bank. 1998a. "National Nutrition Program (NNP) Identification Mission, July 4–16, 1998." Aide-mémoire. Dhaka: World Bank.

————. 1998b. *Project Appraisal Document on a Proposed Credit in the Amount of SDR 185.5 Million (US$250 Million Equivalent) to the Government of the People's Republic of Bangladesh for a Health and Population Program Project*. Report No. 17684-BD. Washington, DC: World Bank.

World Bank and Bangladesh Centre for Advanced Studies. 1998. *Bangladesh 2020*. Dhaka: University Press.

World Health Organization. 1995. *Global Programme on Vaccines and Immunization Information System*. Geneva: World Health Organization.

Wyon, J. B., and J. E. Gordon. 1971. *The Khanna Study: Population Problems in the Rural Punjab*. Cambridge: Harvard University Press.

3 The Comprehensive Rural Health Project in Jamkhed, India

Mabelle Arole

The Jamkhed program in central India represented
the best primary health care model available at the
time of Alma-Ata. Dedicated leadership, strong
community involvement, and self-reliance led to
dramatic declines in mortality, fertility, and malnutrition. Unfortunately, when India tried to duplicate
this program throughout the country, the national
program collapsed due to lack of a full understanding
of the critical elements of leadership, integration
with an effective health care system, and involvement of the people in the community. While Jamkhed
continues, the national expansion was a failure.

—*Jon Rohde*

This chapter is reprinted, with permission, from *Partnerships
for Social Development* (Franklin, WV: Future Generations,
1995). Available at http://www.future.org.

A quarter-million marginalized men and women in Maharashtra, India, realized the potential within themselves to improve their own health. They have learned how to better their lives and those of the people around them. Infant mortality (a standard indicator of health) has been reduced from over 175 to 18 per 1,000 births, and the birth rate has fallen from over 40 to 17 per 1,000 within the last two decades.[1]

Lalanbai Kadam is a woman in Jamkhed, Maharashtra. She says, "I am a Dalit widow. I used to think that I was a nobody. I lived in constant fear because I was treated worse than an animal. My son died when he was less than three years old, and I was blamed for it and sent away by my husband. My parents made me marry an old man who had tuberculosis, and he also died. I returned to the village in shame. I lived in darkness. To support myself, I swept and cleaned the village and did hard manual labor and received a pittance. Even dogs were welcome in the house, but I, as a Harijan, was not. Then, along with many other women, we decided not to accept this anymore."

As young doctors, my husband and I made a commitment to each other that we would devote our lives to improving the health of the poorest of the poor in rural India. After preparing ourselves, we

1. The infant mortality rate in project villages declined from 176 (deaths per 1,000 live births) to 17–20 between 1972 and 1992 (Mabelle and Rajanikant Arole, *Jamkhed: A Comprehensive Rural Health Project*, London: Macmillan, 1994, chapter 16). In 1992, 5% of children suffered from malnutrition (weight for age), versus 40% in the survey 20 years earlier. The crude birth rate in 1992 was 19, compared to 40 in 1972.

worked in a rural hospital in western Maharashtra. We were competent, skilled, and hardworking. The hospital flourished and expanded. We went into the villages and held village clinics. We were successful as professionals.

Our commitment, however, was to the poor, and we asked ourselves constantly if our work and services made a real difference to the health of the people. To my dismay we found that our work was having little impact on the health of the people. Infant mortality continued to be high. Most diseases we encountered were preventable. Children were brought in dehydrated, malnourished, and with diarrhea, and many women had problems such as obstructed labor. Often they came in too late. Further analysis proved that only a few people out of the total population were coming to us. Traditional cultural practices, high cost, poverty, and distrust of modern medicine prevented people from coming to the hospital. We started questioning the top-down, doctor- and hospital-centered approach to health care. This led to a search for a more relevant and equitable health care system. Learning from the collective wisdom of many pioneers with similar concerns, we planned a health program. The program was to be people based, and communities would participate at all stages in its development and implementation. It was to be a health program that would respond to the needs of the people, particularly the poorest of the poor.

THE BEGINNING

As we looked around for an area where people were interested in starting such a health program, an enlightened political leader at Jamkhed (a community development block in Ahmednagar district in Maharashtra) invited us to visit. He and other leaders expressed the need for a hospital to take care of obstetric and other emergencies. They perceived health care to be mainly a provider of relief from pain and suffering. We explained our intention of working with the people to improve health through preventive programs. The leaders were not impressed. However, they emptied a veterinary dispensary in the middle of a cattle market and provided a couple of sheds to start the "hospital." We accepted what the people had and made the place safe for surgical care.

Soon we were called upon to prove our skills. A woman was brought in with a ruptured uterus and we had to operate on her to save her life. This time we were able to follow up by developing direct linkages with villages.

THE STORY

Using curative services as an entry point, we came in more contact with the people. It soon became evident that poor people were not interested in health. They were interested in relief from unbearable pain. Other illnesses were mere irritations. "We need water, we need jobs so that we can buy food to kill the hunger pangs, and then we will not have to migrate to cut sugar cane" was a repeated comment. "You ask us to wash hands, to use soap. Where is the water? Do you know the cost of soap?" they challenged us.

It was we who had to change first. Their questions forced the medical team members to think about poverty. How can we share scientific information in a meaningful way unless we understand people's problems? We decided to live on Rs45 (or about US$7) per month (the prevailing average wage at that time). We were in for surprises. Soap costs almost two days' wages. Water needed to flush a toilet was more than a month's wage. Our eyes were opened to reality. The poor people taught us how they cope with the situation, [through means] born out of experience. Their felt needs of food and water were more relevant than our health interventions.

Setting aside our agenda for health promotion, we responded to the need for safe drinking water. We identified an NGO involved in drilling tube wells and received a grant to drill tube wells. The Dalits were concerned that they would not have access to the water if the well was in the main village. A traditional practice was used to solve the dilemma. A water diviner was taken into confidence and asked to walk through the whole village but divine water only in the Dalit section. Over 150 tube wells were drilled in the Dalit areas of villages. Everyone, rich and poor, needed water, and it was too precious [for anyone] to object! More importantly, we had gained the confidence of the poor people. We were in!

The participation of only leaders was obviously insufficient. Health improvement in the whole village needs total community participation. For example, the physical environment of a village has to be protected by the whole community. Eradication of harmful social practices requires community action. Much starvation and undernutrition were due to social attitudes toward women and children. To change people's attitudes toward women and children, the reality had to be faced that religion, caste, and politics divided both rich and poor people. The device of starting volleyball games solved the problem of getting people to talk together. Socially minded people from all groups and factions were invited to volleyball games in their own villages. After the game, both onlookers and players stood around and talked. It soon became the meeting place for more serious discussions on village development.

Informal groups were then organized into the Farmers' Club. All members were not necessarily farmers. Many were landless poor people. According to their interests, seminars were arranged on subjects such as agriculture, dry land farming, and veterinary medicine. Poor people were more interested in the health of farm animals than [in] their own health or that of their children. In each village men were trained to provide primary veterinary care. Government extension workers helped us in these meetings and training. This led to people becoming interested in human health.

ASSESSMENT AND ANALYSIS BY THE PEOPLE LEADING TO COMMUNITY ACTION

Farmers' Club members, along with project staff, surveyed the health situation. A villager recalls, "The survey helped us to understand the health problems in the village. Five or six of us were involved in the first survey. We realized it was for our own good, so we did an accurate survey. Each of us took one area of the village and filled in all the preliminary information. No family was left out. The questionnaire was not difficult to complete. There were questions about immunization of children and whether they had been ill in the past two weeks. We were to report any child's death in the past 12 months and details of how the child had died. We learned to assess the nutritional status of the child by measuring the arm circumference. To our surprise, many children we thought had severe illness turned out to just lack adequate food!

There were questions on pregnancy and family planning. We knew who was missing at the time of the survey, so we went back and completed the survey.

"We analyzed the results with the help of project staff. We learned a lot and began to understand the causes and effects of disease. We had always believed that children did not thrive because of a curse from God. When we understood that the problem was lack of food and preventive care, we organized a community kitchen. We learned to monitor the growth of our children, by regular weighing every month and plotting weight on a 'road to health' card."

Another action was improving sanitation. Many of the families had repeated attacks of fever and chills. Diarrhea was common. Another villager describes the discussion that took place regarding the frequent attacks of illness. "We discovered that 80% of the families had at least three episodes of fever with chills (which we presume was malaria) in the past year. We realized that if we got rid of the puddles made by wastewater and composted the rubbish heaps, then much of the breeding of mosquitoes and flies would be eliminated and the frequency of diseases reduced. With each attack we spent close to Rs10 to go to a doctor, or Rs30 per year. Imagine the amount we were spending for something we could prevent? Moreover, we learned that even if we did have such illnesses, we did not need injections and expensive medicines to be cured. Why not clean up the village? The social worker showed us several methods of draining wastewater. The soak pit, with water draining underground, appealed to us most. We appointed people to mobilize the whole village to build soak pits. Most families showed interest. We, the Farmers' Club members, dug the pits and the owners provided the filling of sand, broken bricks, and a plank to place over the pit. It made a great difference to the frequency of illness in our village."

In each village, the Farmers' Clubs showed enthusiasm in doing the health survey. It helped the people to assess their own priorities. Such discussions eventually led to a demand from the Farmers' Club members to involve women. They requested us to train their own village women to be health workers. "Educators, professionals from the city do not understand our problems, our traditions. They speak another educated language. Our women have never been to school; they will accept someone from their own community that they trust."

STATUS OF WOMEN AND HEALTH

As the Village Health Workers (VHWs) discussed each health topic, the relationship between women's status and health became apparent. They also realized how much their own lives had been affected by the social pressures and norms imposed on them. Sarubai, a VHW, was particularly vocal when she described her own experience:

"I was married when I was a child. I got pregnant when I was 14, and, as is the custom, I came to my mother's house in Rajuri for delivery. I was in labor for three days. Finally a dai arrived and said that the baby was too big and I would not be able to deliver normally. The only way to save my life was to remove the baby piecemeal. I recovered but remained weak and ill for months. During that time I never heard from my husband. Later he sent word that he did not want a woman who could not produce a living child. As a woman left by her husband, I became an outcaste looked down on by society. I was unwanted, uncared for, living at the mercy of my brother.

"Why did all this happen? All because we women have no value in society. Because I was a girl, my parents were interested in getting me married off as soon as possible. I was not old enough to bear a child . . . I was only 14. Then, like a piece of property, I was thrown off by my husband."

Another VHW replied, *"At least you lost your baby. My daughter has two healthy children. She needed a Cesarean operation and now her husband has sent her away. He feels that she may not be able to do hard manual labor and carry heavy loads because of the operation."* The mother welcomed her daughter home and worked on changing the attitude of the husband.

ORGANIZING WOMEN OF THE VILLAGE AND OVERCOMING CASTE BARRIERS

The village women were not permitted to socialize with women from other castes. They were unwilling to break caste prejudices, since the women were also the keepers of tradition in their society. Centuries of subservience had made them accept their secondary role; they were trained to suffer in silence. This attitude had to be changed. But how could a lone Village Health Worker do it?

The VHWs expressed their conviction that other women in the village should experience the kind of liberation that they themselves had experienced as part of their training. Though the Farmers' Clubs helped them in their work, the VHWs needed the support of other women. A counterpart to the men's Farmers' Club was needed to address women's issues. The Farmers' Clubs supported the idea and encouraged their wives and sisters or mothers to be part of the new women's groups.

The VHWs began to meet with women of their villages once every week or fortnight. In the beginning, only 8 or 10 women in a village were interested in meeting for a couple of hours. They were never sure whether their coming together would raise the wrath of their husband's family, so they made sure to abide by traditional social customs. It was unconventional for women from different castes to meet at all.

Sarubai, one of the VHWs, told how she organized women in her village. *"I was able to convince only seven women to come together in the beginning. We gathered together in one of the women's homes, to sing songs and listen to each other. In between, I taught them child care."*

More and more women began to attend these informal meetings in different villages. They decided to call their informal groups Mahila Vikas Mandals (MVMs, Women's Development Associations). Discussions on health and social conditions were not enough to hold the women's interest for long. The need for money was a constant preoccupation. Sometimes their children needed food or medicines. Older children needed books and school uniforms. They always had to request money from their husband or mother-in-law. They needed their own income and control over the money. The association began to think about income-generating activities.

Traditionally, village women had participated in a self-financing credit plan called a *bhishi*. In the bhishi system, the women in a group each contribute a small amount of money periodically. The contributions are pooled and the person whose name is drawn gets the total amount for a particular period. Ultimately everyone gets her turn. The MVM started a modified bhishi. Instead of having the women draw lots, the MVM gave the money to the most needy in turn. Often the money was used to buy food or treat a sick child. Others used the money to raise poultry, market vegetables and dried fish, or improve a farm. Organizing women around their self-interest in earning money brought stability to the MVMs. The bhishi system built a sense of trust and helped women to be sensitive to one another's needs.

The MVM became a platform on which a VHW could build her health activities. As the members increased and attended meetings regularly, they began to realize they had more power together as a group than as individuals. The VHWs gradually introduced social issues that had affected their health, especially problems of women and girl children. They began to ask questions about why they treated their daughters differently from their sons, or why girls were not fed properly or sent to school like their brothers. They talked freely about alcoholism, wife beating, and harsh treatment of unwed mothers. They discussed how these problems could be solved.

VILLAGE WOMEN UNDERSTAND THE ROLE OF LOCAL GOVERNMENT FUNCTIONARIES

By 1978, 31 villages had such associations. Women used to be afraid of government workers. They feared the government functionaries, who tended to exercise their authority rather than serve. They were terrified at the thought of entering a court, police station, or other government offices. For village women, these officers were the rulers. Various strategies were adopted to remove these fears. We arranged for the women to meet with high-level police and revenue officers, local judges, jailers, bankers, and others. Contrary to their expectations, they found that these well-educated officers were cordial and showed real interest in their work and welfare. These experiences helped women to be bold and confident and to understand their own worth in a free democratic society. Exposure to high officials exploded the myth that village government employees were the rulers. Now, the women understood that these workers were there to serve the village people.

They soon had opportunities to deal with these local bosses. Bank officials in the villages treated women in a condescending and derogatory manner. They were used to providing credit to rich businessmen and farmers. They did not want to bother with the paperwork for small loans to scores of women. However, the Government had a special program for extending credit at low interest rates to women and marginalized people. The MVM members in Rajuri were the first to apply for such credit. They knew the rules and were sure they had met the criteria. At first, the village bankers refused to give the loans. They used many excuses: the women had no property and no collateral security and were illiterate. They harassed the women through bureaucratic procedures, but the women did not give up because, according to government policy, they knew they were eligible for the loans. They would not leave the bank until the banker made a decision to either grant them the loan or give his reasons for refusal in writing. Sensing the power and determination of this organized group, the manager relented and granted the loan.

The women triumphantly shared their story with women in other villages at their regular gatherings. The women used the loans to enhance their incomes. They bought chickens and goats for breeding. Others went into small businesses, buying and selling bangles, dried fish, or vegetables. Some improved their farms by digging wells for irrigation or buying a pump set or a pair of bullocks to help in farming operations. One woman bought a small canopy, loudspeaker, microphone, and record player, which she rented out for functions like weddings, elections, and the numerous festivals that take place in the village. She was able to repay her loan in six months. Lalanbai leased fruit trees that grow by the roadside from the government. During the season she sells the fruit and makes a profit of Rs1,000–2,000 every year. Soon other banks started taking women seriously and extended credit to them.

Access to credit made the MVMs very popular. Over the years, these successes helped women gain self-confidence. Over 3,000 women who had never had any hope of getting out of poverty took out loans and improved themselves economically. Their performance attracted the attention of top bank officials at the state headquarters, and the women were invited to workshops to share their experiences with bankers in other parts of the state.

Women who were once poor, marginalized, and weak became empowered to determine their own lives. Increased food production, safe drinking water, and increased access to money and earning capacity were their primary felt needs. The MVMs had begun with a focus on increasing income and health, which widened into areas of social and ecological development that make healthy lives possible. With funds from their cooperative enterprises, the MVMs increased support for the VHWs. They took more and more responsibility for health in the village. In many villages, the Farmers' Club gave over most of the health responsibilities to the MVM. Planting thousands of trees and [constructing] small dams reduced the frequency of drought and the need to leave the villages during drought seasons to find outside work.

COMMUNITIES TAKE RESPONSIBILITY FOR THEIR HEALTH

Sarubai explains the women's group involvement in health in her village. *"We have divided the village into four sections, and one MVM member is responsible for the health section. She ensures that all the children are immunized and that all the pregnant women are receiving prenatal care. The other women in her section help her in the activities. We have also trained three women to be in charge of deliveries when I am not around.*

"Every year we conduct a house-to-house survey to find out the health and economic status of the village. Both the Mahila Vikas Mandal and the Farmers' Clubs participate in this. The survey helps us plan our program and understand what we have to emphasize."

The MVM has "keep the village clean" drives. They get rid of allergenic weeds that are harmful to people, they construct drainage pits and encourage the use of toilets. They help the VHWs follow up on patients with tuberculosis and leprosy, and assist in the rehabilitation of these patients and their families. Tuberculosis patients need adequate nutrition in addition to medicines. Often such patients starve in the village, since they are unable to work. The MVM members take turns in providing vegetables and grains to patients, based on their needs. MVM members assist with health education. They plan the programs according to special needs and invite health personnel to guide them. In the beginning, the health professionals had to go from house to house and ask mothers to accept prenatal care. Now the women are knowledgeable enough to invite health personnel when necessary.

Most village women had never been to school. They had never been involved in decision-making. Someone else had always controlled their thinking and their time. Now they are beginning to think for them-selves. They have learned to work together to share responsibility and to trust each other.

We have acted as catalysts for the various development activities introduced into the area, encouraging and forging partnerships among people and with different sectors of government. The health center has also functioned as an information bank for the women. Health alone would not have sustained the women's long-term interest.

Every MVM has its own history. It has its own individuality, created by the uniqueness of the women who make up this vital vehicle for social change. Active participation and awareness among men and women have led to a dramatic improvement in the health indicators. Men and women constantly assess, analyze, and act to improve their lives.

EXPANSION

The project team was involved in the first 30 villages. As the village men and women realized the changes taking place in the villages, they con-tacted their relatives and friends and organized Farmers' Clubs and MVMs and selected VHWs to expand the program to 250,000 people. As the people became more self-reliant, over 300 volunteers went to other remote villages to start new programs. In their turn, the village people are becoming facilitators for change. It has become a people's movement, with village people not only encouraging other village peo-ple to start programs, but also training medical professionals and social workers from all around the world to start projects in their own coun-tries. These villages are the base for a training institute that is now run-ning formal courses for people from many countries.

Though it started with health, the program has addressed all aspects of development. Through frequent seminars and meetings, govern-ment personnel interact with the poorest of the poor as they provide services. They work closely with the social forestry department in developing plant nurseries and reforestation. They are involved with NGOs and government in watershed management programs. Health awareness has led both to demand for health services from the govern-ment and partnership with them. Small families have become an accepted social norm, with 70% of couples using family planning.

LESSONS LEARNED

People are the key actors in health and human development. Poor people have coping mechanisms based on collective experience and wisdom. It is important to recognize this and enhance their skills and knowledge so as to increase their choices.

Addressing economic poverty and building large infrastructures alone will not lead to better health. Health depends on individual and community action. The knowledge to acquire and maintain health is a human right. Professionals need to change their attitudes and demystify medical knowledge. They should share knowledge freely, not by providing a few filtered messages that they think are best for the people. Knowledge should be shared in such a way that people can be empowered to assess, analyze, and make the right choices. The knowledge should liberate people and not intimidate them. It should lead to building self-esteem and confidence in oneself and others. It is necessary to address the basic causes of problems and share values leading to greater humanity by showing concern for the dignity of others with equity and justice. It is necessary to respect and trust people and facilitate the process of awareness building.

In the words of a village woman, *"People are like wick lamps, simple, inexpensive, and unattractive. But unlike the expensive chandeliers (which professionals are), the wick lamp has a tremendous energy. It is capable of lighting another lamp and another and another . . . to cover the whole planet."*

Hundreds of thousands of people, not only in Maharashtra but through training and visits to Jamkhed and similar NGOs, have realized this energy and potential and are responsible for a worldwide movement for social change.

AFTERWORD

Mabelle and Raj Arole continued their pioneering
work at Jamkhed, training and inspiring thousands of
villagers, hundreds of health workers from across
India, and scores of visitors from around the world.
Mabelle was convinced to become the UNICEF
Regional Advisor for South Asia and soon thereafter
died a premature death. She is mourned by friends,
admirers, and especially village women, and her
work in Jamkhed is ably carried on by her daughter,
Dr. Shobha Arole.

—*Jon Rohde*

The Impact of Development Interventions on Health in Bangladesh

A. Mushtaque R. Chowdhury

The story of BRAC (formerly the Bangladesh Rural Advancement Committee) is provided in several books and studies documenting the success of national programs in oral rehydration, immunization, treatment of tuberculosis, and dealing with the threat of arsenic in ground water. This chapter evaluates the comprehensive development package aimed at improving the livelihoods of the poor and shows that the provision of rural credit, schools, and empowerment of women have direct and measurable effects on health and fertility. While BRAC is a highly directive and standardized program, it is designed in a culturally sensitive fashion to reach the poorest of the poor and guided by ongoing research and modification of its components.

—*Jon Rohde*

This chapter has two parts: the first presents data from a carefully conducted study of the impact of (nonhealth) development interventions, including literacy, education, credit, and livelihood skills on health. The interventions were part of the standard Rural Development Program of BRAC, carried out in some 65,000 villages and focused on the poorest families.

The second part explores trends in development indicators in Bangladesh since its independence in 1971. There is abundant evidence of a substantial improvement in human development over the past 30 years, a result of synergies between government, nongovernmental organizations (NGOs), and international assistance that have strengthened community action and self-reliance. But much remains to be done to bring the population of Bangladesh to acceptable levels of human development, the "freedoms" described by Amartya Sen.

PART I: DEVELOPMENT FROM THE VILLAGE UPWARDS

Since Bangladesh's independence in 1971, numerous government and nongovernmental organizations have been implementing development programs in various sectors. Many of these programs have earned a reputation within and outside Bangladesh for their innovation, effectiveness, and scale. These programs include the Association for Social Advancement, Bangladesh Academy for Rural Development (BARD), BRAC, Grameen Bank, Proshika, and many others. Evaluations of such programs have traditionally looked at their success in increasing the income levels of participants but less often on the broader goals of human well-being, particularly health. This section looks at the poverty alleviation program of BRAC, a large NGO in Bangladesh, and examines its impact on selected outcome indicators of health.

The BRAC Programs

BRAC started work in isolated rural areas when millions of refugees who had fled to India during the 1971 war of liberation returned. Housing, food, and employment, as well as health, were obvious needs. BRAC workers set out to help villagers reconstruct their lives. While initial efforts were directed at entire villages—providing materials to rebuild homes, supporting fishing infrastructure and agriculture, using locally trained male paramedical workers to provide rudimentary health services—BRAC soon learned that efforts must be directed to the most deprived. In spite of the best egalitarian efforts of BRAC workers, the social structure of rural Bengal society led to exploitation of the poor by those who were better off and to dependency on outside help. Thus, landless women and their families became the focus of BRAC, which established a broad range of development initiatives aimed to empower them as individuals and as an important part of the larger community.

The central effort was called the Rural Development Program. It emphasized group formation, functional literacy using a Freire-type of conscientization (Freire 2000), training in rural income projects, and credit offered without collateral. Today, these efforts have grown to embrace a major rural banking scheme, huge cooperatives in silk production and marketing, milk and other agricultural produce, printing, over 35,000 village schools, and management training on a vast scale. BRAC is now the world's largest NGO in terms of the scale and diversity of its interventions (see Table 1).

The poverty alleviation program functions in over 50,000 of Bangladesh's 84,000 villages and involves over 3.5 million poor women representing as many families. BRAC takes a holistic view of poverty: poverty is not only insufficient income or an absence of employment opportunities but a complex syndrome that manifests itself in many different ways. In the words of Amartya Sen (1995), "The point is not the irrelevance of economic variables such as personal incomes, but

TABLE I
A Brief on BRAC
(August 2000, US$)

Full-time staff	25,378
Part-time staff	29,000
Participants in poverty alleviation program	4.1 million households
Amount of loans disbursed to the poor	$1.3 billion
Percentage of loans repaid	98%
Amount saved by village organization members	$74.0 million
Total primary schools run by BRAC	33,527
Total students enrolled	1.1 million (67% girls)
Mothers taught oral rehydration for diarrhea	13.0 million
Cases of tuberculosis treated in villages	45,377
Total budget (annual)	$152.0 million
Villages with BRAC poverty alleviation program	60,000 of 86,000
Number of field offices	1,070
Number of districts with BRAC program	64 (of 64)

their severe inadequacy in capturing many of the causal influences on the quality of life and the survival chances of people."

In addition to establishing programs to foster income and employment generation, BRAC aids the poor in forming self-help organizations, encourages conscientization, awareness raising, and gender equity, and provides human resource development training. The logic of these programs is the creation of an "enabling environment" in which the poor can participate in their own development and in improving the quality of their lives.

BRAC works through a process of social mobilization, delivery of inputs such as adult education, microfinance, and skills training, and creation of an environment of choice for the poor. Like most other poverty alleviation programs in Bangladesh (Hashemi et al. 1996, Pitt and Khandker 1996), BRAC defines the poor as those having half an acre of land or less. The process of social mobilization in a village begins with the identification of those who fit this definition. As soon as an adequate number of eligible individuals show definite interest, an institution of the poor, called a village organization (VO), is formed. In Bangladesh, about half of the households meet the BRAC eligibility criteria, and about 30 to 40% of the eligible villagers in the areas where

BRAC has a presence have so far joined the VOs. The gender ratio has changed dramatically over time in BRAC: in the 1990s, most VOs were composed of men only, whereas now 98% of the members are women. A VO has 40 to 50 members. Within a month of formation, VO members are allowed to apply for loans. The impressively high proportion of loans that are repaid (98%) is the result of a combination of members' consciousness, peer-group pressure, and BRAC staff supervision. BRAC bank staff are trained as extension agents to ensure the viability of village-based income production projects ranging from fish culture to silk production, from weaving to cattle and milk production, from power-pump rental for small irrigation to the sale of approved medicines by village health workers.

BRAC's education program runs nearly 34,000 primary schools, which enroll a total of 1.1 million pupils. Teachers are recruited from among women in the village, who are provided with a standard curriculum to follow for a three-year course. Two-thirds of BRAC school attendees are girls from the poorest sections of the community, to whom the formal public-sector schools are the least accessible. The effectiveness of the BRAC schools in terms of dropout rates (less than 5% over three years of study), attendance (nearly 100%), achievement (high pass rates on standard exams), and costs (some $18 per child per year) is truly remarkable (Ahmed et al. 1993, Chowdhury, Chowdhury, and Nath 1999).

While improved health of communities has been an objective of BRAC efforts from the start, health care, though important, has been seen as only one element. Although BRAC initially trained paramedics to deliver simple curative care, referring more difficult cases to doctors in fixed clinics, the use of paramedics soon became more prevalent. People neglected prevention. Nonetheless, BRAC areas had the highest use of and continuation rate for family planning, even in the early years. Turning its attention to the largest killer of children, diarrhea, BRAC undertook to teach every household in the country how to make and use oral rehydration therapy (ORT), a technology developed in Bangladesh but not widely known. Over a decade, BRAC workers visited some 13 million households in almost all of the country's 86,000 villages to instruct and demonstrate to each mother how to prepare ORT with home ingredients. This is the largest effort of its kind in the world and has contributed to the fall in infant and young child mortality. ORT has now become a part of Bangladeshi culture (Chowdhury and Cash 1993).

BRAC has applied similar mass approaches to improving immunization levels, in partnership with government health services; improved nutrition through village-based growth promotion; and strengthened the availability in communities of family planning and maternity services for women. Most recently, in response to the arsenic contamination of groundwater in a large proportion of the eight million shallow wells providing drinking water in the country, BRAC has developed field-testing procedures enabling identification of unsafe pumps, which are then painted red to warn villagers not to drink the water. Simple filters have been designed and tested for home use, and patients with symptoms of arsenic poisoning are being treated. The current health program also provides essential health services to villagers through trained women who charge a low fee and emphasize women's health and combating specific diseases such as tuberculosis (Chowdhury et al. 1997, Chowdhury 1999).

Since its early days, BRAC has maintained a research and evaluation division, whose role has been to investigate both the design and impact of BRAC programs. With more than 100 employees at present, it produces 30–40 reports each year, providing a continuous flow of information to modify and strengthen programs. Both qualitative approaches to sociocultural issues as well as quantitative studies of programs' impact are published and used to refine BRAC activities. While most studies are descriptive and not controlled, the collaboration with ICDDR,B has made possible a more rigorous evaluation of the impact of BRAC development efforts on health outcomes.

Studying the Impact of BRAC Programs on Health

Although BRAC works throughout Bangladesh, the data for the present analysis come from one subdistrict called Matlab, the field station of the ICDDR,B. Located 50 kilometers south of Dhaka in a riverine area of Chandpur district, the ICDDR,B has maintained this surveillance area since 1963. The many demographic studies and action research conducted there are testimony to its worldwide reputation (Van Ginneken et al. 1998, D'Souza 1984). Given the high quality of community data collected routinely throughout the Matlab study area, BRAC and ICDDR,B initiated a research project to examine the impact of development activities on the health and well-being of the population. This effort became known as the BRAC-ICDDR,B Joint Research Project.

In 1992, BRAC moved to Matlab, where the population of 250,000 was divided into four study cells. Two cells, one inside and one outside a protective embankment to prevent flooding, received BRAC programs, and two similar cells did not. The BRAC inputs introduced in the villages included VO formation and organization of the poor, microcredit, training of VO members in human and legal rights and vocational skills, and nonformal primary education for children. In the 75 villages where BRAC initially started, a total of 164 VOs were formed with 6,736 members (all women), covering over half of the villages' poor households (all poor households were offered the chance to join). Since 1993, BRAC VO members have saved over $300,000. In addition, a total of $3 million in loans has been disbursed to them, with a 99.7% recovery rate. BRAC opened 81 nonformal schools, which enrolled 2,658 students.

Data Sources

The data used in the present analysis came from the following sources:

Baseline survey. Prior to BRAC's interventions in 1992, a survey of more than 12,000 households (over 60,000 people total) in villages belonging to the four cells referred to above collected quantitative information on assets, expenditures, education, nutritional status, health-seeking behavior, women's empowerment, family planning, and involvement with development activities.

Seasonal surveys. Three rounds of seasonal surveys were carried out in a subsample of the baseline population in 1995–96. These surveys collected the same information as did the baseline surveys.

Ethnographic surveys. Several ethnographic and other qualitative investigations were carried out using in-depth interviews, focus group discussions, and observations focusing on women's status and intra-household food distribution.

Demographic surveillance. The Demographic Surveillance System (DSS) of ICDDR,B provided mortality information on all households in the villages under study. ICDDR,B collects data on births, deaths, in- and out-migration, and marriage through monthly household visits.

Management information. BRAC maintains a management information system for its projects. Information from households joining the BRAC program about the inputs received from BRAC, such as date of joining, amount of loans received, repayments, participation in education or vocational training, is linked with the DSS information.

Figure 1 illustrates the conceptual framework linking expected health impacts to inputs and processes in the BRAC program in Matlab, Bangladesh.

Impact of BRAC Programs on Family Planning

The Matlab area is noted for a highly successful family planning program, based on house-to-house delivery of services and coupled with good health care at the ICDDR,B rural hospital and its outlying clinics. Table 2 shows that the current use of family planning methods is greater among married BRAC members than among poor nonmembers ($p < .05$). BRAC members actually had higher rates of use of family planning than the nonpoor nonmembers did.

Impact of BRAC on Nutritional Status of Children

The BRAC-ICDDR,B project collected data on mid-upper-arm circumference (MUAC) in 1992, when the BRAC intervention was about to start, and in 1995, when the intervention was about three years old. Table 3 looks at severe protein-energy malnutrition (PEM, represented as MUAC < 12.5 cm) in children 6–72 months of age, according to their mothers' participation in BRAC. The prevalence of severe PEM has significantly declined among children of BRAC-member households, but there has been no such change among the children of nonmembers.

The pattern in intrafamily food distribution was explored through observations of 25 households having both girls and boys. It showed that among BRAC-member households, girls more often received equal treatment. Still, boys were more favored in terms of being given culturally preferred/superior parts of the fish, chicken, meat, etc. (Roy et al. 1998). When analyzed by gender, the MUAC data showed a signif-

FIGURE I

Conceptual Framework Linking Expected Health Impacts
to BRAC Inputs and Processes

Inputs

Institution building   Children's education

Health services: Adult education on   Training (skill & human
- BRAC   human and legal   development)
- ICDDR,B   rights

Savings and credit

Processes

Literate self and children

Feeling of self-worth   Better skills

Access to and utilization   More income from employ-
of modern health care   ment, savings, and assets

Control over income   Less hunger
and assets

Health Impact

Intrafamily food allocation   Morbidity
                                   (type, complications,
Nutritional status   resistance to infection)

Mortality   Fertility
(level, cause)   (level, age at marriage,
                                   birth spacing)

TABLE 2

Current Use of Family Planning by BRAC Members

BRAC Membership	No. of Respondents	Current FP Use (%)
Member	500	57.9
Poor nonmember	1,194	49.6
Nonpoor nonmember	1,088	51.3

TABLE 3

Prevalence of Severe Protein-Energy Malnutrition in Children by BRAC Membership Status before and after Intervention

| Malnutrition | Year of Survey | | | | Significance | |
	1992 Baseline Poor Individuals (n = 827)	1995 BRAC Member (n = 273)	1995 Poor Non-member (n = 707)	1995 Nonpoor Nonmember (n = 538)	1 vs. 2	1 vs. 3
% Severe PEM (MUAC < 12.5 cm)	23.2	12.1	21.2	11.5	$p < .01$	NS

Source: Khatun et al. 1998

icantly higher prevalence of severe PEM in females among both BRAC members and poor nonmembers, but not among nonpoor nonmembers. Gender bias is hard to overcome!

Impact of BRAC on Child Survival

Survival rates of children belonging to BRAC-member households in comparison to poor nonmember and nonpoor nonmember households are shown in Figure 2. It shows that survival of children in BRAC-member households is better than that of children from poor nonmember households and is in fact similar to survival of children from nonpoor nonmember households.

The pronounced survival advantage of children of poor members compared to poor nonmembers is seen for girls as well as for boys. It is striking that the survival advantage associated with BRAC member-

FIGURE 2
Life Table Probability of Survival of Children in Households of BRAC Members, Poor Nonmembers, and Nonpoor Nonmembers

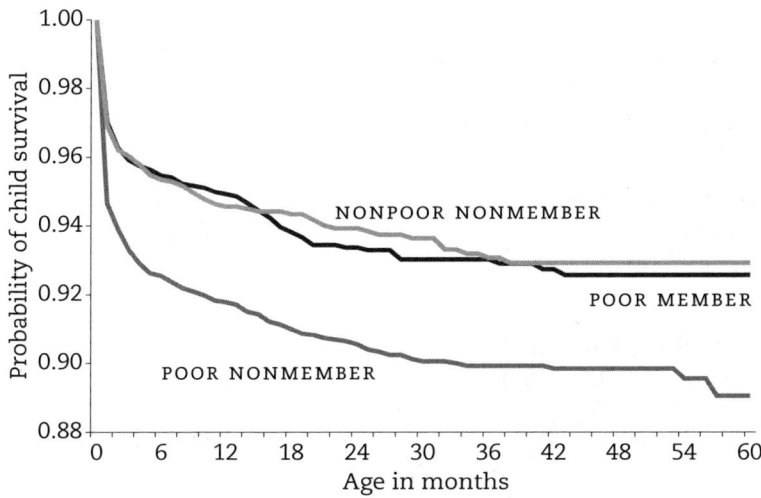

Source: Bhuiya et al. (2001)

ship among the poor was largely the result of mortality differences in the first few months of life, particularly in the neonatal period.

Impact of BRAC on Violence against Women

The prevalence of self-reported violence against women was also studied. A total of 2,038 currently married women aged 15–55 years were interviewed using a structured questionnaire. Each woman was asked about the occurrence of violence in the previous four months. Table 4 compares the incidence of reported physical violence against women in BRAC-member and nonmember households. It shows a higher incidence of violence among BRAC members than among nonmember households. When the incidence figures were analyzed according to length and "depth" of membership (Chen and Mahmud 1995), however, the prevalence of violence tended to decrease with increasing membership length. The peak in violence is reached when credit is introduced but tapers off when other inputs (such as training) are

TABLE 4
Incidence of Violence against Women in Last Four Months
by Characteristics of BRAC Membership, Matlab 1995

	Physical Violence (%)
BRAC Membership	
BRAC member (n = 438)	8.9
Poor nonmember (n = 1,550)	5.8
X^2 significance	$p < .05$
Length of BRAC Membership	
≤ 2 year (n = 185)	10.8
2+ year (n = 260)	7.3
X^2 significance	NS
Depth of BRAC Membership	
Poor nonmember (n = 1,595)	5.6
Only savings (n = 56)	5.4
Savings + credit (n = 268)	11.2
Savings + credit + training (n = 119)	3.4
X^2 significance	$p < .01$

Source: Khan et al. 1998

offered. It appears that the initial "threat" to male hegemony within the family, brought about by women's preferential access to credit, diminishes over time, presumably as the obvious benefits to the overall welfare of the family become apparent.

Conclusions

While BRAC health interventions have been shown to improve survival and nutrition and contribute to reduced fertility in BRAC participants, this study was designed to investigate the health and fertility impact of nonhealth efforts of the overall BRAC Rural Development Program: group formation, credit, schooling, and employment skills. Participants were limited to the poorest households in the communities chosen and were compared to the nonparticipating poor as well as the nonpoor living in the same communities. Survival benefits to children accrued particularly to girls and tended to decrease the typical gender bias that reduces the nutrition and life expectancy of girls. The use of family planning by BRAC beneficiaries was higher, even in comparison to the nonpoor. While women's empowerment, and especially access to credit, seemed to be associated with more acts of domestic violence, this effect diminished over time, as the benefits of the program to the entire family became evident.

The BRAC development efforts clearly contribute to a better life for the poor, even measured by independent survival and quality of life measures.

PART II: NATIONAL TRENDS IN DEVELOPMENT INDICATORS

Having reviewed the evidence of improved health and well-being associated with participation of poor families in the BRAC Rural Development Program, we turn to the broader cumulative impact of development efforts in Bangladesh in the past 30 years.

Poverty Levels

Bangladesh is one of the poorest countries in the world. The GDP per capita (purchasing power parity, or ppp) of US$1,361 is one of the lowest in the world, lower than that of most other South Asian countries. Table 5 compares Bangladesh's per capita income with that of several other countries in the region and with that of the United States.

Whatever pessimistic picture one may draw from Table 5 does not negate the possibility of a better future for this country. In fact, a look at the trends points to a better future. Figure 3 shows the proportion of people in urban and rural Bangladesh who were below the poverty line (the so-called head-count ratio) in various years since independence. This line is based on the "fixed-bundle method"—the expenditure necessary to obtain 2,112 calories per person per day. The figure shows a nearly constant decline in urban and rural poverty, with the improvement in urban areas being faster than in rural areas. This translates into a long-term poverty reduction of 1.55% per year, which is slower than that experienced in East Asian economies but is nevertheless encouraging for Bangladesh (Sen 2000).

TABLE 5
GDP per Capita in Bangladesh and Selected Other Countries

Country	GDP per Capita (ppp US$) in 1998
Bangladesh	1,361
Bhutan	1,536
India	2,077
Nepal	1,157
Pakistan	1,715
US	29,605

Source: UNDP 2000

Economists have also looked at the trends in the depth and severity of poverty over the years. As Table 6 indicates, the depth of poverty, as represented by the "poverty-gap index,"[1] and its severity, as represented by the "squared poverty-gap index,"[2] also decreased, implying improved distribution of wealth as well as a reduction in overall poverty.

Food Production and Consumption

Bangladesh has made commendable progress in food production over the years. In spite of the runaway population growth in the 1970s and 1980s, the average availability and consumption of food grains has remained more or less unchanged (Table 7). This has been made possible by an increase in agricultural production through increased use of technology. For example, between 1984 and 1995, the use of fertilizers in the country more than doubled (from 1.25 million to 2.9 million

1. The poverty-gap index is the mean distance below the poverty line as a proportion of that line. This measure counts the nonpoor as the zero poverty gap.
2. The squared poverty-gap index is the mean of the squared proportionate poverty gaps. The squaring of the poverty-gap index reflects changes in the severity of poverty in the sense that it is sensitive to inequality among the poor.

Trends in Rural and Urban Poverty (1973/74–1995/96)

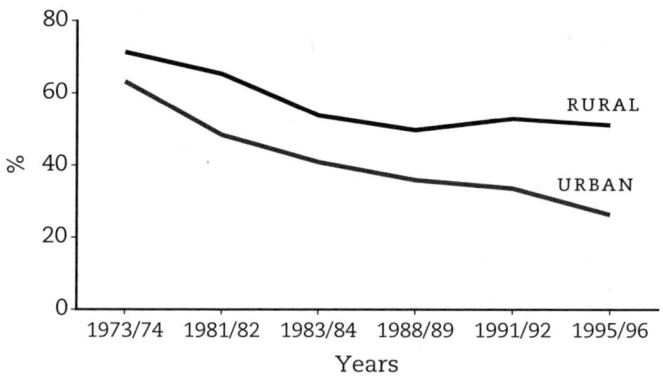

Source: Ravallion and Sen 1996, Sen 2000

metric tons), and the size of irrigated areas also almost doubled. The cropping intensity (the number of times a piece of land is cultivated in one year) also increased over these years, from 168 to 175%. However, the gross cropped area decreased during the same period, from 34.7 million acres to 33.3 million acres, mainly because of population increase and an already low land-to-population ratio[3] (Abdullah and Shahabuddin 1997).

Nutritional Status

Bangladesh also has one of the largest proportions of malnourished citizens in the world. It is estimated that around 80% of Bangladeshi children are malnourished to some degree. Table 8 shows the proportion of children under six years of age who are severely malnourished, as measured by a mid-upper-arm circumference of 12.5 centimeters or less. Nationally, 12.7% of children are severely malnourished, with the situation being worse in rural than in urban areas. The slight improve-

3. Bangladesh is the most densely populated country in the world, with more than 900 people per square kilometer.

TABLE 6
Depth and Severity of Poverty

| Years | ——Poverty-Gap Index—— | | —Squared Poverty-Gap Index— | |
	Urban	Rural	Urban	Rural
1983/84	11.4	15.0	4.4	5.9
1988/89	8.7	13.1	2.8	4.8
1991/92	8.4	14.6	2.8	5.4
1995/96	6.0	14.1	1.9	5.5

Source: Ravallion and Sen 1996, Sen 2000

TABLE 7
Per Capita Daily Availability and Intake of Food Grains (1990–95)

Year	Availability (gm)	Intake (gm)
1990–91	458	461
1991–92	453	451
1992–93	439	449
1993–94	433	440
1994–95	404	434
1995–96	421	432

Source: Abdullah and Shahabuddin 1997

TABLE 8
Nutritional Status of Children
(Measured by Mid-Upper-Arm Circumference) (1985–95)

| Year | ————% Children with MUAC < 12.5 cm———— | | |
	Urban	Rural	All
1985–86	9.90	14.90	14.40
1989–90	8.50	11.00	10.70
1992	8.40	13.20	12.60
1995–96	8.50	13.90	12.70

Source: Bangladesh Bureau of Statistics (1985–86, 1989–90, and 1992), Institute of Nutrition & Food Science (1995–96)

ment from 1986 to 1996 is of little significance and indicates a persisting problem. The country has the highest estimated level of low birthweight in the world: about 50% of newborns weigh less than 2.5 kilograms. These distressing figures are reflected in a secular trend of decreasing adult height in the entire population. This has profound implications for physical work capacity as well as an adverse impact on childbearing.

Health and Fertility

At independence in 1971, Bangladesh was one of the poorest and most unhealthy countries in the world. Nearly 140 of every 1,000 newborns died in their first year, and many more died before age five. Smallpox epidemics ravaged the country, and cholera was endemic. Malaria and kala-azar (an often-fatal tropical fever caused by a blood parasite and spread by a sandfly bite) plagued many areas. The health infrastructure provided care largely in district hospitals. All this fueled one of the highest fertility rates in the world, with over six births per woman.

Extensive external assistance contributed to building *thana* (subdistrict) health centers and, later, smaller clinics in unions (lowest-level administrative units). The global smallpox eradication program concluded its success in Asia with the last case of variola major in Bangladesh in 1975. Efforts to provide safe water through hand pumps were spearheaded by UNICEF and many other donors, as well as by the government. As a result, every hamlet had access to safe water by the early 1980s. In recognition of the role of childhood diarrhea as the major cause of child mortality, BRAC supported a national oral rehydration therapy (ORT) program. Program staff taught a woman in each of 13 million households to make and use homemade ORT—a *labon-gur* (salt-sugar) solution. A coalition of NGOs helped government vaccinators achieve high coverage of routine immunization in infants. A twice-annual dose of vitamin A was added to this regimen. Meanwhile, a major government effort focused on providing modern family planning services, delivered conveniently and reliably in or near women's homes. The combined effect of these health measures is dramatically shown in the decreases in the infant mortality rate and total fertility rate in Figures 4 and 5.

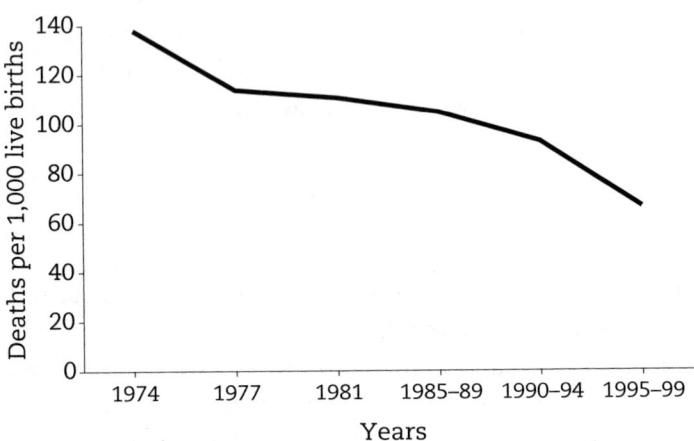

FIGURE 4

Trends in the Infant Mortality Rate

Source: Bangladesh Demographic and Health Survey, Dhaka 2001

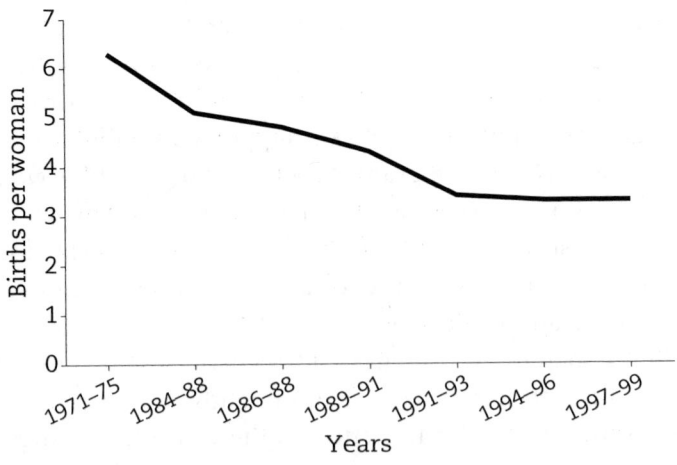

FIGURE 5

Trends in the Total Fertility Rate

Source: Bangladesh Demographic and Health Survey, Dhaka 2001

While mortality appears to be dropping continually, the cessation of the decline in fertility over the last decade is a cause of concern. Bangladesh's demographic transition cannot be considered complete until there is further substantial decline in both these parameters.

Education

Bangladesh is also seriously disadvantaged in terms of the literacy and education status of its population. The country has made progress over the years but at fairly slow pace. As Table 9 shows, the literacy rate rose barely 10 percentage points between 1974 and 1994. The recent claim by the government that it has reached 62% is not borne out by any independent source. On the other hand, the country did make important headway in increasing the access of its children to primary schooling. Recent independent studies show that the gross enrollment ratio (number of children of any age enrolled at the primary level per 100 children) has now reached 107%. The net rate (number of children of primary school age who attend primary classes) has also increased but is still 77%. More significant is the elimination of gender disparity in primary enrollment; in fact, girls now outnumber boys in primary schools. However, the issue Bangladesh still faces concerns the quality of the education. When a very elementary test[4] was administered to children finishing the five-year primary cycle, only 57% qualified, indicating a serious waste of resources and missed opportunities (Chowdhury, Chowdhury, and Nath 1999).

The improvements in both literacy and access to education have been rather slow, and the quality of education is not encouraging. However, when one analyzes such improvements in more depth, important trends surface. Figures 6 and 7 show the share of different socioeconomic groups in the increase in access to primary education. The data show clearly that it is the hitherto-excluded groups that are gaining disproportionately more. The gain has been confined to girls, children from rural areas, and those belonging to socioeconomically disadvantaged groups. This has been possible because the government and NGOs have instituted several policies that favor these groups.

4. Assessment of Basic Competencies (ABC): This measure tests children on basic literacy, numeracy, and life skills (Chowdhury et al. 1994).

TABLE 9
Trends in Adult Literacy Rates and Primary Enrollment

Year	Literacy Rate (%)	Primary Enrollment (Gross) (%)
1971	NA	45
1974	25.8	58
1981	29.2	63
1990	24.8	78
1994	35.3	95
1998	NA	107
2000	62.0	NA

Sources: UNDP (various reports); "Literacy Rates Now 56%," Daily Star 1999; Chowdhury, Chowdhury, and Nath 1999

Environment: Arsenic, Iodine, and Other Issues

Unfortunately, few data are available to evaluate the trend in the environmental situation in Bangladesh. The country has few forests; only 8% of the land is wooded. However, a recent UNDP report (2000) suggests that the annual rate of deforestation in the country declined from 1.8 to 0.9% during the 1980s.

Three decades ago, a national nutrition survey found goiter only in the hilly border areas near India, confirming the classical location of iodine deficiency in high-rain and runoff areas. By the end of the 1980s, goiter was increasingly found on the plains, affecting women and children with predictable effects, including mental retardation, deaf-mutism, and probably lowered IQs. Fortunately, effective measures were taken to iodize all salt at the source from which some 200 distributors supplied most of the country. However, the reasons for this emerging public health epidemic of iodine deficiency have not been fully studied. It appears likely that the intensified agricultural practices of the recent decades have disrupted the replenishment of iodine in the soils through seasonal flooding and silt deposit originating from the high Himalayas. Floods are now controlled by riverine embankments, and most water for irrigation is pumped from the ground. Puddling of

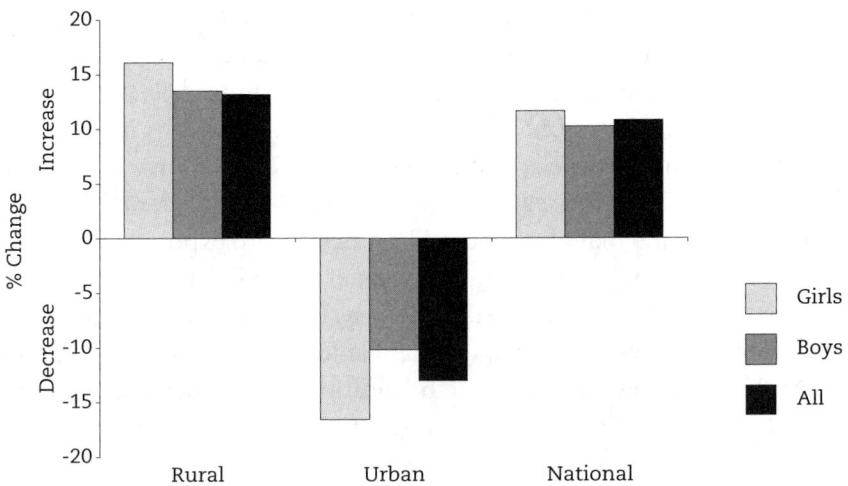

FIGURE 6

Changes in Basic Educational Achievement
by Sex and Residence, 1998 versus 1993

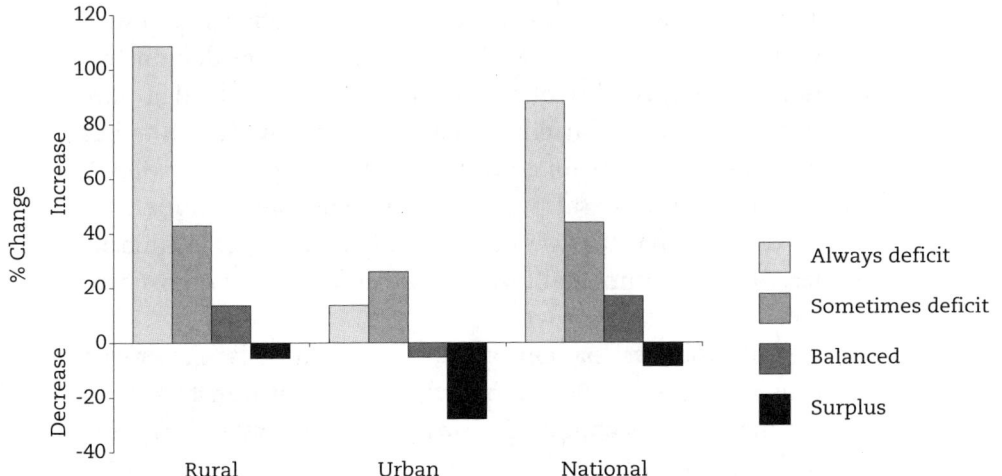

FIGURE 7

Changes in Basic Educational Achievement
by Self-Perceived Economic Status and Residence,
1998 versus 1993

rice paddy fields with tractors effectively washes the soil and may remove other micronutrients as well. The ultimate effects of this intensified agriculture could be far reaching.

Experts foresee other kinds of environmental disasters. Bangladesh was a success story in the provision of safe drinking water to its population. Over 90% of the population had access to tube wells that pumped pathogen-free water out of shallow aquifers. Suddenly, it was found that many of these wells had impermissible levels of arsenic. Arsenic has been detected in areas that constitute about a quarter of the country. This means that about 30 million people are exposed to drinking arsenic-contaminated water. Many experts believe it to be one of the worst environmental disasters in history. Unfortunately, the country is not ready to face this situation. Bangladesh has neither the expertise nor the resources to deal with it. In addition, policymakers are procrastinating. There is a $42-million project supported by the World Bank for arsenic mitigation, but with less than a year to go before its end, only about 10% of the funds have been spent. There are already reports of hundreds of arsenic-related deaths in the country; this problem may increase to epidemic proportions over the next few years. The five main challenges in the arsenic crisis are:

- Find out the reason(s) for the contamination of the ground water; it is unclear whether it is leached from the soils or is related to falling water tables and oxidation of rock layers.
- Test all tube wells for arsenic; there are over eight million such wells in the country. BRAC has conducted a large demonstration of the feasibility of testing and denoting wells that have dangerous levels of arsenic by painting them bright red—thus warning against use for consumption (bathing is permissible).
- Provide alternative safe water options to people; no option has been discovered that is safe, culturally acceptable, technically feasible, environmentally benign, and affordable for most people.
- Identify and treat patients affected by arsenicosis (the disease caused by arsenic poisoning); there is no proven treatment regimen for this condition, nor is the health system prepared to face this disaster.

■ Research the level of environmental contamination of the surface that is caused by arsenic; there are unconfirmed reports that the food chain has already been affected.

Fortunately, there are a few projects that are trying to address these issues, at least on a small scale. Initial results suggest that the arsenic crisis may be tackled successfully if concerted and coordinated efforts are mounted rapidly (BRAC 2000). For now, avoiding use of these wells for consumption is urgent.

Trends in the Human Development Index

The human development index (HDI) is a composite index that measures a society's human development record. Input factors include the expectation of life at birth, adult literacy rate, combined gross school enrollment ratio, and GDP per capita. Of the 174 countries for which the HDI is available, Bangladesh's place is a poor 146th (UNDP 2000). As shown in Figure 8, Bangladesh is making progress in terms of human development, but the country's HDI rank has hovered between 145th and 150th for almost 40 years. This means that other countries have also made comparable progress.

FIGURE 8

Trends in the Human Development Index
(1960–98)

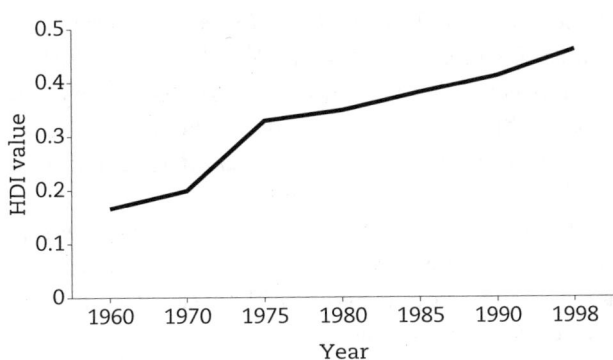

Source: Sen 2000 (for 1960 and 1970), UNDP 2000 (for other years)

Thus, while Bangladesh has made some notable progress in health and education, and held the line against deteriorating nutritional status, there is far more to be done. Many would suggest that persisting poverty is an absolute barrier to further improvement in human development parameters. The experience of BRAC demonstrates, however, that greatly improved human well-being is possible, even in the face of persisting economic poverty. Holistic, community-based strategies that are centered on women and emphasize self-reliance have shown that not only good health but also humane and acceptable living standards can be achieved through decentralized, affordable development.

REFERENCES AND RESOURCES

Abdullah, A., and Q. Shahabuddin. 1997. "Recent Developments in Bangladesh Agriculture." In R. Sobhan, ed., *Growth or Stagnation!: A Review of Bangladesh's Development.* Dhaka: University Press.

Abed, F. H., and A. M. R. Chowdhury. 1997. "How BRAC Learned to Meet Rural People's Needs through Local Action." In Anirudh Krishna, Norman Uphoff, and Milton J. Esman, eds., *Reasons for Hope: Instructive Experiences in Rural Development.* West Hartford, CT: Kumarian Press, pp. 41–56.

Ahmed, M., et al. 1993. "Primary Education for All: Learning from the BRAC Experience." Washington, DC: Academy for Educational Development.

Bhuiya, A., et al. 2001. "An Interventions Study of Factors Underlying Increasing Equity in Child Survival." In Timothy Evans et al., eds., *Challenging Inequities in Health: From Ethics to Action.* New York: Oxford University Press.

BRAC. 2000. *Combating a Menace: Early Experiences with a Community-Based Arsenic Mitigation Project in Bangladesh.* Dhaka: BRAC.

Chabot, C., et al. 1993. *Primary Education for All: Learning from the BRAC Experiences.* Washington, DC: Academy for Educational Development.

Chen, M. A. 1993. *A Quiet Revolution: Women in Transition in Rural Bangladesh.* Rochester, NY: Shenkman Books.

Chen, M. A., and S. Mahmud. 1995. "Assessing Change in Women's Lives: A Conceptual Framework." Working Paper No. 2. Dhaka: BRAC and International Centre for Diarrhoeal Disease Research, Bangladesh (ICDDR,B) Joint Research Project.

Chowdhury, A. M. R. 1999. "Success with the DOTS Strategy." *The Lancet* 353: 1003–4.

Chowdhury, A. M. R., and A. Alam. 1998. "BRAC's Poverty Alleviation Efforts: A Quarter Century of Experiences." In G. Wood and I. Sharif, eds., *Who Needs Credit?: Poverty and Finance in Bangladesh.* London: Zed Books, pp. 171–94.

Chowdhury, A. M. R., and A. Bhuiya. 2001. "Do Poverty Alleviation Programmes Reduce Health Inequity: Evidence from Bangladesh." In David A. Leon and Gill Walt, eds., *Poverty, Inequality and Health: An International Perspective.* Oxford: Oxford University Press, pp. 312–32.

Chowdhury, A. M. R., and R. A. Cash. 1993. "Cultural Incorporation of the ORT Message." *The Lancet* 34: 1591.

———. 1996. *A Simple Solution: Teaching Millions to Treat Diarrhoea at Home.* Dhaka: University Press.

Chowdhury, A. M. R., R. K. Chowdhury, and S. R. Nath. 1999. *Hope Not Complacency: State of Primary Education in Bangladesh.* Dhaka: Campaign for Population Education and University Press.

Chowdhury, A. M. R., M. Mahmud, and F. H. Abed. 1991. "Credit for the Rural Poor: The Case of BRAC in Bangladesh." *Small Enterprise Development* 2: 4–13.

Chowdhury, A. M. R., et al. 1994. "Assessing Basic Competences: A Practical Methodology." *International Review of Education* 40: 437–54.

———. 1995. "Effects of Socio-Economic Development on Health Status and Human Well-Being: Determining Impact and Exploring Pathways of Change." Proposals for Phase II of the BRAC-ICDDR,B Matlab Joint Project 1996–2000 AD. BRAC-ICDDR,B Working Paper No. 6. Dhaka: BRAC and International Centre for Diarrhoeal Disease Research, Bangladesh (ICDDR,B).

———. 1997. "Control of Tuberculosis by Community Health Workers in Bangladesh." *The Lancet* 350: 169–72.

Chowdhury, F. I., and Chowdhury, A. M. R. 1978. "Use Pattern of Oral Contraceptives in Rural Bangladesh." *Bangladesh Development Studies.*

D'Souza, S. 1984. "Small Area-Intensive Studies for Understanding Morbidity Process: Two Models from Bangladesh—The Matlab Project and the Companion Health Project." In *United Nations Databases for Mortality Measurement.* Papers of the Meeting of the United Nations/World Health Organization Working Group on Databases for Measurement of Levels, Trend, and Differentials in Mortality. Bangkok, October 20–23, 1981. New York: United Nations Dept. of International Economic and Social Affairs, pp. 146–58.

Freire, Paulo. 2000. *Pedagogy of the Oppressed.* 30th anniversary ed. New York: Continuum.

Hashemi, S. M., S. Schuler, and P. Riley. 1996. "Rural Credit Programs and Women's Empowerment." *World Development* 24: 635–53.

Husain, A. M. M., ed. 1998. *Poverty Alleviation and Empowerment.* Dhaka: BRAC.

Khan, M. R., et al. 1998. *Domestic Violence against Women: Does Development Intervention Matter?* Joint Project Working Paper No. 28. Dhaka: BRAC and International Centre for Diarrhoeal Disease Research, Bangladesh (ICDDR,B).

Khatun, M., et al. 1998. *Women's Involvement in BRAC Development Activities and Child Nutrition.* Joint Project Working Paper No. 30. Dhaka: BRAC and International Centre for Diarrhoeal Disease Research, Bangladesh (ICDDR,B).

"Literacy Rates Now 56%." 1999. *Daily Star.* Dhaka, June 26, 1999, p. 11.

Lovell, C. H. 1992. *Breaking the Cycle of Poverty: The BRAC Strategy.* West Hartford, CT: Kumarian Press.

Pitt, M. M., and S. R. Khandker. 1996. *Household and Intra-Household Impact of the Grameen Bank and Similar Targeted Credit Programs in Bangladesh.* Discussion Paper No. 320. Washington DC: The World Bank.

Ravallion, M., and B. Sen. 1996. "When Method Matters: Monitoring Poverty in Bangladesh." *Economic Development and Cultural Change* 44: 761–92.

Roy, R. D., et al. 1998. *Does Involvement of Women in BRAC Influence Sex Bias in Intra-Household Food Distribution?* Joint Project Working Paper No. 25. Dhaka: BRAC and International Centre for Diarrhoeal Disease Research, Bangladesh (ICDDR,B).

Sen, Amartya. 1995. *Mortality as an Indicator of Economic Success and Failure.* London: London School of Economics, The Development Economics Research Programme.

Sen, B. 2000. *Bangladesh Poverty Analysis: Trends, Policies and Institutions.* Dhaka: Bangladesh Institute of Development Studies.

United Nations Development Programme. 2000. *Human Development Report.* Oxford: Oxford University Press.

Van Ginneken, J., et al. 1998. *Health and Demographic Surveillance in Matlab: Past, Present and Future.* Special Publication No. 27. Dhaka: International Centre for Diarrhoeal Disease Research, Bangladesh (ICDDR,B).

5 Community-Led Primary Health Care Initiatives: Lessons from a Project in Rural Bangladesh

Abbas Bhuiya, Claude Ribaux, and Peter Eppler

This chapter reports on a rare trial of true community participation, with inputs only in helping the community define its own problems and priorities and possible resources from within and without to meet them. The difficulty of maintaining "restrained generosity" in the face of obvious need results in a program that may indeed be sustainable, beyond the presence of well-meaning outsiders. But how far can such self-reliance meet the needs? And who will be left out? This challenging example leaves some important questions unanswered.

—*Jon Rohde*

A chieving community participation in health matters remains a major challenge. This chapter presents lessons learned since 1994 from indigenous, village-based self-help organizations in Chakaria, a remote rural area of Bangladesh.

There has been a growing realization that the myriad problems which the population of Bangladesh faces, especially in relation to health and environment, may be so large and complex that no governmental or nongovernmental machinery can address them adequately without effective participation from community members. A main tenet of primary health care philosophy, community participation has been on the agenda of health programs of governmental and nongovernmental agencies since the Alma-Ata Conference in 1978 (World Health Organization 1978). Although it was expected that community members would be involved in planning, organizing, and managing primary health care activities, in fact, in the mid-1980s, governmental or nongovernmental agencies planned most such activities with little or no community participation (Morley, Rohde, and Williams 1983). By the early 1990s, community participation in health activities was reported from some places in the developing world (Rohde, Chatterjee, and Morley 1993).

In Bangladesh, community participation has been largely limited to obtaining community support for government immunization drives, providing housing for satellite clinics, and forming village health committees in some localities in response to persuasion either from the government or nongovernmental organizations (NGOs). A systematic attempt to achieve effective community participation in health matters has largely been ignored (Chowdhury 1990, Lovell and Abed 1993).

While most people concerned with health matters see the potential benefit of effective community participation, progress so far has been limited, perhaps due to a lack of understanding about how this can be achieved.

Rural Bangladeshi society has been traditionally rich in community initiatives, in building educational institutions, roads, playgrounds, orphanages, mosques, temples, and cultural organizations. Currently, there are 893 colleges, 9,822 secondary schools, 45,783 primary schools, 5,766 *madrashas* (religious schools), 131,641 mosques, and 58,126 *maktabs* (nonformal religious schools) attached to mosques. Of these, 76% of the colleges, 97% of the secondary schools, 18% of the primary schools, and almost all madrashas and maktabs are managed by the community, with little or no support from the government (Bangladesh Bureau of Statistics 1991). Almost all primary and secondary schools were established by community initiatives. This effort involved over 6,000 registered, village-based, voluntary social welfare organizations, formed and managed by communities (Government of Bangladesh 1985). So far, however, community initiatives for health have been rare, although not totally absent. Despite this social tradition, it is not understood why community initiatives for health have not developed, as have many other aspects of community life (such as education). Health has remained the responsibility of government, outside agencies and, of course, the private sector (both formal and informal), where the provision of medical services is big business.

To examine the possibility and feasibility of activating community initiatives for the improvement of health through existing indigenous self-help organizations (SHOs), the International Centre for Diarrhoeal Disease Research, Bangladesh (ICDDR,B) started a community development-oriented health project in 1994 in Chakaria, a rural area of Bangladesh. The project began its work in three unions (lowest-level administrative units) with a total population of 60,000. Subsequently, the activities were extended to another three unions and now cover a population of 130,000. Two adjacent unions with a population of around 60,000 have been designated as a comparison area. This chapter presents an overview of the achievements of the project since its initiation in 1994, including an exploration of the project's implementation, problems faced, solutions suggested, and lessons learned.

THE STUDY AREA

Chakaria is located on the southeast coast of the Bay of Bengal. Administratively, it is a *thana* (subdistrict) in the Cox's Bazar district, which has a population of 400,000 in 19 unions. It covers an area of 643 square kilometers, including 100 square kilometers of rivers and canals (Bangladesh Bureau of Statistics 1994). The highway from Chittagong to Cox's Bazar passes through Chakaria. The east side of Chakaria is hilly, while the west side is low along the Bay of Bengal.

The climate of Chakaria from May to September is characterized by tropical monsoons and heavy rainfall and is mostly dry during the remainder of the year. Because of its location, Chakaria is very vulnerable not only to regular monsoon flooding but also to cyclones and tidal floods, the most recent in 1991, when a large number of inhabitants and cattle were killed. Innumerable houses and other properties were damaged as well (Hossain, Dodge, and Abed 1992, Cox's Bazar Foundation 1991).

Despite its vulnerability to natural calamities, externally financed development efforts in the area have been scarce. However, after the 1991 cyclone, Chakaria began to receive some attention from development agencies. Efforts were made to improve roads, build cyclone shelters, and plant trees. Traditionally, the main economic activities in the area have been agriculture, forestry, and sea fishing.

The population comprises mainly Muslims and a small number of Hindus and Buddhists. Traditionally, the area is strongly influenced by Islam, and the population is not very open to modern ideas or to outsiders. The nationwide anti-NGO backlash in 1994 originated in this area, occasionally resulting in physical assaults on NGO workers, especially female workers. Security in Chakaria is quite precarious, with incidences of banditry being observed during the study period. Disputes over land sometimes result in violence and murders.

The study area is also one of the poorest performing in the country, in terms of health and family planning indicators. Despite the commendable success of the national family planning and Expanded Programme on Immunization (EPI) efforts during the last decade, the area has lagged far behind the other parts of the country in contraceptive prevalence and immunization coverage. The contraceptive prevalence rate for rural Bangladesh in 1993–94 was 43.4%, but for Chakaria it was only 20.8% in 1994. The coverage rates for DPT1, DPT2, DPT3, and measles vaccination among children between the ages of 12 and 23 months in rural Bangladesh in general during 1993–94 were 82.9, 76.1, 64.5, and 67.8%, respectively. For Chakaria, it was 77.8% for DPT1, 72.5% for DPT2, 66.4% for DPT3, and, for measles, only 47.7% (Bhuiya 1995, Mitra et al. 1994, Bhuiya and Ribaux 1997).

PROJECT STRATEGY AND METHODS OF IMPLEMENTATION

Project Staff

The project started with a team of six community organizers (three female and three male), two self-help trainers, two applied social researchers, and a field team leader. They were supervised by a social scientist, with assistance from an expatriate anthropologist throughout —a trainer at the beginning and a resident anthropologist at a later stage. The project started with nonmedical personnel. This was done intentionally, so that the field staff could in no way start offering curative health services to the community. This would have undermined the promotion of preventive health activities and raised undesired expectations.

After a year of operation, two paramedics and a public health physician joined the team. Six community health workers with a minimum of 12 years of schooling, recruited from the locality, joined the project later. The public health physician was mainly responsible for ensuring the quality of the health messages transmitted and for defining the contents of preventive and curative health initiatives. Subsequently, the number of public health physicians was increased to two, and they began to provide curative services. The paramedics, who started with health education activities, later became involved in running the village health posts. The trainers continued to develop training curricula, as well as train the project staff and volunteers. The trainers were also responsible for conducting People's Participatory Planning sessions. The community organizers were responsible for establishing links with SHOs and the community members for eventual mobilization of the community members through the SHOs. The community health workers have continued to maintain contact with the SHOs and are gradually carrying out the work that used to be done by the community organizers. Now all the female community health workers are trained in community midwifery and in treating diseases with nonprescription drugs; they are emerging as a new cadre of female health workers in this male-dominated society. The applied social researchers have been engaged in monitoring, evaluating, and providing feedback to the program and to community members. The field team leader has been responsible for overall supervision in the field, and for maintaining links with the government and NGO activities in the area.

Training of the Project Staff

All project staff went through an orientation program before starting work in the field. This orientation consisted of a participatory exercise to review the experience of the staff with respect to sustainable development in Bangladesh. The orientation also included discussions about establishing relations with the community, its social and power structures, locating casual meeting places in rural areas, the role of indigenous SHOs in the society, and key people and resource persons. (A key person has power and influence in the community. A resource person is knowledgeable about and interested in community development but does not necessarily have power and influence in the community.) The training program combined various methodologies, including role-playing, field visits, and self-evaluation.

After reviewing the status of initiatives in the villages, all members of the staff reached the conclusion that initiatives taken by the villagers are the only ones sustainable in the long run. Thus, if health can somehow be brought onto the agenda of these existing initiatives, it will not only cause them to initiate health activities, it will also foster adoption of health- and hygiene-related behavior, in turn leading to improved health status of client populations. The issue of creating new organizations and sustaining them—a major concern in any development initiative—does not arise because the village organizations have already been in place for years and are being managed by the community.

During the project orientation, participants also developed a definition of SHOs and an instrument for collecting information about them. Organizations started by the villagers without any external input were considered SHOs. Thus, NGOs were excluded by this definition.

During the training, a consensus was reached for describing the objectives of the project: "We are here to learn about the health problems you face and what you do about them. We are also here to assist you, if you want to do anything to solve your own health problems. We are here for demonstrative purposes only, that is, we will try to provide technical information to you if you would like to take initiatives." The members of the staff were clearly instructed not to say any more than this and to be careful not to create false hopes or raise expectations, since the project was not designed to provide resources or curative services.

Knowing the Community and Building Confident Relationships

After initial training, members of the project staff began visiting villages in Baraitali, one of the unions. They walked through the villages and tried to explain the purpose of the project when asked. They started talking about health problems, the location and number of schools, mosques, clubs, and other community organizations, and key and resource persons in the locality. They also started making maps of the villages. They applied participatory research methodologies to draw village maps and mobility maps showing where people go for health care, to rank diseases, and to carry out group discussions about health problems. These activities helped them to understand the major health problems, health beliefs, care of the sick, and feeding practices of the villagers. Villagers were involved in these activities from the start, enhancing and building a relationship of mutual trust.

During this process, the project staff also participated in a two-week, school-based maternal and child health (MCH) program sponsored by the government. There, they talked about MCH issues with high-school students from the project area. These schoolchildren spoke highly of the project staff and the program to their parents, thereby facilitating access of field staff to the students' families. This experience helped the project staff realize the potential of school-based programs, and similar programs have been incorporated into regular project activities.

Identification of Indigenous Organizations

Data collection. After four weeks of relationship-building activities, the project staff compiled a list of indigenous village organizations and key and resource persons. Detailed information about these people and organizations was collected using a questionnaire developed during the orientation.

Seven college-educated members of the project staff conducted a survey of indigenous organizations. Field visits were made to identify the existing SHOs and initiatives. This was done through discussions with local people casually encountered on the road, at the market, and in restaurants, shops, and educational institutions.

Project staff made a list of the organizations and initiatives mentioned by the villagers and then visited the organizations. Occasionally, new signboards were hung on dormant or newly created organizations. These organizations, which appeared to expect that financial or material help might be forthcoming from the project, were excluded.

Data were collected during visits to individuals whom villagers considered to be associated with or well informed about the organizations. Cross-checks with at least three different sources were made before a final recording of the information. In cases of discrepancies in information from various respondents, attempts were made to cross-check the information with the respondent through repeated visits, before the project staff made a final recording of information.

Data analysis. Fifty-four organizations were listed in one union. However, information from only 45 was collected because the existence of the remaining organizations was doubtful. Almost all the organizations were established locally, most within the last 10 years, by middle-class or upper-class villagers. Their purpose was usually economic improvement, but several had founded schools or programs for religious training. Most had written bylaws and almost all had elected committees, serving up to 5 years. Only 10% had more than 20 active members. Funds were collected from members, government organizations, and other contributors. Most maintained some form of accounting.

Selection of organizations. A one-day workshop was organized with project staff to analyze the data and to select the possible organizations and the key and resource persons for cooperation. After a critical re-examination of all the organizations, four were short-listed for cooperation. The selection criteria included existence of a committee, ongoing activities, and financial resources. From the list of key and resource persons, a list of supportive and neutral (not hostile to modern ideas) key and resource persons was prepared. Project staff also decided to maintain contact with other organizations and with key and resource people. The organizations selected had maximum community representation in terms of membership, community support, regularity in convening meetings, ongoing activities, and resources at their disposal. The four organizations chosen included a mosque committee, two temple committees, and one cultural organization run mostly by youth. Subsequently, project staff continued to maintain a close relationship with the selected organizations and key and resource persons.

Putting Health on the Agenda

None of the organizations had had health on their agenda, so encouraging them to include health issues was a major challenge. The discussion started with the context of well-being, which was a priority for all the organizations: some emphasized economic well-being, others the afterworld, social order, or human values through education. The villagers were requested to identify the most economically disadvantaged individuals and households in the village. Quite often, the most disadvantaged households were those in which family members were in poor health or in which the only wage earner had died young. Those households usually had had to liquidate whatever assets they had to meet the medical costs of their family members. The families fell into a vicious cycle of poverty from which they were not able to emerge.

It was easy to draw the conclusion that, in many cases, poor health was responsible for economic disadvantage. Even the religious groups saw the importance of good health to regular religious activity. The educational institutions too could very easily see a relationship between poor performance at school and the poor health of students. Thus, all the indigenous organizations realized the importance of good health (in its narrow sense—freedom from disease and disability) for human development, be it material or spiritual. However, they had no idea about what could bring about good health. So far, tackling health problems through preventive measures, such as immunization and epidemic control, was viewed solely as a government responsibility. Curative services, on the other hand, could be obtained for a small fee from the government facilities or for a larger fee from private sources. The community members could not identify a role for themselves in health matters.

At this stage, the project staff introduced the villagers to the possibility of prevention by avoiding harmful behaviors. The problem of diarrhea was raised, and an attempt was made to explain its mechanisms of transmission and ways to break the transmission route. Villagers were not aware of the scientific causes and routes of transmission of diarrhea. The need for and advantages of preventive behavior were further emphasized through a participatory discussion about the consequences of illness on health and economic well-being. As one villager said, "This [prevention] is most important for us, especially those of us who are not economically well off. Illness makes one unable to work and dependent on caregivers for treatment, which costs money. Thus we need it [prevention] most."

Thereafter, members of the project staff were invited to participate in meetings held by the organizations. During these meetings, it became clear that an orientation of community members to common health problems, their causes, transmission, and appropriate management would significantly increase the popularity of the meetings.

The project, in collaboration with the SHOs, arranged three orientation sessions in three unions with 15–20 participants from each SHO. Each session lasted one day. The orientation sessions were facilitated by project staff and attended by a medical officer from the *thana* health complex. The representatives of the SHOs were asked to share with the rest of the participants what they considered the major health problems in the locality, what they thought those problems were caused and transmitted by, and what they thought would be the best ways to manage them. Diarrheal diseases, respiratory illness, malaria, complications relating to delivery, and lack of curative services were the most commonly cited health problems.

After explanations from the medical officer, the sessions concluded with an invitation from the project members to the participants to go back and discuss their experiences with other members of the SHOs. If they thought that the knowledge should be disseminated, they should find a way to do this. The project would be willing to provide technical support. The project staff also indicated that they were willing to participate in any meetings that the SHOs might organize.

People's Participatory Planning and Actions

The project staff attended some of the meetings of the SHOs. These discussions were like the earlier ones and focused on major health problems, the importance of maintaining good health, the possibility of preventing disease through behavior modification, and the role of individuals and the community in improving health. The project staff mentioned that if the SHO members decided to take any initiatives, the project could provide technical assistance. If they met again to discuss the matter among themselves, the project staff would be happy to be present, if invited. They requested that the project staff talk to some of the female members of the community about a strategy for disseminating health messages to women. Eventually, commitment from a number of male and female volunteers was obtained, and the project started training these volunteers at the village level. The only material support provided by the project was to cover the cost of tea and lunch on the days of training.

A similar exercise has also been carried out in secular primary and high schools. Progress has been limited in religious educational institutions, due to their lack of interest in the activity. In the high schools, the students in each class have chosen 1 volunteer per 10 students. One teacher was put in charge. In primary schools, the volunteers came from classes four and five only. Formal approval from the thana education officer was obtained to carry out these school-based activities.

ACHIEVEMENTS

During the first six months of the project, members of the staff were able to establish a good relationship with the villagers. In the beginning, villagers resisted allowing female community organizers even to meet village women. The situation improved significantly over three to four months, so work could proceed. Participatory research methods could be used and group discussions on health issues could be held. During the first six months of field operations, a quantitative baseline survey was also carried out in the three intervention and two comparison unions by locally recruited female field workers. The villagers cooperated fully, with a few isolated exceptions.

Regular contact with key personalities in the union was established. Representatives of the self-help organizations participated in health orientation sessions organized by the project. Staff of the project and the SHOs jointly organized more than 50 People's Participatory Planning sessions. Participants discussed health issues and possible solutions. The sessions were held mostly at night. Action plans were developed for implementing health education programs by village health volunteers, female health volunteers, and school health volunteers. During the first two years, the SHOs and neighborhood clusters of women nominated more than 1,000 volunteers. Most of them participated in training programs organized by the project, without receiving any material or cash incentives from the project.

Currently, volunteers disseminate health messages to the community, school volunteers communicate health messages to fellow students, and both groups take the messages to their homes and share information with their family members and immediate neighbors. The male village health volunteers disseminate health messages in mosques during Friday prayers and in informal gatherings at tea stalls and at other casual meeting places. Female volunteers share health information with women in nearby households through cluster meetings.

The SHOs have also started to engage in health matters beyond simply the dissemination of health messages. In three villages, the SHOs, in collaboration with government health authorities, have implemented a program to control malaria by using insecticide-impregnated mosquito bed nets. The project facilitated this government-community collaboration. The project helped the SHOs obtain free growth monitoring charts from the government's Institute of Public Health and also provided them with locally made weighing scales. Members of the project staff trained the volunteers to weigh children, record weights in the chart, interpret the results, and provide nutrition counseling to the mothers.

At the end of the first year of collaboration with the project, five organizations took initiatives to establish village health posts. The local people provided the space and furniture. The SHOs selected one village doctor (allopathic practitioner) for each village health post to provide services with assistance from the volunteers. Currently, there are seven health posts in six intervention unions. Weekly service sessions are carried out by qualified medical doctors, with assistance from a paramedic, community midwife, and SHO volunteers. A family health card system has been introduced whereby a family can buy a card for US$1 that entitles family members to consultation with a medical doctor once a week in the health post for US$.50. For individuals without a health card, a consultation fee of US$.80 is charged. Drugs are available at a price 7% higher than cost and 7% lower than the market price. All the money generated from the operation is being deposited in the bank accounts of the health posts. Recently, a lower level of health post serving a population of around 6,000 has been established. These sub-health posts are staffed by paramedics and operate five days a week. Figure 1 presents the numbers of patients attending the health posts in different quarters since the beginning of the health post services. Women have been the dominant users of the health posts.

By 2001, nearly 33% of the families had subscribed to the health card. After realizing that the family health cards were being disproportionately procured by rich people, the health posts' committees arranged to provide health cards at a lower fee to poor families (13%), and visits to the doctor are provided free to the poorest members of the community. Currently, 8% of the poorest families use the health post services. A health fund for the poor has also been launched to support drug costs for the poor. All these have improved the utilization of the health post services by patients from socioeconomically disadvantaged families.

By the first quarter of 2001, a total of US$7,500 had been earned and saved by the health posts through their services. In each of the six unions, land for the health posts had been either bought or donated by the members of the community. Of the six posts, three are now permanent structures with brick buildings constructed with resources from the community.

In terms of immunization coverage, the intervention areas have been doing better than the comparison areas. Figure 2 presents the per-

FIGURE I

Number of Male and Female Patients Attending Village Health
Posts, 1998–2000

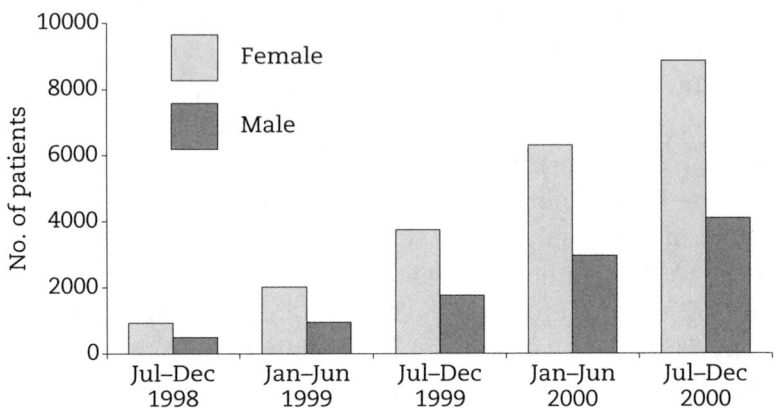

centage of fully immunized children aged 12–23 months before (1994)
and after (1999) the initiation of self-help health activities in the intervention and comparison unions. Over the years there has been an
improvement in both areas; however, the improvement has been much
greater in the intervention areas than in the comparison areas (52%
and 15%, respectively). It should be mentioned that despite the high
level of awareness about immunization among the villagers (dissemination of information about immunization was one of the activities of
the project), immunization coverage could not increase further, due to
the constraints of public-sector service delivery (government program
personnel delivered EPI services).

PROBLEMS FACED AND SOLUTIONS OFFERED

During the first two years of operation, the project confronted many
problems. These included keeping the project personnel centered on
the project philosophy, maintaining the project philosophy in the face
of the current development trends emphasizing external material support, and responding to the needs of the community without creating
dependency on the project in the community. A description of these
problems and the strategies developed to address them follows.

FIGURE 2

Percentage of Fully Immunized Children Aged 12–23 Mos. in Comparison and Intervention Areas before and after Intervention

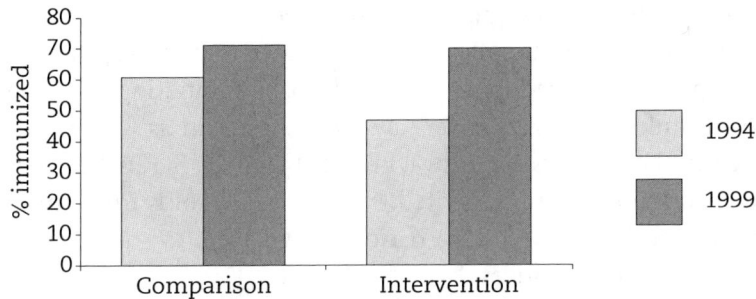

Morale of Project Staff and the Need for Philosophical Clarity

Despite the project's philosophy of promoting self-help, some members of the project staff were apprehensive that nothing much would happen without material support from the project. Given these circumstances, it was necessary to reassure the staff that the process would likely be slow at the beginning. It was also reiterated that if the project provided material support, it would be like any other development activity in the country and would suffer from similar limitations, thus encouraging dependency. The activity would have little chance of becoming sustainable. Staff were further assured that even if the project failed, the documentation of the procedures adopted and reasons for failure would be a valuable contribution. Thus, slow and/or minimal achievement of goals, or even failure, would not result in early closure of the project, and no one would be held responsible for it.

Distrust among Villagers and the Need for a Slow, Transparent Approach

Since the project is located in a very conservative, Muslim-dominated area with a history of opposing development NGOs (especially around the time when this project was launched), it was particularly difficult to earn the trust of the community members. Project personnel were challenged on many occasions about their intentions, and health was seen by some community members as a means for the project to enter into the community and eventually to engage in antireligious activities, as the East India Company did before the British colonized the country. Obviously, this was quite serious and led to discouragement, especially among expatriate colleagues who wanted to visit the project area.

The project adhered to its philosophy of not initiating anything on its own, and the villagers never saw the project staff as very proactive. The control of all initiatives always resided with the SHOs. Project personnel participated only if invited. Initiatives came only from an SHO's activities, and there was little reason for villagers to suspect outside control or ulterior motives.

Project staff provided training of volunteers only if the SHOs asked them to. Contact was always maintained with key and resource persons, who were often involved with the SHOs. The participation of the project staff in school programs brought student support for the project and helped promote acceptance of the project in the community.

The project's attention to the problems identified by the villagers themselves also contributed to the development of trust and respect. Bringing the government malaria control program into some villages also demonstrated the project's adherence to its philosophy of linking the SHOs with a third party to mitigate health problems. In addition, participation in other government initiatives, such as the national immunization days, MCH fortnight (promotion of MCH services at schools and other community forums), leprosy control program, and disaster relief operation, also demonstrated the acceptance of the project by government authorities and the respect it has earned from government officials.

More recently, the project's commitment to provide technical support in managing the village health posts established by the SHOs has also helped the project earn community trust.

Countering the Relief Mentality by Emphasizing Respect for Self-Help

The expectation of the villagers that they will receive external material support has been a problem to cope with in promoting self-help for health. Because the area has experienced many cyclones and tidal surges in the past, it has often received relief from outside agencies. It was difficult for the villagers to believe that no material support would be forthcoming from the project. They continued to request free tube-wells, latrines, curative services, hospitals, allowances for participating in health education training, and so forth. Project staff politely clarified the project's position in this regard and maintained this position constantly. In one village, the demand for free medicine was strong, especially from a person who had been identified earlier by the project as a resource person. The situation was difficult, because at that time a local NGO was distributing free medicine to the villagers. At a meeting with the mosque committee of this village and some expatriate visitors, the spokesman of the committee demanded two sanitary latrines for the mosque from the project. The project spokesperson responded by making a suggestion that to establish latrines what one needs is labor for digging holes and for constructing wooden or bamboo platforms and fences. Volunteers could complete such a project in a day or two. Occasionally, this kind of intervention had to be made to combat the relief mentality. Nevertheless, the project staff maintained relationships with the committee and the person behind the demand but did not give in to the demand (Lanzenderfer, Boulter, and Yahia 1995).

In addition to maintaining the project's philosophy of not providing financial and material support to the community, the project maintained a very low profile in terms of allowing project staff to use vehicular transportation. The male staff members used motorcycles, and female workers used local public transport and pedal tricycles. This helped limit the expectations of community members.

Staying Out of Village Feuds

At the beginning of the project, internal village disputes did not seem to be a hindrance, especially in initiating health education programs. But later, when there was an effort to establish a village health post in one locality, a conflict between two groups of villagers disrupted the agreement and the initiative failed. An investigation of the causes revealed that there was a long-standing dispute within the village and that the villagers could not work together. Some individuals in the village suggested that the project call a meeting with both parties to help the villagers remove the barriers that had developed. The project strategy, however, has been one of nonparticipation in such meetings. The project viewed the conflict as a lack of readiness of the villagers and decided to wait until the conflict was locally resolved.

Underscoring the Participation of Women and the Poor

Although the strategy of promoting health initiatives seems promising, it lacks participation by the poorest segment of the community, especially women. There is virtually no direct representation of the poor and women in the SHOs. The school health education program also does not cover children from very poor households. The mosque-based program, to some extent, includes male members from poor households. To reach women and individuals from poor households, it was decided to start health education among women in neighborhood household clusters using female volunteers. Women's groups formed by development NGOs for the poorest of the poor have also been brought into the health education program. However, it is not yet clear how effective the village health posts will be in meeting the needs of women and individuals from very poor households.

Explaining What the Demand for Curative Services Entails

During initial discussions with members of the SHOs, participants almost always focused on curative services and asked about the technical background of the project staff. The issue of curative services was their only consideration in mapping the project's role as a promoter of community health. After listening to the participants, project staff sought the opinion of a medical doctor, and he shared scientific concepts about the prevention of major diseases with the participants. It became clear to the participants that, by modifying their behavior, they can avoid diarrheal diseases and that appropriate management of diarrhea with oral rehydration therapy can save lives. It was emphasized that once someone gets sick, he or she loses working days and becomes dependent on healers. This costs the patient in terms of both money and physical strength. Thus, prevention is better than cure for the rich, and even more so for the poor, who have fewer resources. Although the benefit of preventive measures was clear to the villagers, the interest in curative services continues.

During the first year of project activities, the staff did not show any signs of responding to the demand for curative services, despite the finding that there has been a dearth of curative services in most of the villages and that women have been the most deprived. The availability of health facilities and government health personnel was always mentioned in the health education sessions. There has been a growing realization among the villagers that despite all preventive measures, illness will occur and the project will not supply any services. The SHOs, in collaboration with the villagers, have started to come forward with proposals that show they are serious about establishing health facilities in their locality with their own resources, but that they will need technical assistance from the project. (In the meantime, the project also had two paramedics and one public health physician on the project team, to ensure the appropriateness of the contents of the health messages and to continuously orient staff members on health matters.) The project staff responded by explaining to SHO representatives what it means to establish a health post, what is feasible, and what resources are needed. With this detailed picture, if the organization still chose to establish a health post, the project indicated that it would supply technical support by procuring weighing scales, growth monitoring charts, and training for volunteers, and by negotiating with local health authorities so that nominees of SHOs can obtain training in curative services and management.

This process has led to the establishment of a number of health posts in the villages. The villagers themselves have provided accommodations, furniture, and a modest sum of cash for meeting initial expenses. All the health posts are named after the village, and the project does not request any mention of the ICDDR,B contribution. Eppler, Bhuiya, and Hossain (1996) provide a detailed description of the process of establishing the health posts.

CHALLENGES AHEAD

The community initiatives taken by the SHOs hold great promise. Nevertheless, there are many challenges that must be met before they become effective.

Keeping the Wheel Moving by Showing Benefits

One of the challenges will be to sustain the enthusiasm of the villagers to keep the initiatives going. This will not be possible if the villagers do not perceive any benefit from the initiatives. To have significant health benefits, the program, including the health posts, should be effective and well managed. In this regard, technical support from outside will be needed.

Maintaining the Tradition of Linking the Public and Private Sectors

Traditionally, community initiatives in Bangladesh eventually receive partial public-sector support. Schools and roads, which were first established through community initiatives, were later subsidized or fully managed with public-sector resources. Thus, the villagers expect that the health posts they have established will some day receive assistance from the government. One way to achieve this would be to link the village health posts with existing government facilities; another would be to convert them into government community clinics. An example of beginning such a link is the hosting of EPI sessions and satellite clinics run by government workers at these village health posts. Other options may evolve as time passes. This linkage will not only make these initiatives sustainable but will also make the government programs more effective.

Extending the Process by Demonstrating the Example

The replicability of this model beyond the project area is another challenge to be faced. Once these local community initiatives are well grounded, the example can be demonstrated elsewhere, and interested parties can make visits and receive guidance and encouragement to initiate similar activities. Extension of the process will not be difficult.

Another possibility for extension is through the relevant government departments under which the SHOs fall. In most cases, these government departments have their branch offices at the thana level. Thus, the extension activities beyond the project area could be carried out under the supervision of the government departments.

WHAT MADE THIS PROJECT SUCCESSFUL?

Given the current trend in development activities, which are largely implemented by outsiders, the SHOs' achievements in initiating health activities on their own have been impressive. The major factors that made these achievements possible are discussed below.

Not Invitation But Participation

One of the most important strategies of the project was to augment the agenda of the existing SHOs rather than invite the villagers to participate in activities designed, implemented, and managed by outside agencies. The processes of relationship-building, needs assessment, health orientation, planning, and implementation were carried out in a participatory manner, resulting in community involvement from the beginning. Leadership from the SHOs was a precondition for the project to provide technical assistance. Thus, leadership of the initiatives has remained with the SHOs.

Usually, development agencies invite community representatives to participate in development activities by asking them to be members of a committee or to attend meetings. The outside agency, however, designs, implements, and manages the project. In such a model, community members do not learn that they do not have an effective role in program management or in control over resources and that decision-making is always led by the agency. What is achieved in relation to community participation in such a circumstance is, in fact, a kind of politeness on the villagers' part to respond to the request for participation from educated urbanites.

In the approach practiced in this project, the project does not invite villagers to participate in the project activities. Rather, the project participates in the initiatives undertaken by the sustainable SHOs created and nurtured through effective community participation. Thus, sustainability of the organizations and community participation will no longer be issues to look for in the future; rather, they are the foundation of these new health initiatives.

Restrained Generosity

The other important strategy the project adopted while working with the SHOs has been to observe restraint in providing material and financial support even in the face of strong demands from the community. Giving in to such pressure could very easily dampen the self-help spirit of the community and produce a dependent relationship. In this age of resource-driven development assistance, this strategy has been difficult to implement, but it has started to show signs of success.

Not Overtaking But Following the Community

Another essential factor was to allow time for the community to establish its own momentum and then for the project to support this momentum. Allowing the project to overtake the community could overpower community initiatives, permanently damaging the community's will to help itself. The project did not have its own time frame; it was set by the community.

Using Curative Services as a Platform for Health Promotion

Despite the project's best efforts, it was not possible to avoid support to curative services. Ignoring community demand would mean poor-quality service and a missed opportunity to use the momentum generated in the community. It was also observed that clients are treated more respectfully in the community-established health care facilities where practitioners are paid for services provided, than in those of the public sector. Thus, user fees should not only be viewed as a means of cost recovery but should also be viewed as a strategy to ensure effective community participation.

CONCLUSION

During implementation, the project faced minor problems related to motivation of project staff, relief mentality of the villagers, access to women, and suspicion of outside agencies. However, we concluded that existing village-based SHOs can undertake health-related initiatives. Health awareness and knowledge of hygiene and water and sanitation, and management of common illnesses have improved. EPI coverage has also increased in the intervention area compared to a comparison area. The process of generating interest and activities in health is a long one, but self-reliance and sustainability are ensured.

Community-led and self-help initiatives exist throughout rural Bangladesh. At times, community members united in formal or informal organizations undertake health initiatives. These organizations can also be activated through participatory processes to undertake such initiatives. These processes may lead to the community's no longer being viewed as a passive recipient of government and NGO services; rather, the government and NGOs will participate in community-generated initiatives. Activities carried out in this way will have a better chance of sustainability and effectiveness.

ACKNOWLEDGMENTS

The project was implemented by the ICDDR,B Centre for Health and Population Research with support from the Swiss Red Cross (representing a consortium of Dutch, German, and Swiss Red Cross societies). The authors would like to express their gratitude to Professor Demissie Habte, former Director of ICDDR,B, Professor John Caldwell of the Australian National University, and Dr. M. Badrud Duza for their continuous encouragement and support in undertaking this project. The valuable contribution of Dr. Mushtaque Chowdhury, Dr. Petra Osiniski, Dr. Henry Perry, Dr. James Ross, and Mr. Graham Wright in providing intellectual support to the project is also much appreciated. The contributions of the Chakaria Community Health Project staff and the members of the community in making this experiment possible deserve special mention.

REFERENCES AND RESOURCES

Arole, Mabelle, and Rajanikant Arole. 1994. *Jamkhed: A Comprehensive Rural Health Project.* London: Macmillan.

Bangladesh Bureau of Statistics. 1994. *Statistical Yearbook of Bangladesh.* Dhaka: Government of Bangladesh, pp. 537–95.

Bhuiya, Abbas. 1995. *Health Knowledge and Behaviour in Five Unions of Chakaria.* Special Publication No. 52. Dhaka: International Centre for Diarrhoeal Disease Research, Bangladesh (ICDDR,B).

Bhuiya, Abbas, and Claude Ribaux. 1997. *Rethinking Community Participation: Prospects of Health Initiatives by Indigenous Self-Help Organizations in Rural Bangladesh.* Special Publication No. 65. Dhaka: International Centre for Diarrhoeal Disease Research, Bangladesh (ICDDR,B).

Bhuiya, Abbas, et al. 1997. *Community Participation in Health, Family Planning and Development Programmes: International Experiences.* Special Publication No. 59. Dhaka: International Centre for Diarrhoeal Disease Research, Bangladesh (ICDDR,B).

Chowdhury, A. Mushtaque R. 1990. "Empowerment through Health Education: The Approach of an NGO in Bangladesh." In Pieter Streefland and Jarl Chabot, eds. *Implementing Primary Health Care: Experiences since Alma-Ata.* Amsterdam: Royal Tropical Institute, pp. 113–20.

Cox's Bazar Foundation. 1991. *A History of Cox's Bazar.* Cox's Bazar, Bangladesh: Cox's Bazar Foundation.

Eppler, Peter, Abbas Bhuiya, and Moazzem Hossain. 1996. *A Process-Oriented Approach to the Establishment of Community-Based Village Health Posts.* Special Publication No. 54. Dhaka: International Centre for Diarrhoeal Disease Research, Bangladesh (ICDDR,B).

Government of Bangladesh. 1985. *Directory of Voluntary Social Welfare Organizations in Bangladesh.* Dhaka: Bangladesh National Social Welfare Council.

Hossain, Hamida, Cole Dodge, and Fazle Hassan Abed. 1992. *From Crisis to Development.* Dhaka: University Press.

Lanzenderfer, M., Arnold Boulter, and Mohammad Yahia. 1995. "Report: Review of the Improvement of Health through a Community Development Oriented Programme in Rural Bangladesh (Chakaria Community Health Project)." Dhaka: International Centre for Diarrhoeal Disease Research, Bangladesh (ICDDR,B).

Lovell, C., and F. H. Abed. 1993. "Scaling-Up in Health: Two Decades of Learning in Bangladesh." In Jon Rohde, Meera Chatterjee, and David

Morley, eds. *Reaching Health for All.* New Delhi: Oxford University Press, pp. 212–32.

Mitra, S. N., et al. 1994. *Bangladesh Demographic and Health Survey, 1993–1994.* Calverton, MD: National Institute of Population Research and Training (NIPORT), Mitra and Associates, and Macro International, Inc.

Morley, David, Jon Rohde, and G. Williams. 1983. *Practicing Health for All.* Oxford: Oxford University Press, pp. 319–27.

Rohde, Jon, Meera Chatterjee, and David Morley. 1993. *Reaching Health for All.* New Delhi: Oxford University Press, pp. 501–17.

World Health Organization. 1978. *Primary Health Care: Report of the International Conference on Primary Health Care, Alma-Ata, USSR, 6–12 September 1978.* Geneva: World Health Organization.

6 Scaling Up Community-Based Primary Health Care

Carl E. Taylor and Henry G. Taylor

The acknowledged leader of primary health care over the second half of the 20th century, Carl Taylor, describes his experiences at the community level, starting with studies in Nepal in the late 1940s. He proceeds to Narangwal in India, showing how the Bhore Commission model can work, and from there to his years in China promoting UNICEF programs. Then he reviews specific community programs in Tibet, Peru, and Nepal. He advocates using sound epidemiological techniques and evidence gathered by the people and in community surveys. Taylor and his son Henry describe how communities resolve their own problems and how their successes make scaling up to larger populations possible. Patience is required, as he has demonstrated through over 50 years of community practice.

—*Jon Rohde*

A continuing problem in communicating about health work in poor communities is that, in learning from the communities we have been privileged to partner with, each of us has a compulsion to develop new terminology for what we do. It was an advance that, during the past 10 years, under John Wyon's leadership, those of us that he brought together each year[1] to share our interest in this topic agreed to call what we were doing community-based primary health care (CBPHC). The evolution of that term requires clarification of three definitions that cause confusion:

Primary medical care (PMC). This term is appropriately applied by clinicians to first-contact treatment of illness, which is the foundation on which the medical care pyramid is built. Referral to institutional, specialist therapy at secondary, tertiary, and higher levels follows if required.

Primary health care (PHC). PHC is an integrated system of preventive, promotive, and illness care. This term is appropriately used by both clinical and public health specialties for efforts to bridge the gaps separating the two. In the Alma-Ata documents of 1978, we widened the definition to include community participation and intersectoral action. In spite of this expanded definition, most PHC practitioners continue to limit their discipline to activities within the health system, or what health workers do in PMC: treatment plus health promotion and prevention. The term "selective PHC," coined in 1984, led to a wave of single-focus campaigns using specific health interventions. These

1. This committee is the Working Group on Community-Based Primary Health Care, a Committee of the International Health Section of the American Public Health Association. Dr. Henry Perry now chairs this group.

work best when new technology fills a gap in health services, but for cost-effectiveness and sustainability the selective interventions must eventually be integrated into comprehensive PHC.

Community-based primary health care (CBPHC). This term can be defined as two-way action for health, at the interface between communities and health services. It emphasizes that communities must ultimately have joint ownership in their own health care. Health professionals then become partners responsible for building community capacity so people can participate in solving their own problems, while health services also provide timely and cost-effective services and referral within the health system. We have defined community as any group of people who have something in common, a shared identity, and the capacity for joint action.

These definitions lead to a major concern about the current obsession with privatization, promoted internationally by major donor agencies and focusing mainly on primary medical care. Publications on health care reform have been concentrating mostly on financing techniques to cope with the bottomless pit of demand for PMC, especially as populations age and become more affluent. Privatization encourages greed for commercial gain through globalized sales of drugs and sophisticated technological services. Efforts to contain costs are focusing on providing care for those who can pay, mainly through insurance mechanisms. The US health care model is being widely copied in developing countries even though it results in gross inequity and leaves over 40 million Americans with no insurance coverage. These trends are extremely damaging to several decades of effort to build CBPHC in developing countries, especially in association with the disastrous impact of International Monetary Fund economic adjustment policies. The Bangladesh experience emphasized in this book demonstrates a practical alternative through community-based action, as summarized in Henry Perry's book (Perry 2000). (See also chapters 4 and 5 of this book.)

REASONS FOR FAILURE OF HEALTH CARE REFORM EFFORTS

For several decades, we have known how to make CBPHC work in local projects. In the 1930s, John B. Grant, C. C. Chen, and Jimmy Yen gave us the first practical demonstration of CBPHC at Ting Hsien (now Ding Xian, 100 miles south of Beijing). A decade later, the breakthrough concepts were confirmed in second-generation projects such as Pholela in South Africa. This project was transplanted after apartheid became the national policy, and key pioneers started projects for PHC in the Office of Economic Opportunity health centers in the US with Jack Geiger and colleagues, and in Israel with Sidney Kark. There were other projects in Indonesia, Chile, Kerala (India), and Sri Lanka. Most people do not realize that PHC started only seven decades ago, and we have learned much in a very short time about how these field methods work in discrete projects. But, as Jim Grant used to say in defending the campaign approach, "those good local projects don't go to scale." This observation was confirmed in the final chapters of Jon Rohde's excellent casebook on successful CBPHC (Rohde et al. 1993).

This chapter focuses first on some principles that help explain why scaling up CBPHC has been difficult and then briefly describes some successes in scaling up CBPHC. The most consistent reason for failure of PHC has been that public health experts still insist on using a blueprint model of scaling up. We treat human populations as inanimate objects that have no decision-making capacity and that can be manipulated by social engineering. We study successes and impose our findings, while donors provide large chunks of money attached to targets and precise deliverables. But people, in all their uniqueness and perversity, always do something different. There are few silver bullets that will fill gaps in existing services, and for them the blueprint approach may be a little quicker in vertical campaigns than in building them into health systems. But eventually even those must be integrated into comprehensive PHC. The first principle of CBPHC is: *There are few universal solutions that can be applied using top-down blueprints, but scaling up depends on finding a universal process to help local communities apply appropriate solutions to their own problems. The community must participate to develop some ownership of the process.*

Another reason for consistent failure is the tendency of officials and experts to polarize issues as they make decisions about funding. This is especially true of the chronic polarization around the top-down vs. bottom-up debate, which has paralyzed progress. As academics, we mostly do deductive research, polarizing complexities into "either/or" issues, since that yields clear statistics and is easiest to publish. Eventually, we also must make inductive discoveries showing that truth is usually not either/or, but both, and in a shifting balance. A second principle is: *CBPHC requires a flexible partnership balancing bottom-up local control by communities with top-down support by officials and outside-in stimulation by experts (perhaps better called empower-mentors).*

But in our field experience the most important reason for failure in scaling up is the obsessive compulsion of officials and experts to keep total control. Rather than respecting partners in the community, we blame them for our failures. As physicians, our arrogance is particularly destructive of community empowerment as we extrapolate into community relationships the usual practices in clinical doctor-patient interactions and try to exert doctor-population control in public health. A favorite indicator of our relationship with people is that terrible word "compliance." Think for a moment what that means—whether the people we "serve" fully obey what we tell them to do. But the question remains, Do we listen to them? For two decades after Alma-Ata we did quite well in building health systems by extending networks of primary health centers in developing countries, but now the health center movement is collapsing because international funding has shifted primarily to promoting privatization. Instead of community participation, we have become very good at community manipulation. Intersectoral collaboration has always been mostly symbolic in trying to get other sectors to help our services.

That brings us to the principle that a good way for officials and experts to show communities respect and gain trust is to help communities collect and analyze their own data. A consistent finding is that communities get close to 100% coverage in their own household surveys, and they also tend to include the families in greatest need, who are often the non-responders in sophisticated surveys done by professionals because they are remote and difficult to reach. Principle three is: *Communities should learn to use participatory methods to collect and analyze their own data, set their own priorities, do their own causal analysis, organize self-reliant action, and evaluate their own results.* If communities could do all this on their own, they would have become empowered long ago. Officials and experts are essential as partners to build community capacity if they support the empowerment process. What they often do instead is produce dependency rather than self-reliance. Many case studies show that building community capacity to carry out these functions is possible and can happen amazingly fast even in very poor communities.

Another common reason for failure in scaling up CBPHC is that, in acting as though public health depends only on health services, we have not focused enough on how to change behavior in communities and among officials and experts. The fourth principle of CBPHC is: *The most cost-effective and sustainable changes are those that occur in family behavior and community social norms. The most obvious changes are the ones the community has to make, but the most important are the new attitudes and values of officials and experts. Behavior change becomes sustainable when all partners adopt, adapt, and support the new social norms. To achieve the goal of integrated social development, people have to learn to balance the goals and inputs needed for healthy communities in this generation while also protecting conservation of the environment for future generations. This leads to true self-reliance and sustainability.*

Equity as a fundamental principle of social and economic development seems finally to be receiving attention as a core value of CBPHC. The growing disparities resulting from globalization demand forthright advocacy for the human rights that are fundamental for survival and development. The Rockefeller Foundation is leading the way with its Health Equity Initiative (Evans 2001), and Amartya Sen has presented economic justifications for paying primary attention to equity in defining development as freedom (Sen 1999). Therefore, the fifth principle of CBPHC is: *CBPHC must start with the clear vision from Alma-Ata of "health for all." A basic epidemiological principle is that to control a health problem, it is important first to find out who in the population has the problem or is at greatest risk and then focus control efforts on them. That is a simple definition of equity, not as a vague moral concept, but as a practical basis for action through surveillance for equity* (Taylor 1992).

The main theme we stress in this chapter is that a process for scaling up CBPHC is possible. A new book to be published by Johns Hopkins University Press in the spring of 2002 focuses on scaling up social development. The tentative title is *Just and Sustainable Change: When Communities Own Their Futures.* The primary author is Dan Taylor-Ide, whose specialty is environmental conservation. Seven years ago, UNICEF published a small monograph we wrote for the Copenhagen World Summit on Social Development, *Community Based Sustainable Human Development: A Proposal for Going to Scale with Self-Reliant Social Development* (Taylor-Ide and Taylor 1995). Jim Grant wrote the foreword as one of his last gifts to us of his wisdom. Since then it has had five printings. We have also been following a series of prospective case studies that demonstrate scaling up and present three of them briefly here as progress reports emphasizing qualitative rather than quantitative results.

CASE STUDIES

Tibet

In Tibet, the Pendeba Project shows what can be done in a pristine situation in building self-reliance in communities. Dan was asked by Chinese authorities to help develop the Qomolangma National Nature Preserve (QNNP), a national park to protect the north face of the heart of the Himalayas around Mount Everest. As far as we know, this was the first park with no wardens other than the people living there. In exchange, we promised to help the villagers with their priorities in social development. Among their top priorities was health, since Chinese government services had never reached these very remote villages. Two of the four counties were officially listed as the two poorest in China. Conservation successes have been dramatic, and now farmers ask what we will do about herds of Tibetan wild ass that eat up barley fields in the night and snow leopards that carry off sheep.

About eight years ago, Carl started to spend a month each summer training about 20–25 *pendebas*—the name in Tibetan means "a person who helps neighbors." We concentrated on the simplest home-based interventions. For instance, local experiments showed that a beer bottle of water, two match boxes of *tsampa* (the roasted barley flour that is the main staple of Tibetan diets) and a large pinch of salt made an excellent and safe cereal-based oral rehydration therapy (ORT) solution. Diarrhea had been the leading cause of death at the start of this project, but three years later the first two groups of trained pendebas reported that in all their villages there was only one diarrhea death in the previous year. Improvement seemed to be occurring also in pneumonia mortality. Immunization rates exceeded 90%. Family planning was in great demand as part of maternal care, in contrast to before the project started, when the survey we did with an international team showed that only 23% of married women knew that there were methods for family planning.

The total population of the QNNP is about 80,000. After four years, there were 87 pendebas working in the four counties, and when Carl arrived for the annual month of training, he found that the governors of the counties had moved in to take over the workshop. They started by saying we were causing a great political problem. This did not surprise us, because from the beginning of the project, we were aware of the delicate situation of working under the autonomous government in Lhasa. The problem, however, was that over 300 villages in the QNNP were demanding pendebas, and government officials had calculated it would take us over 10 years to meet that demand. They said that was unacceptable. They finally agreed to a plan to use members of the first two pendeba classes as teachers. The next year, when Carl arrived, he was told to sit in the back of classes to advise on how the pendebas could improve their teaching. Their self-reliance is amazing. Three years later, they have at least one pendeba in 223 of the 450 villages in the QNNP.

The government in Lhasa has asked for the program to be extended to help establish the new Four Great Rivers Nature Preserve in southern and eastern Tibet, which includes the watersheds of the Yangtze, Mekong, and Salween rivers, and the bend of the Brahmaputra. There is no doubt that the communities own this project. As mutual trust increases, there seems to be more interest in collecting the kinds of definitive data on impact that most international projects start by setting as a first priority.

Peru

In Peru, the Comités Locales de Administración Salud (CLAS) project is an example of scaling up in spite of initial resistance from the existing and well-established government health system. About seven years ago, Carl had a call from the Minister of Health asking for advice. The Sendero Luminoso (Shining Path) guerillas had just been driven out of the Andean villages they controlled, but the people were not letting the government reopen health centers. Carl, with a small Ministry team, spent a month in the region to gather information. In village meetings, which often lasted until midnight in churches and schools, the people said, "it was not the American helicopters that defeated the Sendero, or the Peruvian army, it was our Ronderos, self-defense teams made up mainly of women, who sat in stone pillboxes around the village to shoot Sendero gangs when they came to kidnap teenagers to make them guerillas." They said, "Now we have shown we can look after ourselves. We don't like the way doctors from Lima treated us and we want to run the health centers ourselves." The plan for CLAS was developed and the Minister got an order passed that permitted a committee to be formed to control the centers under approved conditions.

Two years later, Carl was asked to return. With another team, he spent another month visiting health centers. Over 400 health centers had been taken over by CLAS committees. On the door of one regional health office there was a tremendous poster saying "Health Workers Boycott CLAS." Many middle-level health officials were convinced it was dangerous for them to lose control because quality would be jeopardized and financial control would be impossible. One regional health director, however, decided that CLAS was a good idea and every center in his region had a committee, but considerable control was still held by the regional office. Another regional director said, "I am too busy to try to control each health center. I let the local committees go ahead, but I respond if the committee or the staff say there is a problem." Most impressive was the way that CLASes had followed the suggestion that their first activity should be for the committee and health staff together to do a complete household survey in order to set local priorities.

These surveys often had 100% coverage. After completing the surveys, the committees analyzed their data and, with the help of health staff, planned action programs.

The spread of CLAS was rapid as communities took initiative under the guidance of a small team in the Ministry. In four more years, there were about 1,200 CLASes out of the 5,000 health centers and posts in the country. Four formal evaluations by independent Peruvian experts were done, with uniformly positive reports, especially in the improved equity and the use of health services by women and children. Most CLASes were raising money for expanding services. It was remarkable how the transparency of local financing produced few instances of misuse of funds. But there were problems in getting communities to follow official documentation and legal requirements.

The number of CLASes fluctuates and the future of the program shifts with political transitions. In 1999, we helped with an interregional meeting where committee members and doctors from 25 CLASes met in Trujillo for their first chance to talk with each other. The sense of excitement was palpable as they shared experiences. In May 2000, at another regional meeting in Tarapoto in the upper Amazon, plans were worked out for the next stage in scaling up, to form Self-Help Centers for Action Learning and Experimentation. A network of such centers could do action training for all partners, conduct field research to analyze statistics on factors influencing impact, and adapt methods balancing top-down and bottom-up controls to respond to the extreme diversity of Peru.

Nepal

Carl had the privilege of conducting the first published health survey in Nepal in 1949 as the doctor for one of the first scientific expeditions permitted into the country, three years before it opened to the outside world. Fifty years later, we organized a repeat visit to the same villages to document changes in the half-century since Nepal has been exposed to outside influences such as expeditions, foreign aid, hippies, etc. We walked from India to Tibet along the Kali Gandaki watershed, which in the previous year had seen about 70,000 trekkers in the upper half of the route, but very few in the lower half.

We received a Rockefeller grant from the Health Equity Initiative to find out what happened to care for the poorest people during a half-century of massive efforts to develop health services. The measurable cutting of national child mortality by almost half gives plenty of opportunity for the many vertical programs to document their share of the percentage improvement they could claim but quantifying the contribution of changes really made within communities has been harder.

In general, people with money have access to care and are doing quite well. But the poorest quarter of families have benefited much less. Most unexpected was what happened to the carefully designed PHC system, which has been greatly influenced by privatization in the last few years. Public funds can pay only very small salaries for staff, who are now forced to earn their living by selling medicines. Health posts have very few supplies. Next door, staff members run medicine shops, which are well supplied and provide them income. One sustainable preventive program is the UNICEF demonstration from the 1970s that plastic piping can be used to bring spring water into villages. Now bazaar stores have abundant plastic pipe, which people buy because they save time by not having to carry water. The largest vertical programs now are national immunization days (NIDs) for polio eradication, and vitamin A distribution.

The best hope for health equity in Nepal is the Female Community Health Volunteers (FCHV) Program started about 10 years ago, partly because of concern among donors about the sustainability of vertical programs such as family planning and child survival activities. There were then over 46,000 FCHVs serving almost every village cluster. They are the volunteers most responsible for getting out the long lines of mothers walking mountain trails as they go twice a year to polio NIDS and vitamin A distribution points. But there is great frustration among these wonderfully dedicated FCHVs, who serve without compensation. They expressed strong agreement in focus groups and interviews that without their help the poorest families would get little care. A well-planned hierarchy in the Ministry of Health organizes the initial training with manuals, even for illiterate women. The recruitment and training have, however, sustained little evidence of a community base. FCHVs say they get almost no support from the local Village Development Committees or the health posts. They know that all programs supported by donors will terminate, since the first FCHVs have had to live through such transitions in other campaigns. FCHVs are the best hope for equity, but they need help. Our recommendation is that capacity for sustainable community action be built through a network of Self-Help Centers for Action Learning and Experimentation.

Narangwal

The recent experience in Nepal recalled lessons learned in the Narangwal Project in Ludhiana District in the Punjab between 1962 and 1974. The Narangwal Project grew out of much learning from the Khanna Project, which is described in the introduction. At Narangwal, a five-year study of the rural orientation of physicians in seven of the best medical colleges in India showed that even with carefully developed field-practice training, doctors tended to be overwhelmed by the need for acute medical care and were not reliably mobilizing effective primary care. A highly statistical operations research methodology probed the basic functions required from the health team and the need for role reallocation. To maintain coverage, most activities would have to be moved to the community, home, and family. The Indian Ministry of Health, in the annual conferences held in tents at Narangwal, requested a field experiment to demonstrate the proposed shift to community-based action. Separate sources of funding focused on two parallel field trials to study two high-priority issues at that time: one of the first complete studies of how synergism between care of common infections and child nutrition could be implemented by village workers in practical home-based interventions, and second, whether integration between family planning and maternal and child care might be more efficient and cost-effective than providing separate services (an issue that was not resolved for policy purposes until the Cairo Population Conference in 1994). The community-based field trials were started in the mid-1960s with evolution and testing of specific interventions as they became available and lasted until the project was closed down abruptly in 1974 due to political fall-out after the Bangladesh War of Liberation.

Some of the initiatives that Narangwal participated in are summarized in the two volumes published with World Bank support (Kielmann et al. 1983) and in a more recent review (Taylor and DeSweemer 1997). The demonstration that 90% of both clinical and preventive care could be very well performed by Family Health Workers under supervision was linked to further evolution of the concept at Jamkhed and other projects in India. Definitive findings on synergism between nutrition and infection showed:

- the relative cost-effectiveness of defined packages of integrated interventions;
- entry points where interventions could ease introduction of other interventions;
- interactions building on traditional cultural beliefs;
- that the best ideas usually came from listening to the people.

Practical methodological innovations included:

- the first field use of the verbal autopsy;
- simple laboratory and field procedures for following nutrition, growth monitoring, and child feeding in the home;
- one of the earliest demonstrations of the impact of tetanus toxoid immunization of mothers;
- the fact that the important control of common infections does not need to start by reducing incidence but can focus on reducing prevalence by household surveillance and early treatment in the home and that primary prevention can then follow;
- one of the early demonstrations in total communities of carefully documented growth improvement from nutritional interventions, including especially micronutrients in prenatal care and breastfeeding.

Narangwal had the first published demonstration of a 45% drop in child pneumonia mortality, using what became the WHO/UNICEF case management method by auxiliaries, who learned to observe difficult and rapid respirations. The method was later made more specific by research in New Guinea on actually counting respirations. After the first demonstration of oral rehydration for cholera among refugees in

Calcutta and in parallel with the earliest definitive trials in Dhaka, ORT became routine at Narangwal, with a 50% drop in diarrhea mortality. Similar innovations were occurring in integrating simple methods of family planning, showing the relative effectiveness of combining them with maternal care and with child care. This included carefully calculated comparisons of the total costs of specific alternative packages of interventions when provided separately or together. All these activities were part of the exciting worldwide partnerships in field research that led to the recognition that health for all is indeed possible, with appropriate choices of technology made available to communities through a remarkable spirit of shared understanding. The optimism of Jim Grant's "child survival revolution" was born of the results of field trials based on community action and fueled by simple yet sound information owned and acted on by communities themselves.

CONCLUSION

There is great hope for CBPHC. We have learned much but need to move systematically to not make the mistakes that have been so common in past efforts. Community-based empowerment is fragile.

The best example of that fragility is what has happened in China. Two decades of the Barefoot Doctor system showed dramatic improvements, which surprised outside experts with examples of health benefits almost equivalent to the best rates in the United States (Hinman et al. 1982). The China experience was an important part of the optimistic planning that we wrote into the Alma-Ata documents. Just two decades of rampant privatization have now totally changed the Chinese health system, in spite of intensive international assistance. Last year, in remote areas of poor Western provinces, Carl visited health facilities to personally confirm a concern shared by many that preventive services have been overwhelmed by the need for all health workers to focus on earning income by selling medicines and injectables. Between 1999 and 2000, immunization rates in China as a whole, as reported in the *State of the World's Children* reports, dropped by about 10% for each vaccine (UNICEF 1999 and 2000), and other preventive and promotive activities have fared no better.

The case studies in this chapter show that promoting CBPHC is pos-

sible even under difficult conditions. It has seemed especially important in Tibet to be patient in letting local awareness evolve rather than
aggressively pushing outside interests and priorities. The case studies
show the importance of nurturing the delicate and sensitive relationship between the Pendeba project and official services. Statistics on
results will soon, we hope, become available. As pointed out at the
beginning of the chapter, there are still gaps in knowledge about how to
generate the realistic support by governments and experts for community empowerment that is essential for sustainability.

REFERENCES

Evans, Timothy, et al. 2001. *Challenging Inequities in Health: From Ethics to Action.* New York: Oxford University Press.

Hinman, A. R., et al. 1982. "Health Services in Shanghai County." *American Journal of Public Health* 72 (Supplement): 1–95.

Kielmann, Arnfried A., et al. 1983. *Child and Maternal Health Services in Rural India: The Narangwal Experiment.* Vol. 1, Integrated Nutrition and Health Care. Baltimore, MD: Johns Hopkins University Press.

Perry, Henry B. 2000. *Health for All in Bangladesh: Lessons in Primary Health Care for the 21st Century.* Dhaka, Bangladesh: University Press.

Rohde, Jon, Meera Chatterjee, and David Morley. 1993. *Reaching Health for All.* New Delhi: Oxford University Press.

Sen, Amartya. 1999. *Development as Freedom.* New York: Knopf.

Taylor, Carl E. 1992. "Surveillance for Equity in Primary Health Care: Policy Implications from International Experience." *International Journal of Epidemiology* 21: 1043–49.

Taylor, Carl E., and Cecile DeSweemer. 1997. "Lessons from Narangwal about Primary Health Care, Family Planning, and Nutrition." In *Prospective Community Studies in Developing Countries,* eds. Monica Das Gupta et al. Oxford: Clarendon Press, pp. 101–32.

Taylor-Ide, Daniel, and Carl E. Taylor. 1995. *Community Based Sustainable Human Development: A Proposal for Going to Scale with Self-Reliant Social Development.* New York: UNICEF.

UNICEF. 1999. *State of the World's Children.* New York: UNICEF.

———. 2000. *State of the World's Children.* New York: UNICEF.

7

People, Processes, and Technology: Lessons from Haiti and Vietnam

Gretchen Glode Berggren

While eliminating neonatal tetanus clearly requires the provision of tetanus toxoid to women, this experience in rural Haiti demonstrates the importance of cultural sensitivity for designing programs that will lead to high-coverage adoption of appropriate health technologies. The Berggrens went on to address the more complex problem of protein-energy malnutrition among the poorest in Haiti and Vietnam, showing that consistent consultation with communities can determine what works in the most varied sociocultural settings. This chapter exemplifies the marriage of selective primary health care interventions with good leadership and cultural sensitivity to community needs, in the spirit of Alma-Ata.

—*Jon Rohde*

As my husband, Warren, and I progressed from learning about community-based approaches in the Belgian Congo in the late 1950s, to working with communities in rural Haiti in the 1970s, and then to working with communities around the world under Save the Children, community health volunteers and families living in poverty taught us some lessons that are worth sharing.

Most public health practitioners realize that in each cultural setting, one needs to begin by defining the "community" to be served and then striving to understand it, a continuing process. The ethnic background of the people within the communities, their institutions, traditions, and modes of interaction often dictate how they will interact with a program to improve health and survival. An experienced community health team wrote: "Before we can appreciate the problems of a community we must know something about community structure (demography) and function (sociology). We have to learn about its patterns of disease (epidemiology), and the organization and administration of different services that may be provided for the community (e.g. environmental control, immunization, child spacing, nutrition, and education) or for special groups within the community (e.g. mothers and children, school children, workers and the handicapped.)" (Wood et al. 1984, xi).

Despite this knowledge of the primacy of the community, the Western model of medicine is often imposed. To reach a community, people often think first of building and staffing a health facility and then depending on self-selection to achieve coverage. One is not surprised later to find that less than a third of the group targeted for immunization, for example, were reached by a fixed facility. Such lack of coverage is unacceptable not only to public health practitioners but also to communities, once they understand what is at stake.

A FRAMEWORK FOR COMMUNITY HEALTH INTERVENTION THAT ACHIEVES COVERAGE

To achieve the goal of improved health and survival of mothers and children and indeed of all community members, one useful approach is to better define, study, and understand three entities:

- the people
- the processes
- the technology

One could also discuss the goals, objectives, inputs, outputs, and indicators needed to help communities combat conditions that lead to high rates of morbidity and mortality, especially among mothers and children. But technology-driven community health interventions that ignore the people, their processes, and their practices are unlikely to succeed. One has only to look at the AIDS epidemic as it continues to affect young women desperate to make a living in Africa and Asia, or the continuing deaths of babies due to tetanus of the newborn in many developing countries.

Health educators and public health practitioners often feel driven to impose the technology that will "save lives" rapidly and at any cost. They imagine that it will take too much time to understand the history of a community, the constraints, the good traditions, and what the people themselves think is important. In our experience, using the tradition of exchanging ideas through women's "gossip" at the marketplace in Haiti served to get an immunization message out to women, who adopted the new health-seeking behavior in less than one year. Gossip conveyed a message more effectively than the written or radio messages. Similarly, it took the process of discovering and tapping the knowledge resource of "positive deviant" poor mothers whose children were well nourished to find the best method to combat malnutrition in Than Hoa Province of Vietnam.

Although these examples from Haiti and Vietnam appear to be disease-oriented "vertical programs," they built the fund of goodwill that allowed a more comprehensive, caring community health approach to evolve.

NEONATAL TETANUS IN RURAL HAITI

In Deschapelles, Haiti, from 1956 to 1967 the Hôpital Albert Schweitzer (HAS) pediatric ward faced an increasing number of cases of tetanus of the newborn. Despite recruitment, training, and equipping of traditional birth attendants (TBAs), more and more tetanus of the newborn was seen at HAS, until the numbers reached over 600 cases per year (W. Berggren 1974a). Reproductive histories taken from all mothers in a registered population in 23 villages nearest the hospital revealed that many had lost at least one child to this disease. The rate of hospital admission for neonatal tetanus from within the HAS district of 94,000 was 64 per 1,000 live births in 1967 (Berggren and Berggren 1971). Tetanus had its own name in Creole, "maladi machwa sere ak cour red" (the fixed-jaw, stiff-back disease), and people had their own explanations of its causality.

Health professionals at the Hôpital Albert Schweitzer had been active in their efforts to combat tetanus of the newborn since the opening of the hospital in 1956 (Earle and Mellon 1958). In addition to training TBAs, the HAS staff had:

- produced a movie that showed a home delivery and explained clean delivery practices, using local actors who spoke Creole;
- used the educational movie in the outpatient clinic and in communities;
- immunized pregnant women in antenatal clinics from 1965 onwards, explaining the purpose of the immunization.

All these activities appeared to have had little effect on the traditional practices that continued to put infants at risk for tetanus, and since less than a third of women attended antenatal clinics, often very late in their pregnancies, immunization had not diminished the case load for tetanus. Local TBAs insisted that, thanks to the equipment and training provided by HAS, they accomplished clean home deliveries, cut the umbilical cord in a sterile manner, and applied clean dressings. But they admitted that someone in the family of the newborn would apply an unsterile substance to the umbilical cord stump as soon as the TBA left the scene despite their attempts at education. The result would be another case of tetanus (Marshall 1968, G. Berggren et al. 1983).

Dr. Larimer Mellon, founder of the Hôpital Albert Schweitzer of Haiti, decided in 1967 to implement a community health program to solve problems like tetanus of the newborn. At the time, the infant mortality rate in Haiti was estimated at 125 deaths per 1,000 live births, with neonates accounting for more than half the deaths, many of them due to tetanus (Marshall 1968). It was known through small field trials that immunizing all women would eliminate tetanus of the newborn (Newell et al. 1966). To apply this technology to a larger population, one would need to rely on *people*, their *processes*, and the latest scientific *technology*. The community health team had to develop a clear understanding of the people being affected and how they thought of this disease, whether they would accept vaccination as a preventative once they saw that it worked and, most important, where and how women could be reached.

Resource Assessment in Communities Is More Important Than Needs Assessment

The community health team included experienced Haitian leaders who could accomplish a resource assessment. Dr. Mellon discovered and recruited a local woman leader, a former mayor, who commanded respect in all the communities, was familiar with the habits of women in the area, and understood how to inspire her colleagues. Through her efforts and those of other key informants, community volunteers came forth when it was understood that tetanus could be eradicated through immunization.

The strategy to eliminate tetanus of the newborn was not the only one promoted by the community health department of the Hôpital Albert Schweitzer, where daily admissions for severe malnutrition and tuberculosis were second only to tetanus. But it became a priority *because the technology existed to eliminate it quickly and cost effectively* and because interviews with local residents revealed that women would be likely to comply with an immunization program, once they understood its purpose. The question was where and when? The answer was in the marketplaces of the Artibonite Valley. The life of nearly every Haitian woman dictated that she go to market at least once a week to sell her farm goods and buy provisions for her family. These local markets had a predictable schedule and served rather well-defined communities. Furthermore, there was a great deal of information exchange, often at every crossroads, as women trekked to the marketplace. Rural women would leave their homes before dawn to get a good booth or place to sell and stop along the way to get news. By the time they arrived, they would know the price of corn and beans, and other activities that might happen at the market. As they set out their wares, all this was discussed.

Steps in Planning Marketplace Immunization

- **Meetings with community leaders and key informants.** Community leaders, who are very influential, control local market days. If the market were to have an "immunization booth," then those leaders had to be convinced of its worth and reliability, and were needed to help secure the spot in a convenient place. In addition, community leaders and key informants, such as local schoolteachers, could volunteer themselves and recruit local volunteers to assist the technical support team that would be arriving at dawn to set up the immunization session. Tasks included registering women, supplying them with immunization cards, explaining the purpose of the immunization, ensuring that each understood the date of her next visit, helping to keep people in an orderly line, and cleaning upper arms with alcohol. Offering each candidate for immunization a free photo of herself when she had completed the required number of tetanus toxoid doses was tried and was popular in launching the program, but it was later found unnecessary.
- **Social mobilization.** Our informants and women volunteers got the word out at every crossroads leading to a market. Furthermore, each case of neonatal tetanus admitted to the Hôpital Albert Schweitzer was investigated to find what more could

have been done to help the woman get immunized. The investigators were instructed to pass this word all along the way as they proceeded to the home of the tetanus case. On their return, people came out to hear the result. This generated even more conversation about the marketplace immunizations and their importance.

- **Moving the immunization technology to where the people are.** The process of getting a team on the road to the marketplace before dawn, with cold chain intact, and with all equipment for immunizing women required forethought. Refrigeration, vaccine (alum-precipitated tetanus toxoid), cold boxes, and equipment to give the vaccines had to be in place. An information system was needed as well: Hôpital Albert Schweitzer required not only immunization cards and a register but also the transfer of each immunization record to the HAS chart of every woman.

From among the health volunteers, the community health team chose and trained health auxiliaries. Their training at first was skill-by-skill, on-the-job training focused on immunization. Later, that training was expanded to include a broader spectrum of skills needed for a community health program (G. Berggren et al. 1995). It took a schedule made months in advance to ensure that a dozen different marketplaces would be reached at four-week intervals, often enough that women regularly attending the market could complete the required number of tetanus toxoid doses.[1] The market women pointed out that local trucks plied the dirt roads between markets and could provide inexpensive rides for some of the personnel attached to the community health department. Thus, the purchase of new vehicles and a major delay was avoided. Transport was scheduled by arranging to rent local trucks and use their chauffeurs.

---

1. Based on work supported by WHO in the 1960s in Colombia and in New Guinea, three doses of alum-precipitated tetanus toxoid given at 4–6 week intervals were known to give 95% protection to prevent neonatal tetanus for five years (W. Berggren 1971).

The Impact of Marketplace Immunizations against Tetanus

Marketplace immunizations continued for more than five years, even while the community health team moved toward local interventions to reach all mothers and children in their villages. With the marketplace immunization program, neonatal tetanus admissions declined rapidly. Retrospective fertility histories taken from 100% of women living in 23 villages in the HAS district revealed that women had lost 136.9 per 1,000 live births due to tetanus in the 1950s before the hospital was opened. This rate dropped to 78.9 when pregnant women were immunized and finally to zero by 1971, when all women had been immunized (W. Berggren, Ewbank, and G. Berggren 1981). By 1991, there were no cases of tetanus of the newborn reported from the entire hospital district of over 175,000 people (Menager and Berggren 1992). Tetanus of the newborn had cost HAS $60,000 a year for treatment in the early 1960s; immunization had cost less than one-third of that amount and had saved several hundred young lives per year since.

From Marketplace to Community: Activities and Results

The fund of goodwill built by the tetanus immunization program paved the way for formation of volunteer community health workers in village after village, and a more comprehensive approach. HAS gradually introduced a community health program with paid community health workers (1 per 2,000 people), assisted by community volunteers, who registered their entire populations and organized regular village assembly posts for preventive services. Their trainers taught simple skills: oral rehydration therapy, growth monitoring/counseling for under-fives, immunization and vitamin A distribution, and early recognition of illness for patient referral. Communities welcomed the technical support team to their village assembly posts, where they helped with and followed up on broader community health activities.

The cost for HAS to add community-based services was $1.62 per capita per year (Taylor 1992, W. Berggren, Ewbank, and G. Berggren 1981). This model was widely adopted by private voluntary organizations in Haiti and is still in use (Augustin 1993). In *Why Things Work,*

Walsh describes details of the methodology; the book *Community-Based Longitudinal Nutrition and Health Studies,* edited by Scrimshaw, describes nutrition activities and results in more detail (Halstead and Walsh 1990, Scrimshaw 1995).

The Hôpital Albert Schweitzer now trains volunteer women as a component of the ongoing community health program that has expanded to bring more comprehensive care to local neighborhoods. These volunteer women (1 for every 20 families) proved to be essential, especially in reducing deaths due to malnutrition, diarrhea, and (in the case of women) obstetrical causes.

HAS achieved a significant reduction in infant mortality with its community-based package of services in its census tract: from an infant mortality rate of 110 per 1,000 live births in 1967, there was a decline to 34 by year five of the program. The age-specific death rate for 1–4-year-olds in the census tract declined from 14 to 6 per 1,000 over the same period. The methods now reach a population of 250,000, and HAS is working with partner organizations in its outlying areas. Perry and his coauthors report that, according to recent survey results in this population, the under-five mortality rate is 68.2 deaths per 1,000 live births, compared to 144.3 for rural Haiti, a 53% reduction. The 12–59 month age-specific mortality rate is 73% lower (16.7 versus 60.8). He estimates that 18,810 deaths have been prevented and 1.3 million years of life have been saved (Perry et al. 2000).

USING THE POSITIVE DEVIANCE CONCEPT AND SKILL-BUILDING "APPRENTICESHIPS" IN COMMUNITY-BASED MALNUTRITION PROGRAMS IN HAITI AND VIETNAM: THE HEARTH MODEL

How Hearths Emerged

Mothercraft centers (1961–78). The problem of malnutrition was particularly severe in rural Haiti, and while rehabilitation in the hospital was clinically successful, it was a long and costly process. Furthermore, it was seen as a "medical cure" and the role of mothers and local feeding practices were not appreciated. Even when mothers were brought onto the wards and trained in feeding their sick children, the setting convinced them that the illness and its cure were magical, rather than within their grasp.

The Mothercraft centers established in Haiti and other countries in the 1960s, which were based on local culture and practices (G. Berggren et al. 1984, King et al. 1978), were a dramatic and cost-saving alternative to hospital rehabilitation. They used locally recruited women as paid nutrition educators to care for and feed moderately and severely malnourished preschool children daily in their own villages for three months. To the extent possible, the mothers of the malnourished children took turns assisting in daily food preparation and rehabilitation, learning lessons along the way. The program used inexpensive local foods and avoided the use of medications, so that the recovery of the child (the main demonstration objective) would be attributed to food alone and not to medicines, as was the case if the malnourished child was rehabilitated in a hospital setting. The long-term objective was for mothers to learn to prevent malnutrition in the younger siblings of malnourished children and thus to reduce the rates of malnutrition in a given community. Once this was achieved, the educator closed the center and moved to another community.

The emotional state of the malnourished child changed dramatically in a well-run Mothercraft center. Most children were transformed from apathetic and listless to mischievous and full of life within two weeks. Later changes, such as weight gain, were less impressive to the mothers, who often failed to attend the sessions after the first month (Burkhalter and Northrup 1997).

In evaluating the centers, King et al. (1978), Warren Berggren (1971), and Beaudry-Darismé (1973) reported improvements in food selection and preparation, family diets, the nutritional status of participating children, and the survival of their younger siblings. Gretchen Berggren et al. (1984) found that the weights and heights of children participating in the program improved significantly more than secular improvements countrywide. Although Mothercraft centers reported mostly good results, the programs were eventually abandoned because of the small numbers of children that could be reached in a given year and because the centers were not thought to be cost-effective.

Foyers de démonstration nutritionnelle in Haiti (1974–78 and 1984–94). Haiti's Projet Integré de Santé et de Population (PISP) introduced a modification of the Mothercraft centers that has proven successful in the hands of private voluntary organizations in Haiti. Community health teams had observed that even severely malnourished children show psychological "brightening" by the end of two weeks of successful recuperation. It was reasoned that mothers of malnourished children might be convinced to continue the rehabilitation process in their own homes if a brief "skill-building apprenticeship" was offered to them for the *first two weeks* of a child's recuperation. During that time, a balanced diet, including snacks, could be demonstrated, using local foods made more calorie-dense. The mothers might judge the recuperation successful when they saw the change in the child and might continue it at home, especially if encouraged by local volunteer mothers who would initiate the process in their own home (*foyers de demonstration nutritionnelle* or FDNs). The PISP project implemented such a trial, comparing results from the more costly Mothercraft centers in one area with FDNs in another, and with a third area where dry rations (the most costly approach) were distributed when children were shown to be moderately or severely malnourished.

Community volunteers and paid health workers learned about the FDN and explained it to the community, reaching a consensus about the need to treat malnutrition with local foods in the village itself. FDNs implemented by the PISP Project and by Save the Children/USA got large groups of malnourished children together (20 or 30 at a time) in a nearby church, schoolyard, or volunteer's home. As in the Mothercraft centers, a *monitrice* directed the activities, convinced local mothers to help her, and asked the mothers of the malnourished children to take turns in the daily FDN routine. Local foods were purchased on the local market to make a nutritious snack and a well-balanced meal, so that malnourished children were offered 700–800 extra calories per day. Mothers were asked to contribute foods for the daily menus. The community health team followed each FDN closely, and children were weighed at the end of two weeks in the FDN, and monthly thereafter until reintegrated into the growth monitoring/counseling sessions. Those not doing well would be referred to health centers to look for hidden illness. Progress could be measured by weighing the children at entry and every month thereafter.

Prerequisites to the village-level FDN program included immunizations; semestrial "deworming" of children and health education about parasitic diseases; education of parents about how to use oral rehydration therapy; and regular distribution of micronutrients (especially vitamin A) at rally posts. All these services were also available at health centers, but these were miles away and tended to be underutilized due to geographic and financial barriers. Results revealed the FDN to be as effective as the Mothercraft centers and the method described by G. Berggren et al. (1984).

Neighborhood Hearths or Foyers d'Apprentissage et de Réhabilitation Nutritionnelle in Africa and Haiti. In the Foyers d'Apprentissage et de Réhabilitation Nutritionnelle (FARN) program, which began in 1993, more decentralization and community participation emerged. Volunteer mothers under the supervision of the monitrice use their own outdoor kitchens to begin the rehabilitation process for children in their own neighborhoods (usually three to six children from nearby). They use inexpensive local foods based on a positive deviance inquiry (that is, they observe the caring behaviors of the mothers of well-nourished children living in the same community and what they feed their children—these are "positive deviants" in contrast to the "negative" or malnourished). Each participating mother of a malnourished child is required to attend daily and to contribute some food or fuel, or help carry clean water to the site. The volunteer mothers ask participant caretakers of malnourished toddlers not to deny the child any food from the family pot later in the day. For two weeks, the local volunteer mothers invite malnourished children and their caretakers from nearby homes for a few hours of daily skill-building and feeding sessions, and then follow up for two more weeks, making home visits to encourage their participants to continue the extra meal and nutritious snacks. Children not doing well are referred to health centers for detection and treatment of underlying illness. If possible, all caretakers are invited to participate in a poverty lending program.

COMMUNITY PREPARATION AND USE OF THE POSITIVE DEVIANCE INQUIRY IN VIETNAM

Based on experience in Haiti and Bangladesh, Jerry and Monique Sternin (Save the Children/Vietnam) developed a model that was integrated into a community development, health, and poverty alleviation program in Vietnam. The program's mission was to enhance, measurably and sustainably, the quality of life of women, children, and their families through a commune-level development program that could be widely replicated. Families with a malnourished child were automatically eligible for enrollment in a poverty alleviation program at the same time that their community planned for a local approach to nutrition rehabilitation and education using local foods. A local "positive deviance inquiry" became a key ingredient preceding each Hearth application in every village. Save the Children's Poverty Alleviation and Nutrition Program adapted the Haiti model and used it from 1991 onwards. However, there were two major differences: (1) The positive deviance inquiry in each village was emphasized and the whole village participated in interpreting the key findings and (2) project workers made many visits to a village before the Hearth exercise was begun to ensure consensus on the need for it and to make the community the "supervisor" to the greatest extent possible (Sternin and Sternin 1998).

The Vietnam project worked with local governmental organizations. For example, it worked with the Ministry of Health to enhance and expand local health workers' ability to immunize and deworm children, and refer and treat illness. Many of the features of the Haiti program were already in place; villages were well organized, with women volunteers well distributed. However, growth monitoring/ counseling was reaching only a fraction of children, and village health workers needed rosters to be sure "no child was left out." Mothers needed more encouragement to breastfeed, and the Ministry of Health asked that nutrition education be carried out in the context of their primary health care program, which included family planning. The project found women volunteers already recruited and trained to help their neighbors as part of Vietnam's communal development.

Sillan (2001) writes: "Starting in four villages for a population of 20,000, the program was adopted by the Ministry of Health of Vietnam and now reaches many villages with a population of two million." Fathers and community leaders as well as mothers attended several meetings before the Hearth program began. The whole village participated in the "community diagnosis" of malnutrition, helping to weigh children. The positive deviance inquiry became a key exercise in each village. This inquiry taps the existing knowledge and good traditions that must be preserved and built upon in the fight against malnutrition. Child-caring, not just child-feeding, behaviors were sought out, in keeping with more recent findings (Engle 1995).

Vietnam demonstrated that supportive communities are the key to combating malnutrition and that without community participation the Hearth approach will not succeed. Quoting the Sternins, Sillan (2001) points out:

- A malnourished child raises a flag of dysfunction;
- It often flags a dysfunctional family. Something is not working to keep the child well-nourished. There are adjustments needed in either feeding practices, caring practices, or health seeking practices;
- It may further flag a dysfunctional community.

Applying the Positive Deviant Approach

The questions change when using the positive deviant approach to health (see Table 1). It focuses on strengths rather than problems.

Before the Hearth sessions, all children in a community are weighed and each weight for age is plotted on a community graph so that the community can help tabulate the proportion of children who appear well nourished and the number who need rehabilitation. Community leaders in Vietnam (usually fathers) construct a simple pie chart to demonstrate the proportions in each category. Based on this exercise, volunteer mothers and community leaders identify the *well-nourished* children who come from modest homes, and ask permission to visit their homes, observe the child-feeding and -caring practices, and congratulate the successful families. Under the guidance of a trainer (like the monitrice in Haiti) they meet afterwards to reach consensus and tabulate results. Together they discover the foods and caring behaviors most frequently observed in the homes of successful, positive deviant mothers. The interviewers, usually including the volunteer mothers themselves, look for three "goods": good caring behaviors, good health-seeking behaviors, and good child-feeding practices, including the menus.

TABLE 1
The Positive Deviant Approach

Based on Strengths	...Not Problems
What are your strengths?	What is wrong?
What's working here?	What are your needs?
What are your resources?	What can we provide?
What can we build on?	What is lacking in your community?
What is already present and good?	What's missing here?

Source: Adapted from Sternin and Sternin 1998

A local trainer-supervisor debriefs the community volunteer inter-viewers and helps them draw conclusions about the skills they have observed. They consider together how to teach these skills to mothers of malnourished children. The supervisor-trainers draw up menus for Hearth sessions from the results of this exercise, and modify them, if necessary, to make the daily extra meal and snack more calorie-dense and well balanced, since the goal is not only to nourish but also to reha-bilitate. The poor mothers of well-nourished children have usually chosen inexpensive foods very wisely and have shown that they are sensitive to seasonal availability. In Vietnam, mothers of well-nour-ished children were using shrimp, freely available in nearby canals, as well as more fruits and vegetables in the diets of their children. Thus shrimp were called the positive deviant food by the village workers, who translated the term into their own language and were delighted with their discovery.

The trainer-supervisor identifies and recruits volunteer mothers who have helped with the positive deviance inquiry and who are will-ing to use their own kitchens so that mothers of malnourished children can practice new skills. Volunteer mothers in Vietnam were very dedi-cated to their tasks. They had to be willing to:

- come for training for at least five days in advance of the Hearth sessions for a few hours per day;
- demonstrate their ability to transmit simple messages as well as work with the mothers of malnourished children, so that the rehabilitation process could begin (this means, for exam-

ple, overcoming anorexia by making food more appealing to the malnourished child, who often refuses it at first);

- receive neighboring children in the daily Hearth rehabilitation exercise for a few hours per day for two weeks;
- follow up for two weeks by encouraging the mother of the malnourished child to continue the rehabilitation process in her own home.

The volunteer mother will remain a community resource and is often looked upon as a kind of "auntie" who pays attention to the children in her neighborhood.

At the end of the month (two-week exercise in the daily Hearth and two weeks of follow-up), the community members meet to study their results. How many children gained adequate weight according to the growth chart of each child? How many exhibited catch-up growth? How many did not gain weight? Often in Vietnam, ill children were referred for treatment, and often the community requested that the Hearth exercise be repeated for some of the failing children; Save the Children had the resources to help them do so (Sillan 2001, Wollinka et al. 1997).

OVERALL IMPACT OF HEARTHS

Dubuisson et al. (1994) found, for an area near Maissade, Haiti, that, using weight for age as an indicator, there had been a communitywide decrease of 30.6% in severe malnutrition in a child survival project that used the Hearth method. A two-year follow-up study of the earlier PISP project showed some decrease in malnutrition but a very significant decrease in the mortality of younger siblings of children who had been rehabilitated in Hearths, as compared to the general population of children in that age group in the same geographic area (G. Berggren et al. 1984).

During the 1993–94 Haitian embargo, Menager and Berggren rehabilitated more than 9,000 children in their own villages using the method, with a case fatality rate of less than 1%. Their team trained more than 1,600 Haitian volunteer mothers, each capable of rehabilitating malnourished children in her own home. A retrospective study of children rehabilitated in Hearths during the embargo drew mixed conclusions. Immediate results showed that 60% of children gained weight as fast or faster than the international standard median after Hearths. In the remaining 40%, half were found to have tuberculosis or other chronic illness, and half were found to come from extremely poor families, in need of a poverty lending program.

The results from Vietnam are also very impressive. Over 7,000 children were followed in the first villages where the positive deviant/Hearth method was applied. Using weight for age as a communitywide diagnostic indicator, severe (third-degree) malnutrition disappeared and moderate malnutrition decreased from 25% to 2%; children falling in the "normal" range increased from 38% to 69% at the same time. The effect was still present two years later when the National Institute of Nutrition in Vietnam compared the villages where Hearth had been applied to villages where there had been none.

CONCLUSIONS

Respecting and learning from the people and their processes has contributed to the success of many community health programs and the better use of modern technology. An example from immediate experience is the use of "gossip" as a tool for social mobilization of rural Haitian market women. They proved willing to be immunized against tetanus if technology was brought to them in their rural marketplaces and if they understood the consequences. The application of marketplace immunization reduced in-district admissions for tetanus of the newborn to zero and was cost-effective. The goodwill generated by the activity paved the way for a more comprehensive community health approach that reduced infant and child mortality rates and cost $1.62 per capita per year (Taylor 1992).

Burkhalter and Northrup describe the Haiti model:

> Hearth programs engage parents in rehabilitating their malnourished children . . . using diets based on local knowledge and resources. *The programs are designed to take place in the context of a comprehensive [community-based] nutrition promotion program that includes growth monitoring, micronutrient supplementation, deworming and treatment for infectious diseases.* Essentially, the

146 COMMUNITY-BASED HEALTH CARE

Hearth program arranges for volunteer community mothers to [begin the rehabilitation process by feeding] malnourished children [in their own neighborhoods] one nutritious meal and snack each day for two weeks in addition to their normal diet (Berggren and Burkhalter 1997, 1).

Menus and lessons for the daily Hearth sessions are drawn from local studies of child-feeding practices and caring behaviors of mothers of well-nourished children (positive deviants) in the same village (Zeitlin 1992; Zeitlin et al. 1990; Sternin, Sternin, and Marsh 1997). Mothers of malnourished children participate daily, provide part of the menu, and agree to continue the daily extra meal under the supervision of the volunteer mother.

The positive deviance/Hearth approach to combat malnutrition allows community health practitioners to better understand, document, and build on those good behaviors crucial to raising well-nourished children. Allowing mothers to participate in a community-level apprenticeship to practice good child-feeding behaviors and helping them interpret the change in their malnourished children have brought about changes in child-rearing practices. The effect apparently endures over the long term, and the approach does not create dependency. The National Institute of Nutrition of the Vietnamese government has recognized the method's usefulness, and it now reaches more than two million people.

REFERENCES AND RESOURCES

Africare. 1999. "Guinea Experience with HEARTH." Training video. Washington, DC: Africare.

Alvarez, M., Gretchen Berggren, and M. Gay. 1993. "Evaluation of the CARE Richesse Program in Haiti." Report to CARE. Port-au-Prince, Haiti.

Augustin, A. 1993. "Report to UNICEF on Child Health and Mortality in Haiti." Port-au-Prince, Haiti.

Beaudry-Darismé, M. M. N. 1973. "Nutrition Rehabilitation Centers: An Evaluation of Their Performance." *Journal of Tropical Pediatrics* 19: 299.

Berggren, Gretchen, and Muriel I. Elmer. 1999. "The HEARTH Program: Mobilizing Communities in Developing Countries to Combat Malnutrition Using a Participatory Adult Education Approach after the Example of the Good Shepherd." Proceedings of the Ninth World Congress of the International Christian Medical and Dental Association. Durban, South Africa: International Christian and Medical Dental Association.

Berggren, Gretchen, and M. Favin. 1992. "Social Mobilization for the Elimination of Tetanus of the Newborn." Working Paper of the Mothercraft Project. Boston: John Snow, Inc.

Berggren, Gretchen, J. R. Hebert, and C. M. Waternaux. 1985. "Comparison of Haitian Children in a Nutrition Intervention Programme with Children in the Haitian National Nutrition Survey." *Bulletin of the World Health Organization* 63: 1141–50.

Berggren, Gretchen, et al. 1983. "Traditional Midwives, Tetanus Immunization, and Infant Mortality in Rural Haiti." *Tropical Doctor* 13: 79–87.

———. 1984. *The Nutrition Demonstration Foyer, A Model for Combating Malnutrition in Haiti.* Hoviprep Monograph Series No 2. International Food and Nutrition Program of MIT. Cambridge: MIT Press.

———. 1995. "A Prospective Study of Community Health and Nutrition in Rural Haiti from 1968 to 1993." In N. Scrimshaw, ed. *Community-Based Longitudinal Nutrition and Health Studies.* Boston: International Foundation for Developing Countries, pp. 143–73.

Berggren, Warren L. 1971. "Evaluation of the Effectiveness of Nutrition Rehabilitation and Education Centers." In P. L. White, ed., *Proceedings of the Western Hemisphere Conference on Nutrition III, Division of Scientific Activities.* Chicago: American Medical Association Press.

———. 1974a. "Administration and Evaluation of Rural Health Services: A Tetanus Control Program in Haiti." *American Journal of Tropical Medicine and Hygiene* 23: 936–49.

———. 1974b. "The Control of Neonatal Tetanus in Rural Haiti through the Utilization of Medical Auxiliaries." *Bulletin of the Pan American Health Organization* 8: 24–29.

Berggren, Warren L., and Gretchen Berggren. 1971. "The Changing Incidence of Fatal Tetanus of the Newborn: A Retrospective Study in a Defined Rural Haitian Population." *American Journal of Tropical Medicine and Hygiene* 20: 491–94.

Berggren, Warren L., Douglas Ewbank, and Gretchen Berggren. 1981. "Reduction of Mortality in Rural Haiti through a Primary Health Care Program." *New England Journal of Medicine* 304: 1324–30.

Berggren, Warren L., and Barton R. Burkhalter. 1997. "Introduction." In Olga Wollinka et al., eds. *Hearth Nutrition Model: Applications in Haiti, Vietnam, and Bangladesh.* World Relief Corporation and the BASICS Project. Arlington, VA: BASICS.

Burkhalter, Barton R., and Robert S. Northup. 1997. "Hearth Program at the Hôpital Albert Schweitzer in Haiti." In Olga Wollinka et al., eds. *Hearth Nutrition Model: Applications in Haiti, Vietnam, and Bangladesh.* World Relief Corporation and the BASICS Project. Arlington, VA: BASICS, pp. 13–42.

CORE (Child Survival Collaborations and Resources Group) and NGO Networks for Health. 2000. "Community Centered Approaches to Behavior and Social Change." Working Paper for USAID. Washington, DC.

Dubuisson, S. E., et al. 1994. "Impact of Sustainable Behavior Change on the Nutritional Status of Children." In D. Storms, C. Carter, and P. Altman, eds. *Community Impact of PVO Child Survival Efforts: 1985–1994.* Proceedings of USAID-sponsored conference in Bangalore, India, Oct. 2–7, 1994, pp. 51–53.

Earle, A. M., and W. L. Mellon. 1958. "Tetanus Neonatorum: A Report of 32 Cases." *American Journal of Tropical Medicine and Hygiene* 7: 315–16.

Engle, P. L. 1995. "Child Caregiving and Infant and Preschool Child Nutrition." In Per Pinstrup-Andersen, David Pelletier, and Harold Alderman, eds. *Child Growth and Nutrition in Developing Countries.* Ithaca, NY: Cornell University Press, pp. 53–77.

Finlay, S. 1990. "Report on Neonatal Tetanus in Haiti: Special Report to PAHO." Washington, DC.

Halstead, S. B., and J. A. Walsh. 1990. *Why Things Work: Case Histories in Development.* New York: Rockefeller Foundation.

Harvard Center for Population Studies. 1993. "Sanctions in Haiti: Crisis in Humanitarian Action." Progress on Human Security Working Papers. Cambridge: Harvard Center for Population and Development Studies, pp. 5–7.

King, K. W. 1964. "Development of an All Plant Mixture Using Crops Indigenous to Haiti." *Econ. Botany* 18: 311–22.

King, K. W., et al. 1978. "Preventive and Therapeutic Benefits in Relation to Costs: Performance over 10 Years of Mothercraft Centers in Haiti." *American Journal of Clinical Nutrition* 31: 679–80.

Marshall, F. N. 1968. "Tetanus of the Newborn with Special Reference to Experiences in Haiti." *Advances in Pediatrics* 15: 65–100.

Menager, H., and Gretchen Berggren. 1992. "Preliminary Report on the Result of Community Health Outreach Programs at the Hôpital Albert Schweitzer (HAS) in Haiti." Paper presented at the HAS Alumni Association Meeting.

Newell, K., et al. 1966. "The Use of Tetanus Toxoid for the Prevention of Tetanus Neonatorum: Final Report of a Double-Blind Field Trial." *Bulletin of the World Health Organization* 35: 863–71.

Perry, Henry, et al. 2000. "Report to the Grant Foundation on Community Health Impact of Activities of Hôpital Albert Schweitzer." Sarasota, FL: Grant Foundation.

Research Corporation, ed. 1970. Chapters by Warren L. Berggren, W. Fougere, and K. W. King. In *A Practical Guide to Combating Malnutrition in the Preschool Child.* New York: Appleton-Century-Crofts.

Scrimshaw, N., ed. 1995. *Community-Based Longitudinal Nutrition and Health Studies.* Boston: International Foundation for Developing Countries, 1995.

Sillan, Donna. 2001. *The HEARTH Nutrition Model Using the Positive Deviance Approach: An Implementor's Handbook.* Washington, DC: CORE (Child Survival Collaborations and Resources Group), USAID.

Sternin, Jerry, and Robert Choo. 2000. "The Power of Positive Deviancy." *Harvard Business Review,* January-February.

Sternin, Monique, and Jerry Sternin. 1998. *Designing a Community-Based Nutrition Program Using the HEARTH Model and the Positive Deviance Approach: A Field Guide.* Westport, CT: Save the Children/USA.

Sternin, Monique, Jerry Sternin, and David L. Marsh. 1997. In Olga Wollinka et al., eds. *Hearth Nutrition Model: Applications in Haiti, Vietnam, and Bangladesh.* World Relief Corporation and the BASICS Project. Arlington, VA: BASICS, pp. 49–61.

Taylor, Carl E. 1992. "Surveillance for Equity in Primary Health Care: Policy Implications for International Experience." *International Journal of Epidemiology* 21: 1043–49.

Wollinka, Olga, et al., eds. 1997. *Hearth Nutrition Model: Applications in Haiti, Vietnam, and Bangladesh.* World Relief Corporation and the BASICS Project. Arlington, VA: BASICS.

Wood, C. H., J. Vaughn, and H. de Glanville. 1984. *Community Health.* Rural Health Series No. 12. Nairobi: African Medical Research Foundation.

Zeitlin, Marion. 1992. "Child Care and Nutrition: The Findings from Positive Deviance Research." Medford, MA: Tufts University School of Nutrition.

Zeitlin, Marion, et al. 1990. "Positive Deviance in Child Nutrition: With Emphasis on Psychosocial and Behavioral Aspects and Implications for Development." Tokyo: United Nations University.

8 Two Decades of Community-Based Primary Health Care in Rural Bolivia

David S. Shanklin and Nathan Robison

The experience of a community-based nongovernmental organization (NGO) in Bolivia demonstrates the potential for reaching dispersed rural populations with equitable primary health care services that result in measurable and sustained improvements of coverage and impact. This account also highlights the contrast between this more flexible, culturally sensitive NGO model, and more typical national public health approaches. These often neglect difficult-to-reach rural populations, or when attempted, tend to emphasize the provision of a minimum set of standard services in fixed facilities by health professionals who come from outside the community. The NGO model described here emphasizes outreach into the community by local paramedical staff, an approach both possible and affordable. Good record-keeping, family visits, and measurement of health needs are important elements of this vision. Patience, adaptability, and attention to community values and inputs are essential to long-term success.

—Jon Rohde

W hat is today the Consejo de Salud Rural Andino (CSRA) in Bolivia was born as Andean Rural Health Care (ARHC), a nonprofit organization based in North Carolina. ARHC began community-based health work in the highlands of Bolivia in 1981. As of 2001, CSRA supported five Bolivian community health programs, with over 68,000 participants in the highlands and tropical lowlands. In this chapter, we discuss the development of this community-based health care system in Bolivia and its challenges and successes.

THE BACKGROUND OF ANDEAN RURAL HEALTH CARE

"Lost in the wilderness" would be an apt description of our tentative first steps in community-based health care, although our journey resulted finally in the development of an effective methodology of community-based health care: the census-based, impact-oriented (CBIO) approach.

Initially, Dr. Henry Perry, ARHC founder, consulted with Dr. John Wyon, then faculty member at Harvard's School of Public Health, to develop a health project to serve widely dispersed Aymaran Indians living in and around Ancoraimes, a small municipality near Lake Titicaca. They recognized that their approach would need to be a decentralized effort, based on both the measured and the locally perceived health needs of the service population. Primary health services would be based on proven and readily available technologies, and they would be provided by the lowest-level competent health providers whom they could identify and train. These indigenous health providers, in turn, would be supervised by public health-oriented physicians, preferably

Bolivian, who would care for the more seriously ill patients or evacuate them to secondary and tertiary care facilities, with which ARHC would have established written agreements.

Since most people in this region had never experienced reliable access to Western medicine, the services had to be presented in a way that was acceptable to them. Aymaran cultural preferences and beliefs would have to be acknowledged and respected. Because medical practitioners in La Paz, the closest large city, often treated *campesinos* (people of the countryside) with disdain, and because most health services were perceived to be either too costly or of low quality, the rural poor rarely used public hospitals except as places to die. In turn, public hospitals were grossly underfunded, underequipped, and underutilized by those who needed health care most.

For the community health program to work effectively, motivated individuals had to be found in the areas where they intended to work. These community health workers (CHWs) would need to be literate and to have received at the least basic Ministry of Health (MOH) training as auxiliary nurses. Further, their MOH-approved curriculum would have to be extended to include the fundamentals of epidemiology and public health practice, including community health assessment and outreach. A simple model was developed to guide the work of CHWs.

This methodology provided a means of focusing health education, promotion, and prevention, as well as curative services, to the highest-priority unmet needs. These needs were identified both by community members and through epidemiological surveillance. Program staff analyzed the data collected and solicited input from community members in order to adapt program initiatives to the real and locally perceived health needs of their service areas. (Measured and locally perceived health needs were frequently *not* the same.)

Community leaders identified the first group of CHWs.[1] Fifteen individuals were identified and given scholarships to attend MOH training. Upon their return to their community, they received more

1. ARHC now seeks CHWs who present themselves locally through volunteer activities, demonstrating their motivation and interest in community health. ARHC then provides low-cost scholarships for their training.

training and hands-on practice in community health assessment, data collection and recording, and health education techniques.

THE TRANSFORMATION OF ANDEAN RURAL HEALTH CARE INTO CONSEJO DE SALUD RURAL ANDINO

By 1991, the United States-based board of directors of ARHC had decided that its international health programs should be structured for long-term self-direction and corporate autonomy. As a first step, ARHC staff in Bolivia formed the Consejo de Salud Rural Andino (CSRA), which became a nonprofit national organization in 1995, with its own volunteer board of directors and its own corporate identity. ARHC thereafter signed an agreement with CSRA transferring its Bolivian assets and liabilities to that organization.

Since that time, ARHC, on the other hand, has transformed itself from a direct health service provider into an agency whose goal is to equip, train, and assist in-country organizations that wish to replicate the CBIO methodology. With this shift in strategic focus, ARHC has expanded into three additional countries. In 1997, the US Agency for International Development (USAID) awarded its first Child Survival Mentoring Grant to ARHC and three partner organizations working in Haiti. The combined service population of these three partners is now about 70,000 women and young children. In 1999, Rotary International awarded ARHC a grant to support a project in Rio Bravo, Mexico, on the Texas border. The population will reach more than 10,000 individuals by the end of the first three years of project activity. Most recently, ARHC began USAID-supported work in Guatemala in 2000.

THE EVOLUTION OF CONSEJO DE SALUD RURAL ANDINO

Currently, CSRA, the Bolivian NGO, describes its mission as saving lives, by knowing people and working with them to improve their health and well-being. Its managers aim to be the best managers of local primary health care systems in Latin America. Their five-year goal is to achieve health indicators equal to those of Cuba in one rural health district, one urban health district, and five rural municipalities in Bolivia.

Initially, CSRA had envisioned that the MOH would eventually assume management of the local nonprofit health programs, adopting the principles of the census-based approach. Eventually, however, CSRA's leaders realized that the MOH would persist with its traditional means of providing primary health care: through sporadic nationwide vaccination campaigns, occasional growth monitoring with no follow-up, and provision of all other services in health centers. In addition, there was constant turnover of MOH personnel at all levels. Most damaging was the turnover in leadership of local health systems, a role usually assumed by a physician or a licensed nurse. Finally, MOH officials displayed a lack of confidence in the activities of the auxiliary nurses, CSRA's first-line health care providers.

After 10 years, it became clear to CSRA that NGOs could play an important, permanent role in the management of local health systems. NGOs have a crucial role not simply because the census-based approach is somewhat complicated to sustain, but because the Bolivian MOH has not proven itself interested in or capable of sustaining quality health services in isolated rural areas. As these concepts emerged within CSRA, changes began to appear in the national health sector that supported the view that long-term NGO involvement could benefit communities and be financially sustainable.

The first of these national changes was the passing in 1994 of the Ley de Participación Popular, or Law of Popular Participation. This law devolved to municipal governments across Bolivia federal funds to be invested in health, education, sports, and culture and productive infrastructure. In the case of health, it was expected that municipal governments would invest not only in water and sanitation, but also in improving and maintaining health infrastructure, as well as covering certain health system operating expenses (except salaries).

The second major change in the sector came with successive measures to decentralize government services, including health care. Regional governments received increased funding for new salaried positions and increased regional discretion related to their allocations.

The third major change came with the decentralization of decision-making mechanisms. In particular, new legislation created Local Health Boards at the municipal level. CSRA has made great efforts to promote and strengthen these boards, working with municipal governments to help them understand issues of public health, human development and management, administration roles and responsibilities, and improvements in service quality and access. The Local Health Boards include not only elected municipal authorities and MOH representatives, but also representatives from the communities through the newly created municipal oversight committees (Comités de Vigilancia) and the traditional small farmers' organizations (*sindicatos agrarios*).

The fourth change related to decentralization is the Bolivian government's process of "municipalizing" health services. The municipalization of health (and education) services is controversial, but CSRA is well positioned to offer a model and to provide management services in health to municipal and regional governments. These services include the census-based methodology as a key tool for achieving and demonstrating the results expected.

Under these new circumstances, progress has been made in the joint "management" of the local health systems, or *cogestión*,[2] with the municipalities and the MOH health districts. Bolivian rural municipalities had never before had the resources or the authority to participate actively in local health issues. The new laws and decentralized environment provide CSRA with a legal and institutional framework in which to implement its philosophy of greater community participation in the decision-making processes of local health services.

Six years ago, no more than 10% of ongoing operating expenses were covered through income from local sources in the Bolivian highlands. Now, approximately 55% of recurring operating expenses come from local sources. Over the next five years, coverage for 100% of operating expenses is expected to come from a mix of in-country sources, including municipal funds, regional funds, fees for services, and other NGO-generated income.

Today CSRA maintains written agreements with three rural municipal governments for the management of their health systems. Three more are actively seeking CSRA's services.

2. Cogestión comes from *gestión*, which means "to take steps or measures to obtain," in this case to take steps jointly with the municipal and regional governments to obtain a working local health system. This concept does not mean co-administration of the system.

BASIC CENSUS-BASED, IMPACT-ORIENTED SERVICES

The CBIO approach involves the implementation of each of the five steps outlined in Figure 1 and includes visits to each home in a service area, the use of a health information system that allows program staff to track service delivery and vital events by household, the use of community health workers hired to serve their own communities, and multiple locations for service delivery (Perry 1999).

Step 1: Establish a relationship between the program and the community is normally realized through a series of meetings, discussions, and visits between health program leaders, and (usually political) community leaders who solicit the entry of the NGO into their area. These activities frequently take many months or several years to complete. Mutual trust and confidence are prerequisites for progress. This step is formally established through the signing of a time-limited, renewable agreement between representatives of the NGO and the municipality, and separately with the MOH.

FIGURE I

The Census-Based, Impact-Oriented Approach

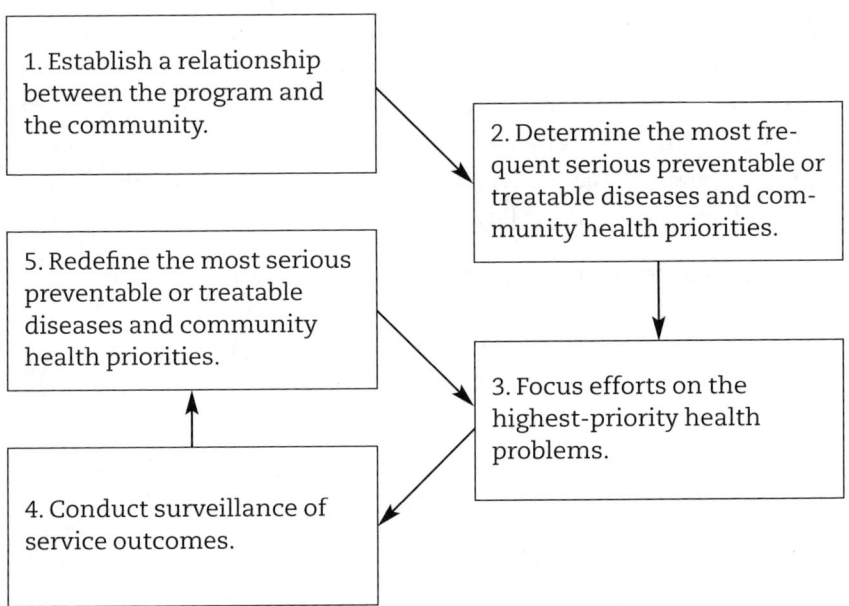

Step 2: Determine the most frequent serious preventable or treatable diseases and community health priorities is achieved through activities that vary from one service area to another but include most or all of the following: a health census of the service area; structured interviews and focus group discussions with local residents and traditional and political leaders; standardized surveys of knowledge, practices, and coverage rates of families, especially mothers; and reviews of existing local health data and published regional and national data. Data are analyzed, results presented to NGO staff and community leaders, and decisions made about which services will be offered to address the local health conditions identified. The range of services proposed is often limited or expanded depending on the priorities of funding agencies supporting the health program.

Step 3: Focus efforts on the highest-priority health problems generally is accomplished by implementing services that include preventive health education, and using medical protocols and treatment regimens standard to the country where the program is being implemented. Health education and preventive and curative services are offered through a system of home visitation (described below), and in small health clinics and remote health posts.

The targeting and frequency of home visits is based on a general risk profile that is developed and applied to each household, using the previously collected census and health data, and the priorities established for the community. (During the process of collecting census data, all homes are numbered, local area maps drawn, and household health folders created.) CHWs then visit most frequently the families at greatest risk of preventable or treatable illness or death. In Bolivia, ARHC eventually developed the following guidelines for visitation:

- six visits per year for any family with children under two years of age;
- three visits per year for families with children aged two to about five years and for families with women of childbearing age;
- one visit per year for all households to update the census for use in planning and evaluation.

A set of additional schedules was locally established for selected health conditions, such as childhood malnutrition (every two weeks) or pregnancy (every month). In addition, CBIO programs offer health education and basic services within group settings (such as mothers' club meetings), at health fairs held at weekly community markets, and in small clinics and remote health posts. The NGO has also collaborated with communities to sponsor complementary community development activities that respond to health-related needs, such as improved access to potable water, and sanitation management.

While home visits remain an important aspect of the Bolivia program, especially to follow up on nonpresenting cases, families are encouraged to seek health care, to reduce the labor costs of home visits. Seeking care is also important for some illnesses, such as pneumonia, when prompt identification of danger signs and appropriate treatment are often essential for survival. Recently, steps have been taken to reduce the number and frequency of home visits, but the impact of this reduction on program coverage rates and impacts has not been measured.

Step 4: Conduct surveillance of service outcomes is a logical extension of the field activities described above and depends on the routine monthly reporting of health service provision and the collection of data on vital events (births, deaths, and migration). Coverage rates and mortality reduction are also periodically assessed, usually within the context of local staff meetings on quality assurance. In addition to other, regularly scheduled reviews of program data (established as part of an annual planning and evaluation process), less frequent surveys and special studies permit the measurement of changes in key behaviors of interest to the program.

Step 5: Redefine the most serious preventable or treatable diseases and community health priorities results from the sharing of the products of Step 4 with community members and leaders, and the development of new initiatives based on perceived and measured health needs of both the NGO and the community. The Bolivian CBIO programs began with a focus on child survival due to the high rates of infant and childhood mortality in the project areas. ARHC has added interventions over the years to address additional unmet health needs. The programs now include health education and promotion on topics such as nutrition, personal and family hygiene, and family planning; preventive services, including childhood and adult immunizations, growth monitoring for infants, and prenatal care; and curative services such as oral rehydration therapy, emergency obstetrical interventions, and treatment of acute respiratory infections.

Other high-demand health services, including dental and eye care, have been added over time. These services help defray overall program costs. In the program areas of the Bolivian highlands, such added services have had a negligible impact on overall program cost recovery, since most residents' ability to pay fully for health services is limited. In the lowland urban service areas, cost recovery from fees for services and sale of medicines is now about 40% of total program costs.

Local program staff have supported health-related services by providing training on health leadership to incoming municipal leaders, activities to improve water and sanitation facilities, and establishing village banking services for women. Regularly responding to the community's unmet needs is at the core of the CBIO approach.

RESULTS OF THE CENSUS-BASED, IMPACT-ORIENTED METHODOLOGY

Reductions in childhood mortality have been documented in communities where the CBIO methodology is being applied. A 1994 study of three established intervention sites showed child mortality rates that were 49% lower than those in geographically adjacent comparison sites (103 for the ARHC program sites versus 202 for the comparison sites). The child mortality rates were also 35% lower than the estimate of 159 from the Bolivian Demographic and Health Survey (Shanklin 1994). Both analyses were based on estimates of probability of death, and the reported differences were statistically significant ($p < .05$).

In 1998, Shanklin reported a reduction in childhood mortality rates within five years of start-up of the child survival program. Infant mortality dropped by 74% in two of the program areas but did not decrease in the third area. This reflected a clear dose-related impact; programs where prenatal care and delivery services were available and used experienced much greater reductions in infant mortality than programs where such services were not well utilized. Among one-to-five-year-olds, mortality dropped by 83% in the three program areas. The overall childhood mortality rate dropped from 164 to 63 deaths per 1,000 live births, or 62%, in the program areas over five years. There was no change in the similar, adjacent comparison areas.

Delivery rates for health services and participant behavior change have also exhibited improvements in the service areas. For example, coverage for full immunization of children between 14 and 23 months was high or much improved in two of the longest-running project sites: 87% in Carabuco and 65% in Ancoraimes (both in the highlands; Espada 2000). This compared favorably to the initial 1992 baseline immunization coverage rate for Ancoraimes of 2% (Perry 1993). The percentage of mothers who introduced solid foods to infants at six months was also high: 86% in Carabuco and 67% in Ancoraimes (compared to 48% at 1992 in Ancoraimes). Likewise, the proportions of mothers who knew about oral rehydration therapy, knew how to prepare the solution properly at home, and had used it recently to treat a child's diarrhea ranged from 60 to 82% in these same two areas during 2000. This compared favorably with the 1992 baseline measure in Ancoraimes of 18%. Meanwhile, in Montero, in the tropical lowlands, program coverage rates for at least one prenatal visit had reached 93% by 1997 (Espada 1998). In the same year, 79% of Montero service area deliveries were attended by a health professional.

SOME LESSONS LEARNED FROM WORKING WITH COMMUNITIES

Over the years, CSRA has pursued two interrelated but separate goals: to improve the health of communities, and to enable communities to improve their own health. Each of these goals requires a different set of strategies and activities. However, CSRA has not been equally successful in meeting both goals. As shown by the key health indicators, CSRA has been relatively successful in improving the health status of communities. Its efforts to enhance the capacity of communities to improve their own health have not been nearly as successful, and they have come up against numerous difficulties, including the following:

- A first principle of empowering communities is that an organization and its staff must respect and proceed at the rhythm of the communities. However, there are important costs associated with proceeding at this pace, and there appears to be little patience within funding agencies for doing so. Many of CSRA's donors are oriented toward rapid improvements in quantitative goals and coverage, not in the development of the slower community processes necessary for sustained long-term change. For example, representatives of one major funding source recently expressed interest in strengthening community processes, but their internal policies did not allow more than a single four-year funding cycle, a period too short to consolidate and extend the desired results.

- A second principle of empowerment is that it implies change. Change requires that community members take risks (for example, attempt unfamiliar behaviors or assume new responsibilities). The willingness of communities to take such risks is often a function of their perception that so-called change agents (including health programs and their staffs) share these risks. However, government authorities, health system practitioners, auxiliary nurses, and even most NGO employees are generally uninterested in or unable to share those risks. Although CSRA has made progress in making empowerment one of its most important organizational values, it still has much to learn about it, particularly in terms of what it means during day-to-day contacts by staff with community members.

- Most government, church, and NGO interventions remain paternalistic. Their policies have conditioned communities to expect primary health care to be provided, usually free of charge, by entities outside the community. PHC is then perceived to be an external agenda, perhaps tied to some hidden agenda. Furthermore, there is still a surprisingly large number of giveaway programs directed at getting communities to accept health care interventions in exchange for donated commodities or other material incentives. CSRA considers it a major accomplishment to have achieved and maintained high levels of coverage without resorting to these types of programs.

- The paternalism of many organizations is reinforced by the expectation of many communities and individuals that it is the obligation of government and other outside agencies to provide free or highly subsidized health care (and other social services). It is as though Bolivia's traditional *padrino-ahijado* (godparent-godchild) relationship plays itself out under conditions of dependency rather than the original, more enlightened, concept of mutual reciprocity. In this light, communities continue to look at most NGOs as wealthy outsiders to be squeezed for all they are worth for as long as possible. CSRA continues to foster local ownership of the organization and to be a part of local civil society.

PRELIMINARY CONCLUSIONS

The single most important determinant of whether clients will use health services, both clinical and preventive, is the client's *confidence* in the practitioner. The *effectiveness* of community-based care is improved by using a census-based methodology like the one used by CSRA. This methodology promotes equity by reaching every family, particularly those at highest risk. In addition, it fosters trust between participants and practitioners.

In working within communities, it is essential to share risks with them to engender trust and co-responsibility for change. At the same time that a community-based organization is seeking greater local participation, however, it must still assume responsibility for specialized tasks (such as providing vaccinations) by offering training, support, and supervision. The sustainability of these elements requires an organizational framework that guarantees continuity. Within this framework, issues of ownership, leadership, accountability, stability, and demand for services are at least as important as financial security and technical know-how.

CSRA found that two factors in particular can enhance the long-term sustainability of care. First, mid-level, paid health workers (usually auxiliary nurses) who come from the communities they serve can provide essential technical support and leadership in isolated rural areas, where MOH-sponsored professional health workers typically change frequently. Second, integrating different levels of curative care with preventive care and health promotion contributes significantly to the long-term impact of primary health care.

In the experience of CSRA, decentralization provided an important opportunity for local authorities to become sensitized to the issues of public health and human development. Once authorities' awareness is raised, their commitment to public health and development increases.

Finally, in any health initiative, expansion occurs only with the development of a skilled and motivated work force. This includes, at a minimum, personal commitment, appropriate technical knowledge, and an understanding of the communities' and NGO's goals and strategies.

IMMEDIATE NEXT STEPS

In early 2000, it became clear that CSRA needed to take a fresh look at its future. A consultant who was hired to facilitate the development of a new strategic plan promoted the idea that CSRA needed a new and ambitious view of its future. CSRA decided to create a vision powerful enough to motivate the organization, all the way from the board of directors and management and operational staff to government and local authorities, communities, and families. Further, CSRA has decided that two key strategies will be necessary to reach its goals. First, CSRA will approach its goals like a business, striving for efficiency and quality. Second, it will mobilize communities, families, and authorities by developing and sharing a vision that is common to all.

THE STATUS OF COMMUNITY-BASED PRIMARY HEALTH CARE

Enormous challenges face community-based health care. Most fundamentally, despite clear evidence of success, epidemiologically informed, community-based local health care programming is still not widespread and is the exception rather than the rule. ARHC's nearly 20 years of experience have consistently demonstrated that the causes of preventable and/or treatable disease and death are usually similar in poor communities, but those most at risk must be identified house by house, and the solutions must be tailored to local circumstances. Even in those countries where the public health system recognizes the need for seeking out those most in need for health services, most, if not all, do not have, nor have they attempted to develop, the mechanism for such outreach.

In reality, community health solutions do not come from top-down approaches. Frequently, those who are most ill do not present themselves to clinic health providers. They suffer and die in their homes, unknown to and unrecorded by the local health system. They often perceive that they will not be welcome at the health facility; they fear that the services will be costly and beyond their means; and they often doubt the quality or efficacy of the services offered. The more traditional way of coping with illness is to "wait and see" or consult family members, friends, or the local healer. Without repeated educational messages from trusted local health providers in a culturally "safe" environment, old behaviors will remain, and unnecessary suffering, sickness, and death will continue.

Related, perhaps causally, is the nature of international and national health funding, which remains focused on a wide range of intervention-specific, vertically funded programs. These programs often do not adequately support community-based health care, the *vehicle* of their intervention. That is, a "vaccination person" (interested in preventing selected communicable diseases) seeks increased recognition and funding for that program. Generally, the person is not concerned so much with *how* these services will be provided, as with *how many* units will be delivered. Further, in any developing country, such a vertical program (whether HIV/AIDS, family planning, or malaria) may compete directly with community-based health care for scarce public health funding. Those in public health often fight for scarce resources for specialized health programming at the expense of the very mechanism that would provide numerous programs in a cost-effective, high-quality, and ongoing fashion.

Another significant barrier to effective community-based health care is lack of community participation, an essential element of the local health system. For health care to be effective locally, the system must have strong ties to the community it serves. Such ties *must* include community assessment and evaluation, community participation in health planning, community feedback about and oversight of services, and open debate about health service alternatives. ("Community" is defined here to include at least the local political and traditional leaders, as well as the health service clients themselves, especially women.) ARHC has found that working with community-based or indigenous nonprofit organizations helps build local capacity for long-term provision of health services.

For various reasons, working within MOH systems is a much less productive and sustainable means of improving community health, at least in the countries where ARHC has operated. To begin with, MOH-supported health personnel frequently come from outside the communities they serve, are perceived as outsiders, and may not be trusted. The turnover of both MOH health service providers and their superiors is high, leading to what one might describe as "permanent institutional amnesia." This means that training or technical assistance provided to MOH health workers is often lost within a few months or years. In addition, MOH-directed health staff frequently do not hold themselves accountable to communities for service quality, further alienating the community from its assigned health provider.

Working with local nonprofit groups provides a way around these structural problems of MOH-led health care. Health workers can be selected from the communities they serve. They are accountable locally and institutionally for the quality of their work, and they have a long-term commitment to the communities they serve. The CBIO methodology is a professionally rewarding process, once health providers have experienced its effectiveness and see real changes measured in their communities. In this model, the MOH would better serve as the *guarantor* of public health coverage and equity. The MOH could also play important and active roles in providing funding, medicines, and equipment and in offering training to health workers to strengthen the quality, uniformity, and range of local services provided.

By applying the values, principles, practices, and tools of good public health within the context of the CBIO methodology, ARHC and its local nonprofit partners are able to efficiently guide local health assessments and develop effective local health strategies. The top-down and bottom-up approaches meet in a mutually respectful dialogue that allows for modern public health inputs, as well as for local values, sensibilities, and resources. Scaling up, or "going to scale," is possible within this approach and is not the monolithic, one-size-fits-all approach that many national health planners too often prefer. Rather, the process encourages appropriate local variation in public health programming, management, and support. Ultimately, we believe that this will be the most cost-effective and sustainable means of radically improving global health. In fact, it may be the only way that community-based health will ever really occur.

REFERENCES

Espada, Sara. 1998. "Three-Year Evaluation of the Montero Health Project." Internal program evaluation report of Andean Rural Health Care and el Consejo de Salud Rural Andino. Available on request.
———. 2000. "Mid-Term Evaluation Report of the Child Survival XIII Project." Andean Rural Health Care and el Consejo de Salud Rural Andino. Washington, DC: USAID, Bureau for Private and Voluntary Cooperation, Child Survival Program, January 10, 2000.
Perry, Henry. 1993. "Notas de la Evaluación, Proyectos de Supervivencia Infantil, Programa de Salud en Carabuco y Ancoraimes." Internal report of Andean Rural Health Care, November 15–20, 1993. Available on request.
———. 1999. "Attaining Health for All through Community Partnerships: Principles of the Census-Based, Impact-Oriented (CBIO) Approach to Primary Health Care Developed in Bolivia, South America." *Social Science and Medicine* 48: 1053–67.
Shanklin, David. 1994. "Estimating the Infant/Child Mortality Impact of a Bolivia Child Survival Program." In *Community Impact of PVO Child Survival Efforts: 1985–1994: Proceedings of a Worldwide Conference Sponsored by USAID.* Bangalore, Karnataka, India, October 2–7, 1994. Baltimore, MD: PVO Child Survival Support Program, Johns Hopkins University.
———. 1998. "Dramatic Reductions of Childhood Mortality in Three Bolivian Child Survival Projects." In *Presented Papers: High Impact PVO Child Survival Programs, Volume 2: Proceedings of an Expert Consultation, Gallaudet University, Washington, DC, June 21–24, 1998.* Arlington, VA: BASICS (Basic Support for Institutionalizing Child Survival) and Washington, DC: CORE (Child Survival Collaborations and Resources Group), pp. 45–53.

9 Decentralized Supervision of Community Health Programs: Using LQAS in Two Districts of Southern Nepal

Joseph J. Valadez and Babu Ram Devkota

Using modern tools of statistical quality control, simple field epidemiology can both motivate and lead community health efforts to achieve higher coverage of essential services. Even basic health workers can measure their accomplishments, which motivates all involved to strive toward agreed-upon goals. This effort at the community level reflects global efforts such as the goals of the World Summit for Children, which are measurable and drive action at all levels. The importance of repeated measurement at the local level is well illustrated in this chapter.

—*Jon Rohde*

Community-oriented approaches to organize health programs have been advocated for more than 75 years (Taylor-Ide and Taylor 2002). In the 1980s and 90s, national and international health and development agencies increasingly promoted decentralized service delivery and health systems management, emphasizing bottom-up, community-oriented methods. Several examples of successful community health programs are documented (Wyon and Gordon 1971, Villegas 1978, Rohde et al. 1993, Arole and Arole 1994, Taylor-Ide and Taylor 1995). While the methods used for bottom-up management are not described in detail, it is clear from those published examples that the programs used data about program progress to show management how to improve effectiveness. Planning and program design also require data to ensure effectiveness. John Wyon and other community-oriented primary health practitioners argue that community health workers ought to use epidemiological information to focus local health programs on the most frequent, serious, and preventable causes of death and illness (see the introduction to this book, and Taylor-Ide and Taylor 2002). In their book, Daniel Taylor-Ide and Carl Taylor list seven steps in a community-oriented approach, of which steps 2–5 and 7 involve data collection and analysis:

1. Create coordinating committees and improve their capacity.
2. Identify successes.
3. Study successes and visit other communities.
4. Conduct self-evaluation.
5. Make decisions based on agreed-upon problem areas and priorities.

6. Involve as many people as possible in decision-making.
7. Monitor the momentum to identify gaps in action and to make midcourse corrections.

This chapter demonstrates a simple community data-gathering method, which local supervisors used in two districts of the Terai of Nepal (south of Kathmandu) to increase the impact of their health programs. This method, Lot Quality Assurance Sampling (LQAS), represents a practical alternative to cluster surveys (Henderson and Sundaresan 1982), a widely used method, to obtain objective information about community outcomes.

WHAT LQAS IS AND HOW IT WORKS

During the mid-1980s, health system evaluators explored the applications of industrial quality control methods to assess health worker performance (Stroh 1985, Valadez 1986, Reinke 1988). LQAS received considerable attention as a potentially practical and easy-to-use method for assessing local health systems in developing-world settings. LQAS was originally developed in the 1920s to control the quality of industrially produced goods (Dodge and Romig 1944). The principle is that a line supervisor takes a small random sample of a recently manufactured lot of goods from a production unit such as an assembly line or machine. If the number of defective goods in the sample exceeds a predetermined number, then the lot is rejected; otherwise it is accepted. This allowable number is called the *decision rule*. The number of allowable defective goods is determined statistically (Dodge and Romig 1944, Lwanga and Lemeshow 1991, Valadez 1991) based on a production standard and a statistically determined sample size. The sample size is set so that a manager has a high probability of accepting lots in which a predetermined proportion of the goods are of high quality, and a high probability of rejecting lots that fail to reach the production standard.

In health systems, an example of a *production standard* is a predetermined population coverage benchmark for an intervention such as immunization, communications about how to prepare and use oral rehydration solution, the quality of deliveries performed by a medically trained provider, or promotion of contraceptive use. Health system managers at either the national or district level can set such coverage benchmarks or targets.

In health systems, a *lot* can be the defined community or catchment area of a health facility or of a health worker. In this chapter, the lot used in the demonstration is a *supervision area* (SA). The *production unit* is the set of health workers working under the supervisor who manages the SA. In this setting, the purpose of using LQAS is to determine whether a specific SA reaches a predetermined coverage benchmark and to compare the performance of different SAs.

LQAS judgments about supervision areas have a percentage of error, namely, the probability of misclassifying an SA as either having achieved the benchmark or not having achieved it. In standard statistical nomenclature, they correspond to alpha (α) and beta (β) errors. The α error is the likelihood of rejecting a sample incorrectly—in this case, of falsely determining that the desired level of performance had *not* been met when in reality it had. The β error is the likelihood of accepting an SA as performing adequately when it falls short of the expected performance. These errors correspond to the specificity and sensitivity of the procedure.[1]

To use LQAS, health system managers need to identify two thresholds. The first is the *coverage benchmark,* which is the proportion of the community that health workers ought to reach during a predetermined period, such as one year. The coverage benchmark should increase over time as the program progresses and service delivery improves. In public health terms, a threshold can be an *annual coverage*

---

1. The α error is a *health system risk,* since the health program would invest unnecessarily to improve the performance of health workers in supervision areas that have actually reached a coverage benchmark. In epidemiological terms, $1-\alpha$ is equivalent to *specificity,* which is the probability of correctly identifying SAs that reach performance benchmarks. The β error is *community risk,* since beneficiaries would receive health services that leave unacceptably large portions of the population uncovered. In epidemiological terms, $1-\beta$ is equivalent to *sensitivity,* which is the probability of correctly identifying supervision areas that cover an unacceptably low proportion of the population. In traditional industrial terms, *health system risk* and *community risk* are *producer risk* and *consumer risk* (Dodge and Romig 1944).

target. The lower threshold is an unacceptably low level of coverage that should provoke managers to identify the problem causing the failed service delivery and to resolve it with a focused investment of time and resources.

Two characteristics have made LQAS attractive to health system evaluators. First, a supervisor needs only a small sample to judge whether a health worker's performance has reached a predetermined level (threshold). With such small samples, data collection does not seriously compete for time for providing health services. Second, the sampling procedures and analyses are rather simple. Because LQAS was originally intended for use by factory supervisors, these procedures could be carried out by a minimally educated person. Managers of international health workers are typically more educated than the line supervisor of yesteryear. Yet this benefit is still welcome to overworked supervisors and health workers, who need management tools that can easily be understood in their own cultural context and are easy to use. These two characteristics in particular make LQAS valuable as a practical management tool for monitoring and evaluation of community health services that seek to include community members in management.

Another attractive feature of LQAS is that the data from individual SAs can be combined into an estimate of a coverage proportion for an entire program area that includes multiple SAs. Weighting the result from each SA by the size of its population and taking the mean of the program area can increase the accuracy of the estimate,[2] particularly in comparison to estimates obtained with the 30-cluster sampling approach.[3]

The growing interest in using LQAS was captured in a review of 34 LQAS applications assessing immunization coverage, antenatal care,

2. Weighting increases precision by a small amount and is not necessary for most applications, because the precision gained typically does not have programmatic implications. See Valadez 1998 for examples.
3. This coverage estimate usually has greater precision than the one obtained with the 30-cluster method (Henderson and Sundaresan 1982), the other commonly used sampling method, because stratified random (or systematic) samples generally have narrower confidence intervals than cluster samples

use of oral rehydration therapy, growth monitoring, family planning, disease incidence, and the technical skills and knowledge of health workers (Robertson et al. 1997). It has also been used to assess the accuracy of health records, outreach of community health workers, and health worker training programs (Valadez 1991, Valadez et al. 1996, Valadez et al. 1997). In Nicaragua, Malawi, and Armenia, networks of NGOs have used LQAS to track national disaster relief and reproductive health programs (Valadez et al. 2001a, 2001b, 2001c). This chapter focuses on using LQAS to assess coverage of SAs with integrated health services in a maternal and child health project in rural Nepal.

This chapter attempts to advance the development of LQAS methodology for community-based public health practitioners and health system managers by:

- presenting a simplified, field-tested LQAS table that community-based public health practitioners can use in any field setting;
- explaining a case application of LQAS used by local supervisors rather than specialized interviewers;
- showing how LQAS can be applied for regular supervision or monitoring;
- summarizing LQAS results collected at four time points to monitor a community-based NGO program in Nepal for maternal and newborn care, child survival, and family planning interventions;
- presenting a cost analysis of LQAS compared to cluster sampling;
- discussing the utility of this system to practitioners.

(Note 3, cont.) of the same size. As others have pointed out, "stratified samples often have narrower confidence intervals than simple random samples. This is because some subjects are selected from each and every strata [*sic*], making it impossible to miss some strata completely" (Robertson et al. 1997, 201). In operational terms, the strata are the SAs. Also, LQAS does not have a design effect, which for cluster samples is usually assumed to be two, due to the intra-cluster correlation resulting from choosing contiguous households within clusters (Henderson and Sundaresan 1982).

PROGRAM AREA: RAUTAHAT AND BARA DISTRICTS, NEPAL

The program area, in the Rautahat and Bara districts, is contiguous with districts in Nepal's Narayani Zone of the Central Development Region in the Terai, south of Kathmandu. The districts border India to the south and include communities of 33 Village Development Committees (VDCs) in Rautahat District and 17 VDCs in Bara District. The VDC is the basic unit of community organization. One VDC contains nine communities or wards. The total beneficiary population in the program area is 140,021 people, including 52,896 women of childbearing age, 39,557 children under five years of age, and an estimated 47,568 newborns expected during a four-year cycle of the program.

The health program is supported by Plan International's field office for the Rautahat and Bara districts of Nepal. Plan International is a child-focused international NGO working in more than 40 nations. It will continue supporting the health program beyond four years because it has long-term commitments to the communities with which it works.

During 1996, the national under-five mortality in Nepal was 118 per 1,000 live births, with an infant mortality rate of 79 per 1,000 live births. Mortality was consistently higher in rural areas. The maternal mortality rate in Nepal was 539 per 100,000 live births (Pradhan et al. 1996). Only 10% of births are attended by medically trained personnel (World Summit for Children indicator, Nepal 1996).

According to Plan International's 1995–96 situational analysis, the under-five mortality rate in the program area was identical to the rate determined by the national Demographic & Health Survey. Among the leading causes of child death listed by the Ministry of Health (MOH) and cross-validated with local clinic records were diarrhea, pneumonia, perinatal causes, malnutrition, and measles. Plan International worked with all 50 VDCs to identify local health priorities. VDCs, district MOH managers, and local Plan International health system managers selected four interventions to implement in the two selected districts: diarrhea case management, pneumonia case management, family planning, and maternal and newborn care. They also agreed to support the MOH to enhance Expanded Programme on Immunization (EPI) and vitamin A coverage.

PROGRAM MANAGEMENT

The program supported services at both MOH health care facilities and the community level by improving supervision, case management, monitoring, drug supply, and community mobilization. This chapter focuses exclusively on the community-level activities. The program area consists of 50 VDCs, each one comprising 9 wards or communities, for a total of 450. Each VDC has one MOH health facility. Each facility has one village health worker (VHW), who is supervised by a senior manager (Health Post In-Charge). Each VHW supervises nine female community health volunteers (FCHVs) and trained traditional birth attendants (TBAs). Supervision of VHWs at the community level had been weak due to lack of transport, incentives, and management systems. Plan International's program was designed to improve community-level supervision and management.

The program area was organized into seven SAs, each one managed by a Plan International field area supervisor (FAS). Each FAS has experience working in the MOH community health system and is qualified as a nurse, midwife, or health assistant. These supervisors work with the MOH district health officer to train VHWs; then they aid the VHWs to train and supervise FCHVs and TBAs. Each FAS trains and supports 7 to 8 VHWs, each of whom is in turn responsible for 9 FCHVs. Therefore, on average, each FAS has at least 63 FCHVs and additional TBAs in his/her supervision area.

FASs train VHWs in management, leadership, and supervision skills, and update VHWs' clinical skills for each intervention. FASs are trained to use a simple supervision checklist to observe FCHVs and TBAs. These checklists determine whether the FCHVs and TBAs are implementing planned interventions, have basic equipment and supplies, and use focus groups to assess community satisfaction. Each FAS aids the VHWs to carry out joint supervision visits two to three times a month to FCHVs as a part of competency-based training.

The program began service delivery in 1997. Plan International introduced LQAS in 1999 for routine community-based monitoring by FASs of mothers, children 0–23 months of age, and women 15–49 years of age to determine whether they received health services and information. All FASs said they would benefit from such empirical information if data collection were not time consuming and results could be rapidly interpreted and used for supervising FCHVs and TBAs.

METHODS: IMPLEMENTING DECENTRALIZED SUPERVISION

This section summarizes the methods used for setting sample sizes, training, questionnaire development, sampling procedures, and coverage benchmarks. FASs collected LQAS data four times at six-month intervals from June 1999 to January 2001. The FASs and the manager chose this six-month sampling interval. The program regularly measured indicators to monitor knowledge and behavior related to diarrhea case management, pneumonia case management, maternal and newborn care, family planning, and EPI. A few of the results from these observations are reported here. Our purpose is to show how LQAS was used and the type of information it provides, rather than to report the program outcomes.

Sample Sizes and LQAS Tables

A sample size of 19 households was selected for this assessment, allowing specificity and sensitivity of greater than 90% (< 10% error). While smaller sample sizes exist for which α and β errors are also < 10% for some coverage benchmarks (e.g., samples ranging from 10 to 18), we do not recommend these smaller sample sizes, despite the improved feasibility of such smaller samples. If an initial rather low coverage benchmark is selected that allows a small sample size (e.g., 40% coverage and n=15, with a decision rule of 8 correct responses) and the coverage benchmark is subsequently changed, requiring a larger sample and a different decision rule (e.g., 65% and n=17 with a decision rule of 11), the data collector would have to return to the SA to collect the additional data from the larger sample. By selecting a sample of 19, the manager can change coverage benchmarks later without having to collect additional data. In practice, supervisors assess several interventions simultaneously with different coverage benchmarks. Using a standard sample size of 19 yields sufficient data to make judgments about all interventions, regardless of their coverage benchmarks. For interventions intended for narrow age groups (e.g., exclusive breastfeeding assesses the 0–5-month age cohort) or for individuals with specific characteristics (e.g., use of oral rehydration therapy for children who have had diarrhea in the last two weeks), LQAS judgments are made with sample sizes other than 19 (see Valadez et al. 2001b).

In practice, FASs have been most interested in identifying SAs that reach a coverage benchmark and those that deviate from it substantially. Table 1 is the basic LQAS tool used for making this judgment. Supervisors have been less interested in lower thresholds and have been satisfied with Table 1's display, which has coverage benchmarks only. This simple format has aided supervisors to select decision rules for a variety of sample sizes and a wide range of coverage benchmarks. In practice, Table 1 has been the most useful LQAS tool for field settings and requires a minimal amount of technical knowledge to use. This table was introduced in Nepal during 2000 and was successfully field-tested in other locations (Valadez et al. 2001c).

In addition to reducing the LQAS decision rules to a single page, Table 1 has another important attribute. While previous tables required counting the number of interviewees who did not receive an intervention, Table 1 embraces the opposite logic, because it requires counting the number who received it. Field staff frequently said that they were used to counting positives for numerators (for example, number of children vaccinated) and that counting negatives was confusing.

A supervisor uses Table 1 by following three steps:

1. Identify the coverage benchmark for an indicator from the top row. However, if the table is used to determine whether an SA is below average, then the average coverage, instead of the coverage benchmark, is located along the top row.
2. Identify the sample size in column 1. In most cases, the sample size is 19.
3. Find the cell where the sample size and the coverage benchmark intersect. That is the decision rule. For example, the decision rule for a coverage benchmark of 80% and a sample size of 19 is 13. A supervisor judges SAs as having reached the benchmark if at least 13 of 19 have the behavior or knowledge stipulated in the indicator.

TABLE 1

Optimal LQAS Decision Rules for Sample Sizes of 12–30
and Coverage Benchmarks or Average Coverage of 20–95%

Sample Size	Annual Coverage Benchmarks (for Monitoring and Evaluation) or Average Coverage (Baselines, Monitoring, and Evaluation)																	
	10%	15%	20%	25%	30%	35%	40%	45%	50%	55%	60%	65%	70%	75%	80%	85%	90%	95%
12	NA	NA	1	1	2	2	3	4	5	5	6	7	7	8	8	9	10	11
13	NA	NA	1	1	2	3	3	4	5	6	6	7	8	8	9	10	11	11
14	NA	NA	1	1	2	3	4	4	5	6	7	8	8	9	10	11	11	12
15	NA	NA	1	2	2	3	4	5	6	6	7	8	9	10	10	11	12	13
16	NA	NA	1	2	2	3	4	5	6	7	8	8	9	10	11	12	13	14
17	NA	NA	1	2	2	3	4	5	6	7	8	9	9	11	12	13	14	15
18	NA	NA	1	2	2	3	5	6	7	8	9	10	11	11	12	13	14	16
19	NA	NA	1	2	3	4	5	6	7	8	9	10	11	12	13	14	15	16
20	NA	NA	1	2	3	4	5	6	7	8	9	11	12	13	14	15	16	17
21	NA	NA	1	2	3	4	5	6	8	9	10	11	12	13	14	16	17	18
22	NA	NA	1	2	3	4	5	7	8	9	10	12	13	14	15	16	18	19
23	NA	NA	1	2	3	4	6	7	8	10	11	12	13	14	16	17	18	20
24	NA	NA	1	2	3	4	6	7	9	10	11	13	14	15	16	18	19	21
25	NA	1	2	2	4	5	6	8	9	10	12	13	14	16	16	18	20	21
26	NA	1	2	3	4	5	6	8	9	11	12	13	14	16	18	19	21	22
27	NA	1	2	3	4	5	7	8	10	11	13	14	15	17	18	20	21	23
28	NA	1	2	3	4	5	7	8	10	12	13	15	16	18	19	21	22	24
29	NA	1	2	3	4	5	7	9	10	12	13	15	17	18	20	21	23	25
30	NA	1	2	3	4	5	7	9	11	12	14	16	17	19	20	22	24	26

NA: not applicable, meaning LQAS cannot be used in this assessment because the coverage is either too low or too high to assess an SA.

Notes: α and β errors < 10% for all decision rules except where noted. Lightly shaded cells indicate where α or β errors are ≥ 10%.

Darker cells indicate where α or β errors are ≥ 15%.

Training and Questionnaire Development

The authors trained the seven FASs and additional support staff to use LQAS to survey 19 households in the VDCs where they supervise FCHVs and TBAs. The manager trained everyone working in the program, including the secretary, accountant, and others, to heighten their involvement. This decision is consistent with the principle of involving as many people as possible in decision-making (Taylor-Ide and Taylor 2002, step 6). Training was carried out over three days, during which time the team reviewed and refined the survey questionnaire and learned LQAS principles, sampling procedures, and how to interpret results. Each FAS or staff person visited 9.5 households on average.

Parallel Sampling and Questionnaire Development

Three short questionnaires were developed, corresponding to the three client groups the program served: women 15–49 years, mothers of children 0–11 months, and mothers of children 12–23 months. Women 15–49 years were sampled to assess their use of family planning methods and to calculate the contraceptive prevalence rate. Mothers of children 0–11 months were selected to assess their knowledge of pneumonia management and maternal and newborn care, including exclusive breastfeeding. Mothers of children 12–23 months were visited to assess EPI and vitamin A coverage, continuing breastfeeding, and diarrhea case management knowledge. Exclusive, complementary, and continuing breastfeeding were assessed with the subsamples of children 0–5 months, 6–9 months, and 12–23 months, respectively. Management of diarrhea was assessed using the stratum of mothers of children 0–23 months whose children had had diarrhea in the last two weeks. The only questions duplicated in the surveys were related to management of diarrhea, because children were needed who had had diarrhea in the previous two weeks; by including related questions in the surveys for mothers of children aged both 0–11 and 12–23 months, sufficient observations were available to measure diarrhea prevalence.

Data were collected using a standard two-stage sampling procedure. In the first stage, 19 wards in each supervision area were sampled in proportion to their size. First, a sampling frame was constructed for each supervision area with VDC and ward names located in column one, with population sizes for each ward in column two, and a running cumulative summary of the population in column three. Second, a sampling fraction was created by dividing the total supervision area population by the LQAS sample size of 19. Third, a random number between 1 and the sampling fraction was selected. The ward having the corresponding person in the cumulative population column of the sampling frame was selected as the first sampling element. The next ward was identified by adding the sampling fraction to the first randomly selected number. All remaining sampling elements were selected by continuing to add the sampling fraction to the preceding sum. The program manager performed all the steps in the first-stage sampling.

In the second stage, households were selected in the identified wards. The FAS and trained support staff visited the sampled wards in their SA and located its geographical center. The FAS divided the ward into three to five segments and chose one randomly, using a random number table. The FAS then went to that segment and divided it into three to five additional segments, choosing one randomly. He or she continued this process until a small number of houses remained—usually fewer than 15. One house was then selected randomly. For the second-stage sample, some supervisors preferred to use the spin-the-bottle method applied in the EPI cluster sample method (Henderson and Sundaresan 1982, World Health Organization 1996).

Once a single house was selected randomly, the interviewer inquired whether a nonpregnant woman 15–49 years of age and in union lived there. If so, she was asked for her consent to respond to the family planning questionnaire. If a woman in the household had a child of either 0–11 months or 12–23 months, she was invited to answer questions in the corresponding questionnaire. Two children, one from either cohort, were never selected from the same household, since the questions about diarrhea case management required analyzing children 0–23 months. All children for this analysis, therefore, had to reside in different households. Otherwise, the diarrhea management practices of a single household would be overrepresented. Therefore, the minimum number of households that an interviewer visited to carry out a survey in any ward was two; the maximum was three. The use of one random point to start a search for households for each of the three questionnaires independently we call *parallel sampling*.

The questionnaires required little time to complete. The family planning questionnaire took 5 minutes, the one for mothers of children 0–11 months took 15 minutes, and that for mothers of children 12–23 months took 10 minutes. Similarly, the search for appropriate households required little time. A woman aged 15–49 years nearly always lived in the first house. One child in either age group could also be located rapidly. The sampling took place during the Nepali monsoon, which exacerbated travel problems. Nevertheless, the total time spent in a ward was about one hour. The entire sample of 399 observations (7 SAs x 3 questionnaires x 19 observations) or 133 sets of 3 questionnaires was collected in 2.5 days. Staff said that because community residents knew them, the women did not resist answering questions. Sampling carried out in an area with dispersed rural populations (Valadez et al. 2001b) or underdeveloped roads to remote areas can take longer to complete (Valadez et al. 2001c).

During June 2000, the FASs used a different approach for data collection. Rather than organizing data collection over an intensive 2.5 days, they decided to collect monitoring data while carrying out their normal work in communities. Therefore, at the beginning of the month they identified the communities to be sampled. They selected houses to interview after they finished other duties in the community, such as providing supplies or competency-based training to the community health workers. While the data collection period extended to as much as 19 days, the evaluation cost less, because the FASs were already scheduled to travel to SAs for supervision. The FASs preferred this approach and continued to use it for subsequent monitoring.

Coverage Benchmarks and Decision Rules

Supervisors assessed the interventions with coverage benchmarks they set, based on the 1997 baseline survey collected with a standard cluster sample method. All FASs used the same benchmarks for a given intervention to permit comparison of SAs. Initial coverage benchmarks and corresponding decision rules for each intervention are recorded in the upper rows of Tables 2 and 3. Only a selection of the indicators is presented here to show how the supervision system works.

RESULTS: HOW DATA WERE USED FOR DECISION-MAKING

Selected results are presented in the four parts of this section to demonstrate how the Nepal team used the new LQAS tools. The first part shows how, at one point in time, FASs judged each SA according to a coverage benchmark. The second section presents LQAS results at four points in time to show development trends in the project area. The third section aggregates data from the LQA samples in seven SAs to calculate coverage proportions for the entire program area at four points in time. The fourth one is a cost analysis of LQAS. All LQAS analyses carried out by FASs used hand-tabulated tally sheets to aggregate the questionnaire data. Project managers cross-checked FASs with tables calculated with EpiInfo 6.04. However, computer-generated results were less useful for immediate decision-making than the hand-tabulated results, which were immediately used for decision-making.

All practices, except exclusive, complementary, and continuing breastfeeding, and diarrhea case management, were assessed in each SA using samples of 19. Because exclusive, complementary, and continuing breastfeeding assessments used small subsamples of children, LQAS judgments were not made, since α and β were unacceptably high. Rather, the data were analyzed only in the aggregated form as coverage proportions. For assessment of the behavior of mothers whose children 0–23 months had had diarrhea in the preceding two weeks, subsample sizes varied from 12 to 18. LQAS decision rules for these sample sizes were taken from Table 1.

Assessing Supervision Areas at One Point in Time:
A Supervisor's Perspective

Table 2 contains the results for six indicators for maternal and newborn care, diarrhea case management, and family planning. Additional indicators were used to review these services (see Child Survival Technical Support Project and CORE Monitoring and Evaluation Working Group 1999, and Valadez 2000 for a full set of indicators). However, only six are presented to demonstrate how the LQAS method was used in Nepal.

TABLE 2

LQAS Judgments for Selected Community Interventions

	Behavior			Knowledge			Total No. of Indicators Not Reaching Coverage Benchmarks or Below Avg.
	MNC Children 0–11 Mos.	DCM Children 12–23 Mos.	FP Women 15–49 Yrs.	MNC Children 0–11 Mos.	MNC Children 0–11 Mos.	DCM Children 12–23 Mos.	
	Assisted delivery with trained TBA or clinician	Correctly prepares ORS	Contraceptive use	Pregnancy danger signs	Postnatal danger signs	Dehydration danger signs	
Baseline Results	Not included in baseline survey	Not included in baseline survey	20.7% §	30.7%	Not included in baseline survey	12.7%	
Coverage Benchmark: Decision Rule	NA	NA	30%:3	45%:6	NA	35%:4	
Avg. Coverage: Decision Rule	43.6%:6	52.7%:8	34.5%:4	51.3%:8	41.8%:6	48%:7	
Supervision Area							
1	7	7*	5	9	5*	6*	3
2	9	7*	3*	8	8	5*	3
3	2*	12	4	(5*)	5*	12	3
4	13	9	(2*)	(5*)	2*	9	3
5	4*	11	4	15	13	14	1
6	15	16	13	16	16	15	0
7	5*	8	7	6*	3*	4*	4
Total Below Avg. or or Substandard FASs	3	2	2	3	4	3	17

Notes: MNC=maternal and newborn care; DCM=diarrhea case management; FP=family planning; ORS=oral rehydration solution. § A cluster sample was used for the baseline survey, which sampled mothers of children 0–23 months of age for all indicators. Therefore, contraceptive use as calculated at baseline is not an accurate measure, since the 15–49-year cohort of women is required. ◯ indicates an SA that has not reached a benchmark. * indicates an SA with below average coverage.

An SA is judged according to whether it has reached the coverage benchmark and whether it has achieved at least average coverage. SAs not reaching a benchmark are circled. Those below average are marked with an asterisk. SAs having both a circle and an asterisk have the highest priority for improvement. Those marked with either a circle or an asterisk (but not both) are the next highest priority.

The first indicator discussed is *knowledge of pregnancy danger signs,* found in column 5 of Table 2. The baseline measure of September 1997 revealed that 30.7% of respondents knew two or more danger signs. The program members planned to increase the proportion to 45% by June 1999. The LQAS decision rule for this coverage benchmark is 6 (see Table 1). In June 1999, the FASs interviewed 19 mothers and then counted the number who knew two or more pregnancy danger signs. The results are in the rows of Table 2 labeled 1–7 for each SA. Of the seven SAs, two (SAs 3 and 4) did not reach the 45% coverage benchmark, since fewer than 6 women knew two or more danger signs. The FASs drew a circle around them to show their status. They then calculated the average coverage, which was 51.3%.[4] The FASs used the decision rule from Table 1 for average coverage to identify SAs that fell substantially below average coverage. The procedure they used was to round up the coverage estimate to the nearest 5% interval. Therefore, 51.3% rounded up to 55%. The corresponding decision rule is 8. Three of the seven SAs were below average and are marked with an asterisk. SAs 3 and 4, marked with both a circle and an asterisk, were the highest priority for improvement, because their populations had the greatest health risks. SA 7 was the next highest priority for improvement. Although it had reached the benchmark, it was substantially below average coverage. The previous indicator, *contraceptive use,* revealed two priority SAs (2 and 4). SA 4 was the highest priority, however, because it had not reached the coverage benchmark and had substantially below average coverage.

The indicator *knowledge of dehydration danger signs* revealed a different pattern, because all SAs had reached the coverage benchmark of 4.

---

4. This coverage is actually a weighted coverage calculated by a computer. However, an unweighted or crude coverage calculation done by hand would have been sufficient.

Nevertheless, three SAs (1, 2, and 7) exhibited below average coverage and were thus the areas where improvement would most increase the overall impact of the program. The remaining three indicators did not have baseline values, because the FASs had decided they were important indicators to track after the baseline had been completed. Therefore, the monitoring data were used to identify SAs that were below average. They are identified with asterisks in Table 2.

The marginal totals in Table 2 reveal that SA 7 was identified as a priority four times, and four other SAs were priorities three times. *Knowledge of postnatal danger signs* had the largest number of priority SAs (four), while *assisted delivery, knowledge of pregnancy danger signs,* and *knowledge of dehydration danger signs* were priorities for three SAs. By using these results, the manager knows both which interventions and which SAs should be given time and resources to address community health needs most effectively and efficiently.

Assessing Supervision Areas at Four Points in Time:
A Supervisor's Perspective

Table 3 tracks the program's performance for two indicators at four six-month intervals ranging from June 1999 to January 2001. These indicators were introduced after the program began in September 1997, so there are no baseline measures. Nevertheless, a row is included in the table where the baseline value would go. In June 1999, all SAs were assessed to determine whether they ranked below average. Two SAs were below average for *correctly prepares oral rehydration solution* and four were below average for *knows postnatal danger signs.* These SAs hence became the priority SAs for supervisors to focus on to enhance the performance of community health workers. After the first monitoring, the FASs established performance benchmarks for the next six months. In general, they raised the benchmark by about 10–20% above the average coverage. For example, at Time 2, average coverage for the first indicator was 68.2%; FASs set the coverage benchmark for Time 3 at 80%, which is about 10% higher. At each time period, the manager met with FASs and jointly decided on benchmarks for the next period based on what they thought was feasible to achieve.

It is interesting that the SAs that did not reach performance bench-

TABLE 3

LQAS Judgments for Demonstrating Correct Preparation of Oral Rehydration Solution and Knowledge of Postnatal Danger Signs (June 1999–January 2001)

	Correctly Prepares ORS: Children 12–23 Months				Knows Postnatal Danger Signs: Children 0–11 Months			
Dates Monitoring Data Were Collected	June 1999	January 2000	June 2000	January 2001	June 1999	January 2000	June 2000	January 2001
Baseline Results	Not included in baseline survey				Not included in baseline survey			
Coverage Benchmark: Decision Rule	NA	65%:10	80%:13	95%:16	NA	55%:8	70%:11	95%:16
Avg. Coverage: Decision Rule	52.6%:6	68.2%:11	85.7%:15	91.3%:16	41.8%:6	59.6%:9	83.9%:14	92.2%:16
SA 1	7*	(7*)	(12*)	17	5*	17	16	19
SA 2	7*	(9*)	17	18	8	12	19	19
SA 3	12	14	17	19	5*	(7*)	18	17
SA 4	9	13	17	19	2*	19	(10*)	(13*)
SA 5	11	17	18	18	13	15	18	19
SA 6	16	19	19	19	16	14	18	18
SA 7	8	12	15	(13*)	3*	8*	12*	16
Total Below Avg. or Substandard FASs	2	2	1	1	4	2	2	1

Notes: ◯ indicates an SA that has not reached a benchmark. * indicates an SA with below average coverage.

marks for the first indicator were not necessarily those that did not reach it for the second one. For example, for the first indicator, SA 1 was below average for three of four time periods. However, it was below average for only the first time period for the second indicator. In another example, SA 7, for the first indicator, was below average for the last time period only; however, for the second indicator it was below average for three time periods. The assumption is that the service problems in an SA are not necessarily associated with any other intervention. Therefore, all critical parts of the community health program should be monitored at each point in time.

During the last three monitoring periods, coverage benchmarks were established for all indicators. SAs during those time points were judged both on whether they reached benchmarks and on average coverage. SAs displaying both a circle and an asterisk for an indicator are the highest priorities for improvement.

The final observation is that both indicators show a continuous increase in performance over the four time periods. Problems are evident at each point in time but did not persist, very likely due to interventions by the supervisors in response to the data. Each of the key community health indicators can be tracked using a table like Table 3 to manage the program, identify the location of problems, track progress, and identify SAs that excel.

Assessing Supervision Areas at Four Points in Time: A Manager's Perspective

The preceding sections displayed how FASs used LQAS data to identify their SA problem-solving priorities and the performance of each SA relative to other SAs. Both applications helped the FASs and their manager to determine which interventions and locations needed technical assistance. This section shows how the program manager or district health officers can use the same data to track the entire community program over time. The main difference is that the data are aggregated; Table 4 displays the weighted coverage proportions of seven indicators with confidence intervals.

Indicators for safe motherhood, diarrhea case management, and family planning interventions are included. As in the previous section,

TABLE 4

Coverage Proportions and Confidence Intervals
for Selected Indicators

Indicator	—Weighted Coverage Proportion and Confidence Interval—				
	Baseline	—————————Monitoring—————			
	Sept. 1997	June 1999	Jan. 2000	June 2000	Jan. 2001
Delivery assisted by clinician or medically trained TBA	NA	43.6% (± 7.9%)	59.2% (± 8.3%)	64.5% (± 8.3%)	53.0% (± 8.8%)
Knowledge of two or more pregnancy danger signs	30.7% (≤ 10%)	51.3% (± 8.6%)	77.9% (± 7.1%)	93.5% (± 4.2%)	98.6% (± 2.1%)
Knowledge of two or more postnatal danger signs	NA	41.8% (± 8.5%)	59.6% (± 8.4%)	83.9% (± 6.3%)	92.2% (± 4.6%)
Demonstrates correct ORS preparation	NA	52.7% (± 8.6%)	68.2% (± 8%)	85.7% (± 6%)	91.3% (± 4.9%)
Knowledge of two or more dehydration danger signs	12.7% (≤ 10%)	48.0% (± 8.6%)	75.3% (± 7.4%)	93.7% (± 4.2%)	94.1% (± 4.1%)
CPR, modern method**	20.2% (≤ 10%)	33.4% (± 8.5%)	38.0% (± 8.8%)	61.7% (± 7.7%)	53.4% (± 9%)

Notes: *Baseline data were collected using an EPI cluster sample for which the confidence interval is assumed to be ≤ 10%. Any indicator not included in the baseline is marked as NA.
** The standard EPI cluster sample includes mothers of children 0–23 months for all interventions. Therefore, the baseline measure of the contraceptive prevalence rate is of that group of women, as well, which is not a true CPR estimate, since the family planning method use of that group of women cannot be assumed to be the same as among women 15–49 years of age. The latter group was sampled during June 1999–January 2001.

only a selection of indicators is presented to demonstrate the use of the LQAS data. Three indicators did not have a baseline measure, because they were introduced after the program began. All interventions display an increase in coverage by January 2001, although assisted delivery and contraceptive prevalence showed slight declines between June 2000 and January 2001. However, the confidence intervals do not indicate slippage.

FASs think that coverage decreased for assisted delivery because priorities during June 2000–January 2001 had shifted from safe motherhood to other interventions. In earlier years, all FASs had made it a priority to increase assisted delivery. By June 2000, FASs were satisfied that pregnant women and their families were embracing this practice and shifted attention to other priorities. However, based on the January 2001 results, FASs concluded that safe motherhood interventions needed to be emphasized continuously for the improvement to be sustainable. This may be because there is little transfer of information between different cohorts of pregnant women and their families. Therefore, FASs need to promote the use of trained health workers during delivery for coverage rates to be maintained.

The contraceptive prevalence rate also decreased slightly during January 2001;[5] however, even at that time, a person was 3.75 times more likely to use a family planning method as compared with baseline.[6] In June 1999, most family planning users sought permanent methods (47.5% = tubal ligation, 5% = vasectomy). Twenty-five percent chose hormonal methods (12.5% = injectables, 7.5% = pill, 5% = Norplant), 20% selected condoms, and 2.5% practiced lactational amenorrhea. By January 2001, the pattern of use of family planning methods had changed. A smaller percentage selected permanent methods (21.7% = tubal ligation, 1.4% = vasectomy). Larger proportions of the women used hormonal methods (injectables = 27.5%, pill = 14.5%), and 33.3% used condoms. Only 1.4% said that abstinence was their chosen family planning method. Both the increase in the contraceptive prevalence rate, and the changed pattern of method use, may be due to the increased availability of family planning methods in the program area. Before family planning became a community priority, procurement of family planning methods had been a major challenge that FASs and their manager had to overcome.

FASs also cited another reason for the decreases in assisted deliveries and contraceptive use in January 2001, namely, the political instability

5. The reduction in CPR in January 2001 could be a regression effect. See Campbell and Stanley 1966 and Valadez and Bamberger 1994.
6. This odds ratio was calculated as part of a trend analysis, not reported here. Because LQAS data, in aggregate, are a stratified random sample, statistical tests can be used, since each observation is independent of every other observation.

FIGURE I

Exclusive Breastfeeding of Infants 0–5 Months and
Complementary Breastfeeding of Infants 6–11 months

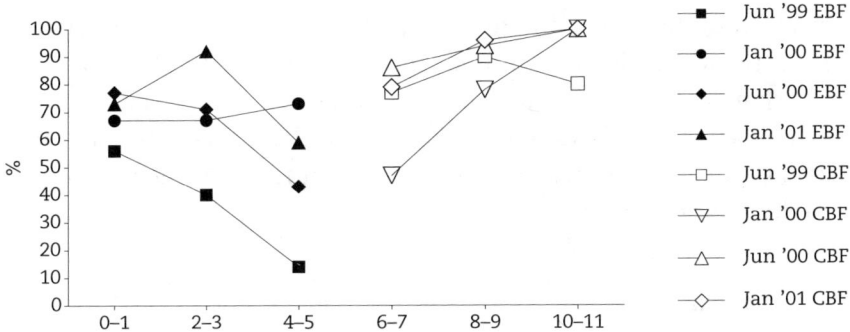

and violence in Nepal at that time. These factors could have prevented women from obtaining assistance for deliveries and made family planning methods unavailable.

The final key intervention category is breastfeeding. Figure 1 tracks exclusive and complementary breastfeeding practices at each of four time points. The data show that, at Time 1, only 56% of women exclusively breastfed infants aged 0–1 months. By the time these infants reached 4–5 months of age, only 14% of the cohort was exclusively breastfed. However, by Time 4, 73% of infants 0–1 months were exclusively breastfed, with 59% of the 4–5-month-old cohort being exclusively breastfed. Although the trend lines fluctuate over the four time points, the trend suggests that, by Time 4, more infants in the older stratum were exclusively breastfed. Some of the variation in breastfeeding results over time may be due to the small sample sizes of each monthly cohort. When data for children 0–11 months are broken down into six two-month cohorts, each one has, on average, 22 children. While the confidence interval for each point estimate is wide, some trends are nevertheless evident.

The right-hand portion of Figure 1 displays complementary breastfeeding. Little change is evident when Time 1 and Time 4 are compared, except in the 10–11-month cohort. This result also suggests that women are breastfeeding their children longer.

Other analyses examined exclusive breastfeeding among infants 6–11 months. Results suggest that a reason complementary feeding was low among infants 6–7 months is that 26.7% still exclusively breastfed; 8% of infants 8–9 months also still exclusively breastfed. This practice may suggest either resource deprivation in these communities or lack of knowledge about the need to provide supplementary food when infants reach 6 months of age. Interestingly, the trend lines with the highest proportions of exclusive breastfeeding of infants aged 0–11 months are in the January measures. This may suggest a seasonal influence.

In conclusion, this section has illustrated the diverse uses of LQAS data at both the community and managerial levels. Some were quite simple, while others were more sophisticated.

Cost Analysis

The total field costs for the cluster sample used at the baseline was $6,548, while the initial LQAS application cost $2,947. The second LQAS application cost $1,180. The baseline and initial LQAS applications included training costs, while the recurrent application included refresher training at lower cost. See Table 5.

However, because LQAS uses FASs who are already employed rather than special interviewers, many costs, such as salaries, were already being paid by the program. If the supervisors had not been participating in this assessment, they would have been carrying out other essential tasks. These represent opportunity costs. The marginal costs columns shows additional money spent for LQAS in both its initial use ($1,585) and recurrent use ($456). None of the cluster sample costs are considered opportunity costs.

The main savings in recurrent costs is the elimination of training costs. The team also reduced costs by shortening the questionnaire. The costs of using expatriate trainers are not included in this analysis of both the cluster sampling and LQAS, because those costs can vary substantially across different organizations. The January 2000–2001 applications included no outside technical assistance.

The total cost for each questionnaire set of the recurrent application of LQAS is equivalent to a 1986 application that estimated $9 (in 1999 dollars) (Valadez 1991). However, the application in Nepal cost substantially less than the $5,000 to $8,000 reported elsewhere, both for other LQAS applications and for cluster sampling (Singh et al. 1996).

TABLE 5

Comparison of the Costs of Cluster Sampling for a Baseline
and the Costs of LQAS for Monitoring

	September 1997 Cluster Sample Baseline Costs	June 1999		January 2001	
		LQAS Costs	Opportunity Cost = Marginal Cost	LQAS Costs	Opportunity Cost = Marginal Cost
Salaries	$2,498	$1,328	$0	$724	$0
Transportation	$673	$420	$420	$413	$413
Materials	$816	$403	$403	$43	$43
Food/Accommodation	$2,561	$796	$762	$0	$0
Total Costs	$6,548	$2,947	$1,585	$1,180	$456
Total Cost per Set	$21.83	$22	$12	$9	$3
Total Cost per Observation	$21.83	$7.39	$3.97	$2.96	$1.14

The lower costs of this study are probably due to two factors: (1) the monitoring system is decentralized, which minimized travel costs, including food, accommodations, and transport, and (2) local supervisors are able to work more rapidly in their communities than interviewers not known by residents.

Collecting the baseline data for this project using cluster sampling cost more than twice as much as collecting the LQAS data. When only marginal costs are considered for this decentralized LQAS application, then cluster sampling was more than four times more expensive than this decentralized application of LQAS. The reasons are: More data collectors are required for the cluster sample; and centrally organized teams travel to 30 clusters, which results in considerably higher transportation, food, and lodging costs than when seven FASs travel locally to their own communities to visit 133 households. This analysis shows that decentralized monitoring and supervision systems are substantially more cost effective than centralized approaches.

The costs of LQAS were recently analyzed in Armenia, where three organizations used LQAS in a baseline study for their reproductive health program. The average total cost per organization was $2,740, which is comparable to the initial application of LQAS in Nepal ($2,947) (see Valadez et al. 2001a).

DISCUSSION

During the 1990s, LQAS was used for two different management purposes:

1. to collect *population-based data* with a known confidence interval. Health system (α) and community (β) risks were less emphasized. Professionals working in the EPI have driven this development (World Health Organization 1996, Robertson et al. 1997, Bhattacharyya et al. 1998). WHO's training manual embraces this approach (World Health Organization 1996);
2. to assess supervision areas with known health system and community risks. This community-oriented approach emphasized decentralized data collection and analysis using LQAS. Calculating coverage proportions was a secondary interest. *Community-oriented* health practitioners have written about this approach (Stroh 1985, Valadez 1991, Vargas 1998).

This chapter describes a community-oriented application of simplified LQAS tools used by local supervisors at four points in time to improve their programs. Supervisors did not find the concept of coverage benchmarks difficult to grasp, as they already had established coverage targets for the project. Table 1, which displayed decision rules, was more acceptable to field supervisors than other LQAS tables that also showed α errors and β errors. Although the latter (more standard) tables are preferred by epidemiologists and some managers (Lwanga and Lemeshow 1991, Valadez 1991, Valadez 1998), they were confusing to field supervisors.

Training in data analysis used examples such as the results presented in Table 2. FASs saw the benefits of identifying both specific program interventions and SAs that were performing at substandard levels. Pinpointing program interventions that were not successful highlighted the topics on which health workers needed retraining, while identifying SAs that needed specific technical support indicated which supervisors needed this support. Both of these analyses are necessary to improve the management of decentralized health systems.

After data are collected, each FAS and support staff tallied the results from their SA by hand and shared the results in a joint meeting with other supervisors and support staff. It took approximately one-half day to complete this task and to double-check tallies. The joint meeting provided a forum for discussing results and to assist supervisors to observe the performance of their SA vis-à-vis other SAs. Group discussion helped FASs to plan programmatic changes for their SAs and to request technical assistance from other FASs and the manager. Discussions also helped the program manager identify systematic problems that affected multiple FASs and identify specific SAs needing attention. The program manager was also able to identify the supervisors whose SAs exhibited the fewest substandard interventions and use them as technical advisors for other SAs with program problems. Supervisors were motivated by seeing how their SAs compared to those of other FASs.

In our experience, a factor that constrains program monitoring is the time required to collect data. Overworked local staff may view data collection as a waste of time. For this reason, independent interview teams are often employed to carry out surveys. However, the local supervisors participating in this decentralized application of LQAS did not have this reaction. They agreed that the LQAS sample of 19 was small and did not compete with other responsibilities. Also, in the first application, they noted the importance of visiting beneficiaries in the age ranges of the interventions and hearing for themselves responses to survey questions. By so doing they were able to judge the strengths and weaknesses in their programs and had already begun the reform process before all the data were collected.

From 1999 to 2001, Tables 2 and 3 were the most useful analyses for supervisors and their staff. They also provided the most useful inputs for immediate decision-making by supervisors and the program manager. Table 4, with the aggregate measures of coverage, was useful to the manager to judge the overall progress of the project and to report to his donor and supervisors. It also provided measures to compare with baseline information. However, the coverage proportions did not prove to be of immediate interest to field supervisors, because these figures did not reflect their own individual work in their SAs, as did the LQAS results.

Cost analyses indicate that this decentralized application of LQAS is inexpensive relative to cluster sampling, and when applied regularly, the marginal cost was less than $500. In January 2001, FASs said they would use LQAS as part of their ongoing supervision system every six months and that LQAS has enabled them to steadily improve each intervention.

The Taylors' Seven Steps for Developing Community-Oriented Health Programs

This chapter demonstrates how important a practical and inexpensive yet highly scientific method for gathering, analyzing, and using data at the community level can be for effective supervision and management. The use of LQAS in Nepal resulted in ongoing improvements in the performance of health workers and ultimately in the health of communities. While the LQAS approach was not developed in response to the Taylors' seven steps emphasizing community participation, those seven steps and the LQAS approach can be linked, as follows:

1. **Create coordinating committees and improve their capacity:** In Nepal, these committees included the FASs at a program level.

At an SA level, they included community health workers. Our next task is to involve the community more in using LQAS.

2. **Identify successes:** This is one purpose of using LQAS.
3. **Study success and visit other communities:** FASs who were not reaching coverage benchmarks were able to visit FASs that were successful. However, in most cases they preferred to understand for themselves first why they lagged behind other FASs. Often visiting other communities was not necessary.
4. **Conduct self-evaluation:** This is a central purpose of the community-oriented version of LQAS, as it was applied in Nepal: workers evaluate themselves objectively.
5. **Make decisions based on agreed-upon problem areas and priorities:** FASs met to discuss LQAS results and to identify priorities. Managers used the data as the basis for allocating their attention to priority interventions and supervisors.
6. **Involve as many people as possible in decision-making:** All FASs were involved in decision-making. We have yet to learn how to include community members in the actual decision-making. However, local people were informed of the results and of the priorities for the next six-month period. In this manner, many people were involved.
7. **Monitor the momentum to identify gaps in action and to make midcourse corrections:** The six-month assessment ensured periodic review and revision of action strategies to achieve agreed-on benchmarks, which were progressively raised.

In the context of this collection of experiences with community-based health care (CBHC), this experience in Nepal shows clearly how critical the effective collection and use of data is to improving CBHC services. Because of its low costs, ready acceptance, and ability to be understood by field workers, we think the LQAS approach offers great promise in making ongoing collection and use of data part of the delivery and management of CBHC, rather than being confined to academic studies and generally ignored in the field. Now more long-term applications of LQAS are needed so that additional refinements can be identified and cost analyses can be replicated. We also need to engage communities more actively in using the data to understand and improve the health of their members.

ACKNOWLEDGMENTS

This chapter would not have been possible without the support of Plan International in Nepal and the United States. The authors thank Plan's dedicated local staff (Y. Thapa, N. Shrestha, K. Achhame, D. P. Raman, B. Khatri, S. Bista, Y. Giri, S. Singh, H. Sah, S. B. Rana, S. Kharel, S. Gurung, R. P. Sah, and S. Khanal) and senior management (Dr. Rishi Adhikati, Dr. Kedar Baral, Ramrajya Joshi, and Durval Martinez). We thank Jennifer Luna, Dr. Pierre Marie Metangmo of Plan's international headquarters, and Kate Jones of USAID/BHR/PVC. Our deep gratitude goes to Corey Leburg for participating in the data analysis and to Dr. Mandy Rose, who aided in the development of the training curriculum. Corey Leburg and Nancy Vollmer also deserve recognition for assisting in the refinement of the LQAS tables. In conclusion, we are deeply grateful to Dr. Eric Starbuck, who participated in the fieldwork in June 1999, and whose collegiality and imagination aided the study immeasurably. We also thank Dr. Robb Davis of Freedom from Hunger, who facilitated the testing of the training curriculum in Kenya in 1998. This work was supported by USAID through Child Survival Grant XIII from BHR/PVC (Cooperative Agreement FAO-A-00-97-0042-00) and the NGO Networks for Health Cooperative Agreement (HRN-A-00-98-0001-00).

REFERENCES

Arole, Mabelle, and Rajanikant Arole. 1994. *Jamkhed.* London: Macmillan.

Bhattacharyya, K., et al. 1998. "Community Assessment and Planning for Maternal and Child Health Programs: A Participatory Approach in Ethiopia." Arlington, VA: BASICS (Basic Support for Institutionalizing Child Survival), Partnership for Child Health Care, Inc.

Campbell, Donald T., and Julian C. Stanley. 1966. *Experimental and Quasi-Experimental Designs for Research.* Chicago: Rand McNally.

Child Survival Technical Support Project and CORE Monitoring and Evaluation Working Group. 1999. "KPC-2000: Knowledge, Practices and Coverage Survey." Calverton, MD: Child Survival Technical Support Project and CORE Monitoring and Evaluation Working Group.

Dodge, H. F., and H. G. Romig. 1944. *Sampling Inspection Tables: Single and Double Sampling.* New York: John Wiley & Sons.

Henderson, R. H., and T. Sundaresan. 1982. "Cluster Sampling to Assess Immunization Coverage: A Review of Experience with a Simplified Sampling Method." *Bulletin of the World Health Organization* 60: 253–60.

Lwanga, S. K., and S. Lemeshow. 1991. *Sample Size Determination in Health Studies: A Practical Manual.* Geneva: World Health Organization.

Pradhan, A., et al. 1996. "Nepal Family Health Survey: 1996." Kathmandu, Nepal, and Calverton, MD: Ministry of Health (Nepal), New Era, and Macro International.

Reinke, W. A. 1988. "Industrial Sampling Plans: Prospects for Public Health Applications." Baltimore, MD: Institute for International Programs, Johns Hopkins University School of Hygiene and Public Health.

Robertson, S. E., et al. 1997. "The Lot Quality Technique: A Global Review of Applications in the Assessment of Health Services and Diseases Surveillance." *World Health Statistical Quarterly* 50: 199–209.

Rohde, Jon, Meera Chatterjee, and David Morley, eds. 1993. *Reaching Health for All.* New Delhi: Oxford University Press.

Singh, J., et al. 1996. "Evaluation of Immunization Coverage by Lot Quality Assurance Sampling Compared with 30-Cluster Sampling in a Primary Health Care Centre in India." *Bulletin of the World Health Organization* 74.

Stroh, G. 1985. "Rationale for the Development and Trial of Q.C. Sampling Designs in Program Evaluation." Personal memo to Donald Shepard.

Taylor-Ide, Daniel, and Carl E. Taylor. 1995. *Community Based Sustainable Human Development: A Proposal for Going to Scale with Self-Reliant Social Development.* New York: UNICEF.

———. 2002. *Just and Lasting Change: When Communities Own Their Futures.* Baltimore, MD: Johns Hopkins University Press, forthcoming.

Valadez, J. J. 1986. "Lot Quality Acceptance Sampling for Monitoring Primary Health Care Coverage." Washington, DC: Pan American Health Organization.

———. 1991. *Assessing Child Survival Programs in Developing Countries: Testing Lot Quality Assurance Sampling.* Cambridge: Harvard University Press.

———. 1998. *A Manual for Training Supervisors of Community Health Workers to Use LQAS: A User's Guide.* Arlington, VA: OMNI Research.

———. 2000. "NGO Networks for Health: Detailed Monitoring and Evaluation Plan." Washington, DC: NGO Networks for Health.

Valadez, J. J., and M. Bamberger. 1994. *Monitoring and Evaluating Social Programs in Developing Countries.* Washington, DC: World Bank.

Valadez, J. J., et al. 1996. "Using Lot Quality Assurance Sampling to Assess Measurements for Growth Monitoring in a Developing Country's Primary Health Care System." *International Journal of Epidemiology* 25: 381–87.

————. 1997. "Assessing Family Planning Service-Delivery Skills in Kenya." *Studies in Family Planning* 28: 143–50.

————. 2001a. "NGO Network for Health in Armenia: Baseline Survey Report for Three Partner Organizations." Washington, DC: NGO Networks for Health.

————. 2001b. "NICASALUD Baseline Survey Results for Eight Partner Organizations." Washington, DC: NGO Networks for Health.

————. 2001c. "Umoyo Network Malawi: Baseline Survey Results for Six Partner Organizations: Adventist Health Services, Blantyre Christian Centre, Ekwendeni Hospital, MACRO, Malamulo Hospital, and St. Anne's Hospital, April–June 2000." Washington, DC: NGO Networks for Health.

Vargas, W. V. 1998. "Assessing Community Based Coverage of Nutritional Interventions in Sri Lanka: An LQAS Assessment." Arlington, VA: OMNI.

Villegas, H. 1978. "Costa Rica: Recursos Humanos y Participación de la Comunidad en los Servicios en el Medio Rural." *Buletín de la Oficina Sanitaria Panamericana* 84: 13–24.

World Health Organization. Global Programme for Vaccines and Immunization. 1996. *Monitoring Immunization Programmes Using the Lot Quality Technique.* Geneva: World Health Organization.

Wyon, John B., and John E. Gordon. 1971. *The Khanna Study: Population Problems in the Rural Punjab.* Cambridge: Harvard University Press.

10 Resources to Get the Job Done: The Sustainability of Community-Based Health Care

William Newbrander

How do we pay for it all? This chapter derives principles from many countries and contrasts the experiences of poor and rich countries. Developing countries that have obtained resources from donors and government are often pressured to shift financial responsibility to users, while in rich countries, foundations and private grants try to shift responsibility to routine government budgets. The author cites important principles of affordability and recommends programs that start small and scale up to ensure that financial constraints do not ultimately bankrupt successful health projects.

—*Jon Rohde*

The community-based health care (CBHC) model is built upon the premise that community-based mechanisms for providing health care must be based on need and provide appropriate technology that is available and affordable in an integrated system of services using qualified, local personnel. The experiences from different countries that are presented in this anthology reaffirm the value of the CBHC model.

CBHC AND SUSTAINABILITY

For the CBHC model to succeed, the resources to implement it must be adequate and reliable over a period that will allow delivery of high-quality services (preventive, promotive, and curative) to which there is equal access. Sustainability requires more than adequate financial resources, however. The sustainability of CBHC comprises two elements, one micro, because it relates to the application of a specific model, and the other macro, because a CBHC model can be reproduced in many places and become the basis for expansion. The micro element focuses on the human, financial, and physical (facilities) resources required over time to keep a particular CBHC model functioning well (as compared to merely surviving). The macro element involves scaling up current models and replicating them in a series of communities. The desired cumulative effect is that CBHC covers large segments of a population.

THE SUSTAINABILITY OF CBHC MODELS IN DEVELOPED AND DEVELOPING COUNTRIES

Current models of CBHC in developed and developing countries have similarities as well as differences, particularly with regard to sustainability. The following principles, based on the experiences presented in this book, must be considered with caution because they are derived from comparing experiences with CBHC in the United States with those in developing countries.

Common characteristics of sustainable CBHC programs in the United States and developing countries include (1) founding by visionaries, (2) funding from many small sources, (3) insufficient human resources, and (4) lack of financial resources to support the use of appropriate technology. These features, discussed below, threaten programs' long-term survival and success.

Founding by visionaries. CBHC programs are usually started by people with a vision of something different from the norm. As the former CEO of Pepsi and Apple Computer, John Sculley, stated: "The future belongs to those who see possibilities before they become obvious" (quoted in Maxwell 1999, 148). CBHC programs are often started by someone, or a small group (like the Aroles), who is dedicated to turning a dream into a reality (see chapter 3). However, visionaries, while setting into motion the operationalizing of a new structure or way of doing things, often have problems with generating sufficient resources to expand the vision or program. After launching a program and making it work, the visionary leader must eventually pass on to others the management and marshalling of resources. The program also becomes too large for one person to adequately manage. A CBHC program started by one person often requires another person or group of people to manage its growth and take it to the next level.

Resources from many small sources. The experience of CBHC programs in both developing- and developed-country settings is that the financial resources needed for not only start-up but also continued operation and expansion require the cobbling together of multiple sources of funds, most of them small relative to the total need. These funds often cover only short periods and the program has to reapply for grants every one to three years. Much of the time of managers is devoted to evaluations and grant renewal applications, often at the expense of program activities. It is common for community-based programs, even those with a demonstrable impact on the target population, to go out of existence because their grant is terminated. A foundation may choose to fund another agency, even one carrying out a very similar program with the same target population, to "diversify its grant recipients." There may be little concern about the cost of starting up a new operation or about the monetary and social costs of closing down an existing program.

For example, the PACT Project, a community program in metropolitan Boston, has been important and successful in providing health and social services to HIV/AIDS patients in poor communities. (See chapter 14.) Yet its survival is threatened because there is no sustainable funding stream. A former staff member recently articulated her frustration with the resulting situation: "They put us in a position in which, instead of doing our work, we are worrying about money. It takes so much time to look for money and it's so frustrating" (Contreras 2001). This situation is common and poses real sustainability problems, since a program must have an adequate and reliable source of funding to be sustainable.

Insufficient human resources. A CBHC program uses various workers, often volunteers as well as regular staff. Employing volunteers may make it difficult to have an adequate and reliable source of human resources. This reliance on volunteers may mean there are not always appropriate workers for a task. Those who volunteer from poor communities and live at the limits of subsistence cannot afford to volunteer many hours. In Indonesia, for instance, village volunteers in *posyandus* (health posts) are asked to give only one or two days per month, to ensure that they are not overburdened.

Lack of appropriate technology. Most CBHC programs seek to use the most appropriate and affordable technology, rather than technology that is more sophisticated than that needed (but is often used) for the services or programs offered. In many instances, however, lack of financial resources and other constraints may mean that the most appropriate, or even sufficient, technology may be too costly for the program. For example, optimal drug requirements for tuberculosis often exceed communities' resources, even when people are willing to pay for them. Outside resources are essential to achieve public health control of TB in this situation. Vaccines and family planning supplies are also often considered a legitimate cost to governments or donors to support CBHC.

Three differences between sustainable CBHC programs in the United States and developing countries are (1) their origin as public-

or private-sector initiatives, (2) their initial funding source, and (3) their approach to financial sustainability.

Public- or private-sector origin of CBHC. Developing-country CBHC programs often start with encouragement from the public sector and international donors. They seek community input and usually wish to shift the CBHC program from the public to the private sector over time. The public sector is involved initially because essential public health services are considered governments' responsibility. For example, the Basic Minimum Needs approach of Thailand in the 1980s, which included health care, was an initiative of the government to involve communities in their own development and well-being. The government understands that CBHC has a role to play in extending the activities of the health sector in developing countries. It often sees that CBHC can mobilize material and human resources in rural communities, which the formal health system has difficulty in reaching. Hence, public-sector encouragement and involvement in starting CBHC in developing countries is a means for increasing access in the long term through means other than the public-sector health system. By contrast, in the United States, most CBHC programs start as private endeavors. Because they have to assemble grants from foundations and government agencies, they tend to attempt to move into the public sector to guarantee a regular source of resources for their programs.

Initial funding source. CBHC programs in developing countries often receive their initial funds from a single source, often an international donor. In the United States, CBHC programs seek their initial funds from private sources. They may also seek government funding by applying for grants. Since government grants and contracts are usually competitive, these funds cannot be considered regular and will not provide 100% of the programs' funding. Hence, there is the need to cobble together many sources of money and develop staff (specialists in finance, human resources, contracts, proposal management, writing, and editing, as well as support staff) who are expert in developing and producing proposals.

Approach to financial sustainability. In developing countries, the idea of financial sustainability is that most of the finances for the CBHC will eventually come from the community itself or the users of the services or both. The concept of financial sustainability in the

United States is very different from the understanding of sustainability in developing countries. In the United States, there are very few instances in which user fees are charged for services for low-income populations, particularly in community-based programs. These services are covered through government-funded insurance programs, such as Medicaid, special government grants and contracts, and grants from private foundations associated with corporations or wealthy individual benefactors.

Private foundations in the United States believe that sustainability implies a shift to the government sector. Foundations will support a project for a limited time, with the expectation that the project will eventually be included in a local, state, or national government budget. This conviction often leads private foundations to support lobbying by community-based organizations to fund their programs through government budgets. While this approach should also apply in poor countries, their government budgets are generally reserved for government-run services, leaving NGOs to seek sustainable financing from fees and donations for CBHC. This leads to the paradox of the rural poor receiving the least help from government while urban dwellers have access to more costly and sophisticated government-funded services.

CHALLENGES FOR THE SUSTAINABILITY OF CBHC MODELS IN THE FUTURE

Several challenges face CBHC programs seeking to become sustainable: (1) going to scale, (2) integrating CBHC services, (3) training, supervising, and motivating personnel, (4) generating financial resources, (5) managing resources wisely, (6) setting up monitoring and evaluation systems, (7) managing the growth of services, and (8) finding and nurturing effective leaders.

Going to scale. The objective of most CBHC programs is to cover the population they have targeted for the services they provide. After that objective has been achieved, the programs may plan to expand their scale at that location or to offer services in additional locations. An example is PROSALUD, begun in 1985 as a public-private partnership to establish and operate primary health care services in Bolivia. It has evolved through the collaboration of the public and private sectors to respond to the unmet needs of Bolivia's low-income populations, and it enjoys the active participation of the communities it serves. Today it is a nonprofit organization that manages an innovative network of high-quality, low-cost, client-focused services. Since 1985, it has grown from 2 health centers to 33, which employ more than 580 people and serve over half a million low- and lower-middle-income Bolivians, most of whom are underserved by public and private health services, in nine cities (Cuéllar, Newbrander, and Price 2000).

Integrating CBHC elements. The easiest way for CBHC to become established and obtain funding is to develop vertical programs that address one disease or health condition, especially one of concern to large donor agencies. Vertical programs rarely become independent. However, as the experience of the Bangladesh Rural Advancement Committee (BRAC) has demonstrated, even programs begun as vertical interventions can expand into a wider set of services that can meet an expanding array of community needs. These services may eventually provide the breadth of services and interventions needed by the community. This was the strategy behind James Grant's GOBI (growth monitoring, oral rehydration, breastfeeding, and immunization) initiative for UNICEF.

Sustaining human resources. The human resources of a community-based scheme are just as important as financial sustainability, if not more important. Human resource sustainability requires training, supervision, and motivation of staff and volunteers involved in the CBHC program. Without them and their continued growth and satisfaction, the community-based scheme will not be able to operate even if it has sufficient financial resources. BRAC has shown how continued staff development in skills and knowledge leads to sustainable health activities and an increasing array of services. Posyandus in Indonesia started as nutrition promotion activities, then after several years expanded to include family planning, immunization, and treatment of common ailments, adding one function every year or two. Some posyandus have even started monitoring chronic ailments of the aged, such as hypertension.

Generating financial resources. A CBHC program has to be creative in obtaining financial resources. It will need to combine different financing mechanisms. For example, it should consider the possibility of community financing, which is a local risk-sharing scheme in which the community manages health services while raising financial resources and promoting community responsibility and self-reliance. Such community financing or insurance schemes can provide a portion of the resources needed. The Dana Sehat (local health insurance) program in Indonesia has paid government PHC charges for the rural poor for three decades. Similar schemes have worked in Bangladesh (Gonoshasthaya Kendra) and Bolivia (PROSALUD).

In other cases, community financing may involve targeted user fees. But if a program chooses to use such fees, managers should consider the following principles in establishing them:

- Services should be provided to community members based on need, not ability to pay.
- There should be equity in both the receipt of services and the burden of financing them.
- User fees should not be the only source of revenues for the program.
- People should not have to sacrifice meeting other basic needs to pay for PHC services.
- The quality of services must be the same for all, whether they paid for the services or not.

Another means of encouraging certain services for which fees are charged is cross-subsidization. This financing mechanism involves collecting a fee that, although affordable, is greater than the actual costs for certain services for which there is high demand. Then the excess revenue is used to subsidize the costs of necessary services whose actual costs would make them unaffordable for most members of the community.

Managing resources wisely. Community-based programs can offer comprehensive services without an extravagant amount of financial resources. But to do so they must make the best use of their existing resources. This requires properly allocating those resources and then making the most productive use of them for the purposes for which they were allocated—that is, being efficient. Efficiency depends on good management practices. Efficiency gains mean that a CBHC program can provide more services, or services to more people, for the same amount of financial and human resources. For example, in Haiti the Hôpital Albert Schweitzer found that it was less expensive to provide tetanus toxoid to all women than to manage the consequences of tetanus forever (see chapter 7). In urban India, hospitals in the Baby Friendly Hospital Initiative changed their policies to encourage breast-feeding and then maintained it at no ongoing cost. In reality, it saved the cost of formula, even for the hospitals. Oral rehydration of diarrhea cases, developed in Bangladesh and popularized in every household throughout the country by BRAC, is a campaign that cost $25 million over 12 years. But it saves its entire cost in hospitalization (including IV fluids) every year, as well as saving lives.

Measuring the effectiveness of the system. A CBHC program requires a continuous monitoring and evaluation system so its manager can track the resources being used and their impact, and identify new priorities. As part of effective management and stewardship of community resources, CBHC programs also need adequate information systems so they know whether these resources are improving the well-being of the community. Such a system allows the program to ascertain the cost-effectiveness of various interventions or services when there are different options.

Expanding services incrementally. The CBHC program will seek to expand its services to provide a comprehensive package of services that meet the needs of the community. This package must be balanced with the resources available if it is to be sustainable. Hence it is important that program managers not make promises they cannot keep about the services the program will provide when it begins or as it expands. This will help ensure that costs do not outstrip revenue growth. One strategy is to keep costs and expectations reasonable from the start and add services only as they can be paid for. In the beginning, it is useful for the CBHC program to pick interventions it can afford and which have a high probability of success. For instance, choose an intervention such as the eradication of a disease like guinea worm, which has been eliminated in India and Pakistan, or like BRAC, finish teaching everyone how to manage diarrhea at home.

Finding effective leaders. Community-based schemes require leaders who not only have a vision of where the CBHC program is going but who are also committed to the principle of equity for the members of the community. The leader is needed to galvanize the human and financial resources to move the organization forward but must be flexible enough to share power and eventually vest it in other leaders.

While many governments seek alternative sources of revenue for health services, the ultimate responsibility, especially for promotive and preventive activities affecting the entire population, belongs with government. One of the greatest limitations of community-financed health services lies in their inability to bring about greater equity in health care. Simple fee-based payment systems can exacerbate existing inequities within communities, between communities, and between regions. While cost sharing by individuals and communities can reduce the financial burden on government, tax revenues are generally the most equitable source of funding. Governments must guarantee that receipt of health care is based on need rather than ability to pay. Responsibility for equitable access to health services, especially for the poorest, must not be relinquished in enthusiasm for privatization and the market economy. So even with widespread expansion of CBHC, there remains a major and significant role for the public sector in health care. Health for all remains a public good.

REFERENCES AND RESOURCES

Abel-Smith, B., and A. Dua. 1988. "Community-Financing in Developing Countries: The Potential for the Health Sector." *Health Policy and Planning* 3: 95–108.

Aubel, J., and K. Samba-Ndure. 1996. "Lessons on Sustainability for Community Health Projects." *World Health Forum* 17: 52–57.

Contreras, Maria. 2001. Telephone conversation with Gail Price. W. Roxbury, MA.

Creese, A., and S. Bennet. 1997. "Rural Risk-Sharing Strategies." World Bank Discussion Paper No. 365. Washington, DC: World Bank.

Cuéllar, Carlos, William Newbrander, and Gail Price. 2000. *Extending Access to Health Care through Public-Private Partnerships: The PROSALUD Experience.* Boston: Management Sciences for Health.

Konradsen, F., et al. 2000. "A Village Treatment Center for Malaria: Community Response in Sri Lanka." *Social Science and Medicine* 50: 879–89.

MacIntyre, K., and D. Hotchkiss. 1999. "Referral Revisited: Community

Financing Schemes and Emergency Transport in Rural Africa." *Social Science and Medicine* 49: 1473–87.

Maxwell, John C. 1999. *The 21 Indispensable Qualities of a Leader.* Nashville, TN: Thomas Nelson Publishers.

Mburu, F. 1989. "Whither Community-Based Health Care?" *Social Science and Medicine* 28: 1073–79.

Moskalewicz, J., and G. Swlatkiewicz. 2000. "Malczyee, Poland: A Multifaceted Community Action Project in Eastern Europe in a Time of Rapid Economic Change." *Substance Use and Misuse* 35: 189–202.

Preker, A., et al. 2001. "A Synthesis Report on the Role of Communities in Resource Mobilization and Risk Sharing." CMH Paper Series, Paper No. WG3:4. Geneva: Commission on Macroeconomics and Health.

Shediac-Rizkallah, M., and L. Bone. 1998. "Planning for the Sustainability of Community-Based Health Programs: Conceptual Frameworks and Future Directions for Research, Practice and Policy." *Health Education Research: Theory and Practice* 13: 87–108.

Zakus, J., and C. Lysack. 1998. "Revisiting Community Participation." *Health Policy and Planning* 13: 1–12.

PART II

EXPERIENCES IN DEVELOPED COUNTRIES

Introduction to Part II

Hugh S. Fulmer and Anthony I. Adams

This book focuses on developing partnerships between medical and public health services, and the communities they serve, to define and solve community health problems. Such partnerships are by no means new, but because of the way in which they have evolved in many parts of the world, they have come to be known by a range of often confusing names. Early efforts to integrate community medicine, public health, and community-oriented primary care (COPC)—and what would fall under the definition of community-based health care—into public policy in both rich and poor countries have borne fruit. However, to reorient medical and public health service institutions, organizations, and agencies to have them view communities as they would individual patients, as fully involved in their own health, a nationwide and global revolution is needed. That revolution would insist that all health workers—physicians, nurses, public health professionals, paramedical specialists—be trained at all levels (undergraduate, graduate, continuing education) through practical experience in the community. The practicum, also called service learning, is a combination of course work and practical, community-based experience guided by academic and field faculty. This concept is hardly revolutionary, since clinicians have always been trained thus in relation to the individual patient.

The community health care movement had several beginnings, ranging from the early work of Sidney Kark (1981) in South Africa and the Arizona-based Navajo-Cornell Field Health Research project (McDermott 1960, Deuschle 1982) in the 1950s, to the innovative domestic and international clerkships at the University of Kentucky in the 1960s (Deuschle and Fulmer 1962, Fulmer, Adams, and Deuschle 1963, Adams 1964, Fulmer 1964, Adams 1965). Many of the graduates from these clerkships have attained very senior positions influencing public health, and all would credit their community experience as the critical influence on their career choice.

A World Health Organization document entitled "The Use of Health Service Facilities in Medical Education" (Deuschle et al. 1967) describes these efforts to integrate community medicine and community-based health care into medical education. The authors achieved a consensus of domestic and international proponents of these similar approaches to education within the broad community-based health care concept. The principles of community-based health care and professional training hold equally well in developed and developing nations.

Yet the need for the community itself to play a role in designing its own services awaited the Alma-Ata conference in 1978. There, the world's attention was drawn to the need to regard communities as important social entities with unique health problems and service needs, both preventive and curative. This deepened understanding of the community's role was followed by a gradual realization that involving the community at all stages of designing, delivering, and evaluating health services could expedite solving community health problems. This is the only environment in which students can learn and assimilate the team approach.

Lashof and Schauffler describe (chapter 11) some of the most important developments in the evolution of community health centers and COPC practice in the United States and bring us up to the contemporary Healthy Communities and "future of public health" movements. They review the principles of COPC, contrasting it with "primary care," and identify key tools of public policy, giving examples of their use. Large hospital-based organizations have learned the necessity of a community-oriented approach, often as a result of well-developed information systems that reveal the social and behavioral determinants of the illness eventually treated in hospitals. The Mayo Clinic (chapter 12) well illustrates the effective marriage of specialized hospital care and community action through a well-developed health information system allowing the study of the natural history of health and disease. Boumbulian and his coauthors (chapter 13) describe how a major public hospital complex, after establishing community health centers, progressed to the formation of community-based HMOs, which can effectively integrate the COPC approach. Their treatment of financing complexities demonstrates the myriad considerations required to make an economically viable, equitable health system that is responsive to the community.

Chapter 14 shows how a case management approach in Boston supports provision of HIV/AIDS services to poor populations that would otherwise fall through the cracks. By working individually with HIV-positive clients, case managers help them to learn about their own health and connect with the resources they need to stay healthy. The viability of such community-based care depends on grant funding, making such innovative and responsive efforts highly vulnerable.

Keck (chapter 15), after summarizing the substantial advances made by the public health system in the United States since the 1988 Institute of Medicine *Future of Public Health* report, demonstrates how an urban health department, in partnership with academic medical centers, can become involved in exciting teaching endeavors in training community-responsive health care professionals. The benefits of such partnerships are mutual, because they provide a teaching and research environment for students while stimulating the innovative and responsive service linkages and problem-solving approaches that communities need.

The same principles can be applied in rural settings. Pearson and Taylor (chapter 16) describe how a remarkable statewide initiative in West Virginia, where leadership emanated from a publicly funded academic health center, grew to include state government, public health, medicine, and community members. This initiative has culminated in a statewide network of clinics supported by academic services providing specialty care designed to meet the commonly defined objectives of *West Virginia Healthy People 2010.*

In chapter 17, Pörksen shows how Germany has moved to a community approach to mental health, reducing both the costs and the stigma associated with mental illness. An array of services has been established, reaching far into the community and emphasizing home care for the ill, and mental wellness.

Much has been written in recent years on the concept of "community orientation" as it applies to the training of health professionals and the delivery of health care (Cashman et al. 1999, Fulmer 1999, Rhyne et al. 1998, Cashman, Bushnell, and Fulmer 2001, Klevens et al. 1992, Thomas, Cashman, and Fulmer 1995). Health services, and thus health status, can be improved if communities are intimately involved in the assessment of community health problems, the development of interventions, and the evaluation of the effectiveness of those interventions.

Some of the most dramatic examples of how successful this approach can be in practice are found in the management of the HIV/AIDS pandemic in different parts of the world. In Thailand, the involvement of the sex worker community helped avert a potential disaster for that country, while in Australia the early involvement of the gay community, the sex workers' union, and the intravenous drug-using community were critical in preventing the spread of HIV into the latter two groups and in effecting a decline in incidence of new infections in the gay community.

A big challenge put forward by this book is how to bring the training of public health and family physicians, nurses, and health workers of all kinds into line with the new approach to delivering community-based health care. In the public health arena, it has for too long been assumed that a master's of public health degree on its own is sufficient, without—for public health physicians—a traditional residency in preventive medicine. While an MPH is essential theoretical grounding, there can be no substitute for practical experience, dedicated supervision, and mentorship. This process can take place in countless settings: health centers, health departments, community-oriented hospitals, NGOs, academic departments of public health or family practice, international aid agencies, and the community itself; the principles are universal although their implementation must be locally relevant. For example, the Harvard School of Public Health, with the global deployment of its graduates through the years, could offer a worldwide practicum with these alumni serving as field faculty, acting as mentors for the new graduates in community-based practicum experiences after they complete their MPH (or other advanced) degrees. If physicians, they could complete preventive medicine training; if nurses or other health professionals, team-training experiences with physicians could lead to new accreditation credentials for each of the disciplines.

In Boston, the 13-year-old Center for Community Responsive Care (CCRC) program, continuing the evolution of its Navajo-Cornell and Kentucky antecedents, has trained over 70 multidisciplinary health professionals, using the one- or two-year preventive medicine residency as a training model, to learn how to work with communities in partnership to identify and address community health problems. Communities, in defining themselves, learn to identify their own resources and strengths and how to evolve toward ownership of the medical/public health system serving them; and the health care system (both medicine and public health), through the catalytic action of its team-trained health professionals, learns how to become responsive to community needs and priorities in health (Cashman, Bushnell, and Fulmer 2001, Klevens et al. 1992, Thomas, Cashman, and Fulmer 1995). Notable examples of transformation processes of this kind that the CCRC training program induced in the late 1980s and early 1990s include the Codman Square, Bowdoin St., and South Boston Community Health Centers (Klevens et al. 1992, Thomas, Cashman, and Fulmer 1995). These sites now offer community-oriented medical education programs that include undergraduate and graduate practicums involving all three Boston-based medical schools and their schools of public health, nursing, and social work.

Yet these changes toward ownership by the community are evolutionary: they have not "arrived." Paul Farmer, in describing Partners in Health's work with community health programs in Boston (chapter 14), indicates that the "bottom-up" approach from the community is essential for the partnership with medicine and public health to become effective in meeting community needs. "Top-down" inducements are insufficient. Recognizing this reality, community health programs affiliated with Partners in Health have partnered with CCRC in providing training at the undergraduate, graduate, and continuing education levels to bring medicine, public health, and the community together to improve community health, combining bottom-up and top-down approaches. Such efforts are essential if the future leaders of community-based health projects are to fully assimilate community members, ownership, and control into the fabric of community-based health care. We hope this book will provide the long-needed impetus for a great expansion of the concept not only in the United States but also around the world.

REFERENCES

Adams, Anthony I. 1964. "Kentucky Medical Students Abroad." *Journal of the Kentucky Medical Association* 62: 378.

————. 1965. "Teaching International Community Medicine." *Archives of Environmental Health* 10: 95.

Cashman, S. B., F. K. L. Bushnell, and Hugh S. Fulmer. 2001. "Community-Oriented Primary Care: A Model for Public Health Nursing." *Journal of Health Politics, Policy and Law* 26: 617–34.

Cashman, S. B., et al. 1999. "Carrying out the Medicine/Public Health Initiative: The Roles of Preventive Medicine and Community Responsive Care." *Academic Medicine* 74: 473–83.

Deuschle, K. 1982. "Community-Oriented Primary Care: Lessons Learned in Three Decades." *Journal of Community Health* 8: 13–22.

Deuschle, K., and Hugh Fulmer. 1962. "Community Medicine: A New Department at the University of Kentucky." *Journal of Medical Education* 37: 434–45.

Deuschle, K., et al. 1967. "The Use of Health Service Facilities in Medical Education." WHO Technical Report Series. Geneva: World Health Organization.

Fulmer, Hugh S. 1964. "Teaching Community Medicine in Kentucky." *Harvard School of Public Health Alumni Bulletin* 21: 2–6.

————. 1999. "Community-Oriented Primary Care: An Approach to Health Care for the 21st Century." *CommonHealth* 7: 10–12.

Fulmer, Hugh S., Anthony I. Adams, and K. W. Deuschle. 1963. "Medical Student Training in International Cross Cultural Medicine." *Journal of Medical Education* 38: 920.

Kark, Sidney L. 1981. *The Practice of Community-Oriented Primary Care.* New York: Appleton-Century-Crofts.

Klevens, M., et al. 1992. "Transforming a Neighborhood Health Center into a Community-Oriented Primary Care Practice." *American Journal of Preventive Medicine* 8: 62–65.

McDermott, W. 1960. "Introducing Modern Medicine in a Navajo Community." *Science* 131: 197–205 and 280–87.

Rhyne, R., et al. 1998. "Community Oriented Primary Care: Health Care for
the 21st Century." Washington, DC: American Public Health Association.

Thomas, C., S. Cashman, and Hugh Fulmer. 1995. "The Cluster Committee:
Setting the Stage for Community-Responsive Care." *American Journal of
Preventive Medicine* 11 (Pt. 1): 9–18.

11 The Evolution of Community Health Centers and Community-Oriented Primary Care

Joyce C. Lashof and Helen H. Schauffler

"Community-oriented primary care," a term used in the United States, is in many ways synonymous with primary health care, as it is used in international health circles. Both address the social, economic, and environmental factors underlying ill health, both emphasize health promotion and disease prevention, and both promote the use of community-based, multisectoral approaches to improving health. Community health centers (CHCs) in the United States have historically tried to add these broader elements to the clinical medicine practiced at these institutions. This has become more challenging as market forces incline the CHCs to turn away from services that fall outside the more narrowly defined clinical medicine.

—Gail Price

This chapter reviews the development of community-oriented primary care (COPC) in the United States. It also presents some of the current trends in both public health and medical care that offer new opportunities to further the practice of COPC.

The term community-oriented primary care, first used by Sidney Kark, was based on his experiences as a primary care physician in South Africa in the 1950s. His assignment was to set up a clinic in a rural area that had no health facilities. First he mapped where the members of his community lived; then he assessed what the prevalent health problems of the community were. Rather than developing interventions independently of the community, he involved community members in setting priorities and enlisted their support in designing specific health programs. It was this model that the early developers of the neighborhood health center movement drew upon in the 1960s. When President Johnson declared his War on Poverty and set up the Office of Economic Opportunity to combat joblessness, lack of adequate housing, and lack of educational opportunities, he also sought new ways to bring health care services to underserved communities. The model that was instituted by Drs. Geiger and Gibson, first at Mound Bayou, Mississippi, and Columbia Point in Boston, and then replicated in New York, Chicago, and Denver, established a neighborhood health center that included the community in its governance. The centers were designed to be more than a place to deliver primary care. They were looked to as social institutions that would address the socioeconomic and environmental problems that were important in determining the health of the community.

For example, the Mile Square Health Center in Chicago, which served a population of 25,000 people living in an area of one square mile, engaged in extensive outreach services to the community using community health aides, public health nurses, and community mental health workers, and a community organization that served as the center's board. Community activities ranged from consultation with the elementary schools to public health nursing visits to the housing projects; from dealing with housing violations to marching to obtain a traffic light at a dangerous intersection. In Mound Bayou, Mississippi, the center took the lead in helping the community develop a farming cooperative and build latrines, and center physicians prescribed food for the malnourished.

The success of these initial centers in bringing culturally sensitive, community-based, and accessible services to previously underserved populations led to the rapid expansion of the Neighborhood Health Center Program and its eventual transfer to the Public Health Service. Initially funded by the Office of Economic Opportunity, the centers were renamed Community Health Centers (CHCs) and came under increasing pressure to become self-sufficient through Medicaid, Medicare, and sliding scale fees. Today, although economic pressures have reduced the array of services and outreach activities, some 670 CHCs serve over 8 million people and continue to provide primary care services. These services are combined with a somewhat more limited public health approach, which continues to offer some "wraparound" services such as translation and social services. Although community boards remain a critical component of CHCs, their responsibility for a defined community is much less clear than it was in the earlier neighborhood health centers. Detailed studies demonstrating the effectiveness of CHCs in improving access to care, reducing infant mortality rates, preventing rheumatic fever, improving the detection of hypertension, and reducing hospitalization rates were published in the late 1960s and in the 1970–80 decade (Geiger 1983, 78–79).

In 1982, the Institute of Medicine sponsored a conference to explore the applicability of COPC to the health care system as a whole. At that conference, Dr. Geiger suggested that COPC is a synthesis in which "all [these] elements of community orientation, demographic study, epidemiologic investigation, personal medical services, environmental intervention, community organization and health education [should] be performed by the same practice or team, or at least by a small number of practices and health agencies acting as a single system (not just coordinated)"(Geiger 1983, 70). Mullan characterized COPC as the reunion of public health and personal clinical health services (Mullan 1987, 29). After this conference, the Institute of Medicine undertook a yearlong study to more thoroughly examine the essential elements and organizational aspects of COPC. Their report, issued in 1984, distinguished COPC from traditional primary care in five ways:

1. COPC is *population based,* defining its community as both active users and nonusers of the clinic, while primary care views patients as individuals.
2. COPC *uses epidemiologic methods* to determine the health needs of the larger community, whereas primary care is case oriented.
3. COPC *includes intervention strategies that address both individual cases and the population at large;* planning for primary care is primarily concerned with utilization.
4. *Service providers play multiple roles* in COPC, whereas primary care is designed to use professional specialties.
5. *Community involvement* in clinic planning and implementation is also an essential ingredient of COPC, which enables the clinic staff to become familiar with community structures and resources that are essential for undertaking broader health promotion and disease prevention initiatives (Institute of Medicine 1984, 1).

The IOM study also developed an operational model of COPC to help centers evaluate themselves and to serve as a model for development of new centers. This model of a primary care practice serving a defined population contains four elements:

1. definition and characterization of the community;
2. identification of the community's health problems;
3. modification of the health care program in response to the community health needs;
4. monitoring of the impact of program modifications.

More simply, COPC represents the integration of public health and primary care with the goal of improving the health status of a community. It emphasizes health promotion and disease prevention in addition to treatment of illness.

Our knowledge of the multifactorial nature of the major killers today reinforces the need for such an approach. A panel of experts assembled at the Carter Center in 1984 examined the 13 leading health problems in the United States. They estimated that 66% of the deaths under the age of 65 that occurred in 1980 could have been postponed if all the social, environmental, and behavioral factors leading to death and disability were effectively controlled.

McGinnis and Foege (1993) looked at some of the underlying causes of death and quantified the major external, nongenetic factors that contribute to death. They developed a list of the 10 leading causes of death and estimated the number due to each cause:

- *smoking* contributes to cancer, heart disease, pulmonary disease, low birthweight, and burns;
- *poor diet and inactivity* contribute to cardiovascular disease, including stroke and high blood pressure; Doll and Peto (1981) estimated that at least 35% of all cancer deaths can be attributed to diet, and approximately half of all Type II diabetes is estimated to be preventable by obesity control;
- *alcohol* underlies 60–90% of cirrhosis deaths, 40–50% of motor vehicle fatalities, 16–67% of home injuries, fire fatalities, and job injuries;
- *microbial agents* are an important cause of death, although they are no longer the threat they were. (This category excludes deaths due to HIV or attributed to alcohol, tobacco, sexual behavior, or use of illegal drugs.) A significant percentage of these deaths are preventable;
- *toxic agents,* including occupational hazards, environmental pollutants, contaminants of food and water supply, and occupational exposures, have been linked to 4–10% of cancer deaths, and 1–3% of cardiovascular and pulmonary deaths;
- *firearms* pose a unique problem in this country for young males, whose homicide rates are 12 to 273 times those in other industrialized countries. In 1986, there were 1,043 homicides among males age 15–19, compared with 6 in Canada and 2 in Japan. Homicides now account for 41% of deaths among black males age 15–19;

- *unprotected sexual intercourse* is associated with excess infant mortality rates among those whose pregnancies were unintended, sexually acquired hepatitis B, and HIV;
- *motor vehicle accidents* result in deaths that could be prevented by seat belts, air bags, and bicycle helmets;
- *illicit drugs* implicated in deaths include those reported to the vital statistics system as drug related as well as those from drug-related HIV infection, automobile injuries, and hepatitis infection.

It is important to recognize that to have an impact on these causes of death we will need to look at a broader array of interventions than that offered by traditional medical care.

Building on these and other data related to social determinants of health, the Public Health Service (2000, 18) in *Healthy People 2010* cited individual behavior and environmental factors, both social and physical, as being responsible for 70% of all premature deaths in the US. The PHS also highlighted the marked disparity in health status between racial and ethnic groups and noted the importance of socioeconomic status and the impact of social environment on health in setting the goal of healthy people in healthy communities.

The Codman Research Group and the United Hospital Fund of New York analyzed hospitalization rates for a series of conditions, including hypertension, cardiac failure, acute asthma, and uncontrolled diabetes, in which early diagnosis and treatment could have prevented hospitalization (Institute of Medicine 1993, 105). A review of these diagnoses suggests not only that early diagnosis and treatment would have prevented the majority of such admissions but also that many of these conditions are the result of modifiable social and environmental factors. Data on hospital admissions for relatively controllable chronic conditions reveals a similar pattern of marked discrepancy between low- and high-income neighborhoods (Institute of Medicine 1993, 13). A COPC practice clearly provides the opportunity to address such issues through provision of comprehensive primary care, careful program monitoring, and outreach activities.

To address the underlying causes of premature death and preventable morbidity, we need to go far beyond the clinical and individual approach. A growing body of literature over the past decade has broadened our understanding of the interrelated behavioral, social, economic, and environmental factors responsible for unnecessary morbidity and mortality. We have come to a recognition that if we are to have an impact on our major health problems we must not only direct a much larger share of our health care resources toward preventive strategies but also expand our vision of what we include in our prevention armamentarium.

Partners for Prevention has defined the essential elements of prevention as falling into three categories: clinical preventive services; community-based health promotion and disease prevention; and public policy for health promotion and disease prevention. An elaboration of this approach was presented in "Health Promotion and Disease Prevention in Health Care Reform."[1] This report discusses the actions that need to be taken to ensure that each of these areas are addressed.

Clinical preventive services are, of course, an essential element of primary care. The US Preventive Services Task Force continues to review and recommend age-appropriate clinical preventive services, including screening, immunizations and counseling based on an evaluation of the effectiveness and cost-effectiveness of these procedures. A COPC practice needs to have a monitoring system to ensure that the age-appropriate clinical preventive services are provided to all members of the population for which they are responsible.

Community-based health promotion and disease prevention present a bigger challenge. The World Health Organization defines health promotion as "The process of enabling people to increase control over, and to improve their health. To reach a state of complete physical, mental and social well being an individual or group must be able to identify and to realize aspirations, to satisfy needs, and to change or cope with the environment"(WHO 1986). This definition requires that we go well beyond the health care system to identify the most effective way to create conditions conducive to health. To accomplish this requires developing partnerships with a broad array of community and social agencies, both governmental and nongovernmental, that can address the underlying conditions that we now know are so important in

---

1. The following section is adapted, with permission, from Helen Schauffler, "Health Promotion and Disease Prevention in Health Care Reform," *American Journal of Preventive Medicine* (1994) 10: 1–31.

determining health status. Effective community-based programs require assessment of community health problems, priority-setting, and collaborative planning. Health departments have the responsibility for collecting epidemiologic data not only on morbidity and mortality but also on the prevalence of risk factors, and for monitoring and evaluating community-based interventions. Public health agencies and COPC practices can play a key role in bringing together the community and voluntary and governmental agencies to set priorities and develop effective interventions. Community-based interventions include such diverse activities as school curricula that include conflict resolution to decrease violence, outreach workers that can provide health education in the home as well as link patients with health care providers, parenting programs for teenage mothers, and antismoking campaigns in the community and in the schools.

The third element that must be part of a holistic approach to disease prevention is the public policy approach. Historically, this approach has been responsible for the major advances in health. The sanitary reform movement of the 1800s was responsible for the early decline in infectious diseases, and the social reform movements of the first half of the twentieth century were responsible for improved working conditions, housing laws, and child protection.

Certain principles must underlie the development of healthy public policy, which must be:

- developed with the understanding that the major determinants of health are behavioral and environmental, including not just the physical environment but the social, cultural, and economic environment. Poverty remains the single most important predictor of health status.
- consistent with national goals, such as those set out in *Healthy People 2010,* "Objectives for Improving Health";
- population-based and grounded in research (there should be more emphasis on epidemiologic research concentrating on underlying causes);
- equitable: designed to reduce disparities in health and recognize the needs of special population groups;
- fair in distributing the burden of responsibility for implementing or paying for a policy and respectful of individual liberty.

A number of policy tools are available and multiple tools appropriate to the specific problem need to be utilized. These tools include:

- *participatory decision-making:* The public must be actively engaged in understanding the factors that are important in their community and developing appropriate policies;
- *public education:* This is essential and must involve all avenues (e.g., schools, media) and be clear, targeted, culturally sensitive, and linguistically appropriate;
- *incentives to promote healthy behavior:* These are difficult to develop and often controversial, but one successful example is providing infant car seats or other infant products to women completing prenatal care;
- *taxation:* The most successful example, of course, is the cigarette tax, which has its greatest impact on decreasing smoking in young people. Many other tax policies to influence behavior can be used;
- *regulation:* This relates to the advertising, sale, and use of various products as well as development and enforcement of environmental standards.

All three approaches—clinical preventive services, community-based health promotion, and public policy—can work together to attack some of our major health problems, for example, smoking. Clinical approaches include counseling by a physician and use of nicotine replacement therapy and other drugs approved by the FDA to treat tobacco dependence. Community-based approaches are school education, making smoking socially unacceptable, and antismoking campaigns such as the Great American Smokeout. Public policy interventions encompass warning labels, taxation, limitations on advertising, restriction of sales to minors, bans on smoking in public places, and antismoking ads.

Similarly, teen pregnancies can be prevented using a combination of approaches: clinical (contraception provided by private physicians, schools, and community clinics), community based (health education, teen social programs, and social support groups), and public policy (increase educational and job opportunities, provide positive role models, and use the media to provide information on contraception).

Nutrition can be addressed in the clinic via dietary advice and counseling or weight reduction clinics; in the community, via heart-healthy menus in restaurants, community gardens, and healthy school lunch programs; and through public policies related to food labels, limitation of advertising of junk food (especially that directed to children), provision of school breakfasts in low-income communities, food stamps, and the WIC program (the Supplemental Food Program for Women, Infants, and Children).

Many more examples of the three elements of prevention could be developed to illustrate ways to address each of the leading causes of death.

Today's health care climate offers opportunities to further the principles of COPC. Although there are many barriers to any single organization embracing all elements of both comprehensive primary care and public health, the potential for collaboration between communities, social and public health agencies, and medical care systems exists. HMOs are being held accountable for providing personal preventive services. The Centers for Disease Control and Prevention, in collaboration with the National Association of County and City Health Officials (NACCHO), has launched an initiative entitled Mobilizing for Action through Planning and Partnership (MAPP). Their recently released field guide (NACCHO 2001) calls for:

- mobilizing the community using a community-driven process;
- actions to access community resources and improve community health;
- collaborative planning, including strategic analysis and ensuring that 10 essential public health services are provided;
- inclusive and accountable partnerships.

The Healthy Communities movement, well described in a number of articles in a recent issue of *Public Health Reports* (2000), also focuses on the broad definition of health and the need to involve all aspects of community life. Much is happening in the private and public sectors that can give us hope that an integrated effort to implement COPC and improve the health of our communities will occur. Unfortunately, the increase in the uninsured, the rising costs of medical care, and the countervailing movement to compete rather than collaborate, to pursue profit, and to capture market share present major obstacles to accomplishing this, but sooner or later this is where we must be.

REFERENCES

Doll, R., and R. Peto. 1981. *The Causes of Cancer: Quantitative Estimates of Avoidable Risks of Cancer in the United States Today.* New York: Oxford University Press.

Geiger, H. Jack. 1983. "The Meaning of Community Oriented Primary Care in the American Context." In *Community Oriented Primary Care: New Directions for Health Services Delivery.* Washington, DC: National Academy Press.

Institute of Medicine. 1984. *Community Oriented Primary Care: A Practical Assessment. Report of a Study.* Washington, DC: National Academy Press.

———. 1993. Committee on Monitoring Access to Personal Health Care Services. *Access to Health Care in America.* Washington, DC: National Academy Press.

McGinnis, J. M., and W. H. Foege. 1993. "Actual Causes of Death in the United States." *Journal of the American Medical Association* 270: 2207–12.

Mullan, F. 1987. "COPC and the Challenge of Public Health." In "Community-Oriented Primary Care: From Principle to Practice." US Dept. of Health and Human Services, Health Resources and Services Administration APE86-1. Washington, DC: US Government Printing Office.

National Association of County and City Health Officials (NACCHO). 2001. *MAPP Field Guide.* Washington, DC: NACCHO. See also their Web site: www.naccho.org.

Public Health Reports. 2000. Special issue on Healthy Communities. Vol. 115, Nos. 2–3.

Schauffler, Helen. 1994. "Health Promotion and Disease Prevention in Health Care Reform." *American Journal of Preventive Medicine* 10: 1–31.

US Public Health Service. 2000. *Healthy People 2010: Understanding and Improving Health.* 2d ed. Washington, DC: US Government Printing Office.

World Health Organization. 1986. "Ottawa Charter for Health Promotion." International Conference on Health Promotion: The Move towards a New Public Health. Ottawa, Ontario, Canada: World Health Organization, Nov. 17–21.

12 The Mayo Clinic's Origins and Contemporary Status as a Community-Based Health Care Model

Philip T. Hagen, Joan M. Altekruse, and Robert R. Orford

Although it is one of the most prestigious academic medical centers in the world, the Mayo Clinic has had, since its founding, a strong commitment to its local community. An early data system allowed the Clinic to collect population-based data from the community. These data were (and are) used to establish local priorities for public health and to develop community-based programs that corresponded to these priorities. The residency in preventive medicine elevated the status of population- and community-based health care, which in many other settings is seen as a lower-priority medical specialty. The tradition of community focus and the blending of population-based care, training, and research with individual patient care have helped the Mayo Clinic maintain a community-based health care model for the residents of Olmsted County, Minnesota.

—Gail Price

A comparison of the history of the Mayo Clinic in Rochester, Minnesota, and that of start-up community-based health care (CBHC) centers, particularly those in developing countries, reveals clear similarities. Resemblances are noted in both the mission and operation of the Mayo Clinic, both in the past and today. The Mayo Clinic has provided and continues to provide care responsive both to the health needs of individuals and of the community, Olmsted County, that surrounds it.

There are also differences between the Mayo story and CBHC programs. The scope of clinical procedures, the large number of staff, and the extensive research and educational programs at Mayo today contrast with the conventional image of a CBHC program. Yet the development of the Mayo Clinic demonstrates that community-oriented values and behaviors can survive in a large and complex academic medical center if it maintains principles and practices consistent with its founding mandate.

THE MAYO CLINIC'S MISSION

Community-oriented care was part of the vision of the founders of the Mayo Clinic, Drs. William J. and Charles H. Mayo. They advocated two complementary objectives:

1. to provide, through coordinated expertise, health care for a defined population;
2. to collect, interpret, and report data to measure community health status and to develop concomitant programs that respond to the priorities of those served.

Succinctly, the mission is to "Heal the Sick and Advance the Science."

A DISPERSED ORGANIZATIONAL STRUCTURE

Various standards have been devised to define CBHC activities (see chapters 11 and 15). Because of the size and diversity of the Mayo Clinic practice, the components of a CBHC program, while present, are not immediately visible. The CBHC is functionally embedded within the parent institution in discrete sites and programs, such as the Division of Preventive and Occupational Medicine. These sites and programs coordinate their efforts with those of partners in the community, such as the Olmsted County Health Department.

In addition to providing consultation, planning, and physician staff for the public health department, Mayo supports community action initiatives, coordinates volunteer care for the uninsured (including primary care and tertiary care), gathers comprehensive data on community health, and conducts research. Participatory teaching/learning programs are associated with each of these components. Because of the historical growth and development of the Mayo Clinic and the Olmsted County community, the Clinic and the community have a symbiotic relationship. The interreliance of the community and the academic health care system reinforces the incentive to develop new programs that benefit the community.

MEETING STANDARDS

Nevertheless, any particular example of CBHC in action must be held to and measured according to the conceptual framework that defines organizations in its category. The core components of CBHC programs are:

- **Purpose.** The central objective is to improve the health of a designated population and its members through access to essential health services encompassing both preventive and remedial care.
- **Defined community.** The participating population is specified by ecological, demographic, and epidemiologic characteristics, or other classifying factors.

- **Data-based formulation.** Community data are collected and analyzed to support planning, monitoring, and evaluation of the effectiveness of the program.
- **Community input into program design.** Community input and data describing morbidity, mortality, health behaviors, and management practices are used to determine needs, plan interventions, and measure impact and satisfaction.
- **Community partnerships.** Collaborative individual and institutional coalitions extend and/or complement community health programs. This includes collaborative activities in social services sectors, economic development, education, and recreation.
- **Evaluation.** Qualitative and quantitative measures of health status, user evaluations of programs, and suggested changes to respond to perceived needs are examined. Operational processes and efficacy in financial and technical performance, organization, service delivery, and, if pertinent, research projects, are evaluated and reports are produced.
- **Leadership education.** CBHC programs in academic health centers in particular must recognize the need for and support academic programs in medical schools and schools of public health to train staff and develop leaders with expertise in the care of communities.

HISTORICAL PERSPECTIVE

The origins of the Mayo Clinic are intriguingly similar to those of CBHC projects of more recent decades. The population focus and community bond at Mayo began with Dr. William Worrall Mayo, who began his medical training in Glasgow. When he moved to the United States, the country was embroiled in the Civil War. He was nevertheless able to complete his training, graduating from Indiana Medical College in 1850. Answering a call to examine military recruits, he was posted to southern Minnesota. He respected and accommodated local cultural standards and habits, and he quickly achieved successful social integration. He also recognized that medical care in the area was insufficient and opened a solo general medical practice in Rochester in

1864. In 1883, after a devastating tornado, the Sisters of St. Francis approached him with an offer to build and staff a hospital, if he would provide doctors for it. He accepted, and a 27-bed hospital, Saint Marys, was built to serve the community.

GROUP PRACTICE AND INDIVIDUAL PATIENT CARE POPULATIONS

Dr. W. W. Mayo and his sons, Drs. William J. and Charles H. Mayo, were blessed with energy, curiosity, and the professional habit of recording demographic and clinical observations. They traveled internationally, researching the best medical practices of the day, and they started the first multidisciplinary group practice in the world. An early innovation of this group was to combine multiple clinical specialties, laboratories, workshops, a library, editorial services, and a business office under one roof. As Dr. W. J. Mayo said, they believe in "uniting for the good of the patient."

In 1901, a young physician and innovator, Dr. Henry Plummer, joined the group practice. He recognized the importance of research based on clinical records. He developed a "unit record," which contained all inpatient and outpatient records of histories, examinations, and test results and findings for a patient. He also started a system of cross-tabulated lists of diagnoses, operations, physicians, and patients. By combining the unit records and cross-tabulated lists, he created the framework for detailed population-based epidemiologic studies of diseases in the community.

MERGING MEDICAL AND PUBLIC HEALTH ROLES

Formal links between the Mayo Clinic and the community were forged when Dr. Charles Mayo was asked to be the first public health officer for Olmsted County. This brought into focus the need to know what diseases affected the community and in what ways, and the necessity of understanding how best to meet those challenges. Dr. Joseph Berkson refined Mayo's data system in the 1930s to help address these two needs. His first innovation was a standardized nomenclature of disease, while the second was automated cataloging of data using keypunch cards.

In 1950, Dr. Leonard Kurland, a neurologist trained in public health, recognized the unique advantages of the Clinic's long history of interaction with the Olmsted County community:

- Defined, stable population
- Limited provider group (two medical practices)
- Good, established relationships with the community
- Longstanding diagnostic database
- Unit medical records
- Ability for longitudinal follow-up

In 1966, the Rochester Epidemiologic Project was started with funding from the National Institute of General Medical Sciences to study community trends in disease incidence.

COMMUNITY-BASED DISEASE PROFILES

Because Mayo's diagnostic records and pathology specimens dating back to the early 1900s were catalogued, it was relatively easy to study community trends in disease incidence, and the natural history of diseases. Through ongoing grant funding from the federal government, the Rochester Epidemiologic Project has evolved to embrace the rapid growth of the population in recent decades and the evolution of the unit record to an electronic medical record. A unique data-gathering tool called Patient Provided Information, developed by Philip Hagen and colleagues, has enabled the community database to combine data on patients' symptoms and behavior with the existing diagnostic and pathologic data. To date, more than 1,200 scientific papers have been published from the Rochester Epidemiologic Project. These articles include descriptive, case-control, and cohort studies on the epidemiology of stroke, transient ischemic attack, dementia, heart disease, cancer, Alzheimer's disease and other neurologic disorders, diabetes, digestive disease, osteoporosis, and arthritis. No other resource in the world exists for studying secular trends of these diseases over as many decades in such a clearly defined population. The comprehensive structure of the data has allowed on-demand queries to rapidly answer clinical questions such as whether breast implants cause rheumatologic disorders. Long-term studies have helped define the natural history and impact of treatments on prevalent high-impact conditions like osteoporosis.

DATA TRANSLATED INTO COMMUNITY ACTION

Disease and practice data are continuously used to improve the delivery of health services in the community. Mechanical innovations, such as pneumatic tubes to speed unit records around the medical center, evolved into motorized underground vehicles connecting clinics, hospitals, and laboratories, and supporting the efficient collection and distribution of medical data. With the advent of the electronic medical record, even greater efficiencies are being realized today. Specialized treatments have been developed, ranging from surgical procedures on patients with goiters (common in the community before iodized salt was introduced) to the development in 1950 of a potent new drug, cortisone, to treat rheumatoid arthritis. The health needs of the community have been recognized and population measures developed, ranging from sanitation in the 1930s to community-oriented reduction of cardiovascular disease in the 2000s through "CardioVision 2020."

EDUCATION AND TRAINING

The Mayo brothers established a tradition of practice, education, and research, which have come to be known as the three shields of Mayo. They established one of the first formal graduate training programs for physicians. The focus of much of this training has been highly specialized care. However, trainees also learn and provide care daily in the community in nursing homes, schools, Salvation Army clinics, and the county health department. Dr. Julie Abbott, a member of the Division of Preventive Medicine, continues the tradition of Dr. Charles Mayo, who served as the county health officer from 1912 to 1937. Preventive medicine fellows provide care in the community through home-based visits with county health nurses, sexually transmitted disease clinics, and immigrant clinics. In 2000, Dr. Abbott worked with Clinic and county data to create a "Community Health Report Card for Olmsted County." The Report Card uses the structure of the Healthy People

2010 goals to analyze and report on the health status of county residents, present information for policy development to improve the population's health, and provide benchmarks to measure progress.

Principles of population-based medicine have been taught and explored at Mayo through the work of Dr. Kurland and his colleagues in the Epidemiology Department. Although the blending of principles of population-based care and individual patient care was born of the Mayo brothers' devotion to the community, formal programs to teach these principles did not begin until Dr. Bruce E. Douglass began the Division of Preventive Medicine at Mayo Clinic in 1963. Now called the Division of Preventive and Occupational Medicine, it employs 20 physicians board certified in internal medicine, family medicine, preventive medicine, public health, aerospace medicine, and occupational medicine. Faculty have worked to define the qualities of specialists in population health and the skills necessary to care for a community and its members.

The early design of the Clinic as a collegial practice that integrates multiple specialties has been effectively applied to the training of specialists in prevention. Preventive medicine fellows rotate through diverse areas, for example:

- specialized medical areas, such as the Breast or Metabolic Bone Clinic and the Preventive Services Clinic;
- the Olmsted County Public Health Department;
- Detention Center clinics;
- treatment facilities for chemical dependency;
- the Health Information Division (where trainees learn how to effectively deliver health information to populations through print, media, and the Internet);
- the Continuous Improvement Office (which shares information about major initiatives and successes, and encourages engagement in continuous improvement activities).

The tradition of effective writing and communication was started at Mayo in 1907, when Maud Mellish (later Maud Mellish Wilson) was hired as librarian. She became the first editor in the Section of Publications. This section continues to support the publication of Mayo research studies. This tradition of communication to a professional audience has grown to encompass a full spectrum of communications to adults and children in the community.

ECONOMIC AND COMMUNITY INTERDEPENDENCE

For a practice to remain viable and support research and educational efforts, it must be financially sound. Mayo's business success was built on expertise from the community. Harry Harwick, who joined the Clinic from the Rochester business community in the early 1900s, designed a business office integrated into the Clinic practice. The financial stability and solidarity of the institution and the community remain tightly entwined. This interdependence is fostered by the fact that the Clinic is the largest single employer of Rochester citizens: the Clinic employs approximately 25% of the local workforce. The Clinic's presence has a positive impact not only on the health of community members but also on the health of the local economy, because many patients come from around the world to this relatively small community of 100,000 people.

The Mayo brothers created the nonprofit Foundation for Medical Education and Research before they retired so that there was no personal gain to individuals from clinical activities beyond their established salary limits and no financial gain to the Clinic beyond what is needed to sustain the practice. All revenues support foundation activities and thus are largely returned to the community.

PREPARING FUTURE PHYSICIAN-LEADERS FOR POPULATION MEDICINE

The preparation of medical personnel to become leaders for the future development of CBHC practice models is demanding, as is the process for entry into a medical specialty. The first requirement is a deep personal and professional commitment to community service. Medical professionals must attain a high order of technical skills in preventive medicine, public health, and population medicine, including an understanding of epidemiology, information sciences, institutional and program management, and sociology applied to communities. And future leaders must have experiential learning in CBHC, preferably with a mentor steeped in community health practice. In this way, trainees can assimilate the traits, perspectives, and skills associated with effective performance.

Although the original medical staff of the Mayo Clinic did not undergo this rigorous program in CBHC, they combined their talents and experience to create innovative programs in clinical medicine, education, and research. Today, the training program in preventive medicine produces residents well prepared to satisfy the credentials required by the American Board of Preventive Medicine. The Mayo Graduate School of Medicine will continue to prepare graduates who bring to their communities the principles expressed in the enduring Mayo mission of community-oriented care, and to extend this mission and practice through Mayo's other practices in Scottsdale, Arizona, and Jacksonville, Florida.

THE APPLICATION OF PRINCIPLES OF COMMUNITY-BASED HEALTH CARE

This book identifies strategies for enhancing interactions between communities and health care providers. Although many CBHC programs, international and domestic, use these strategies, their common applicability does not imply that normative practices are or should be prescribed. Instead, the intent is to respond to locally identified needs, using such methods as:

- engaging a competent staff committed to community-responsive care;
- ensuring patient and community participation in programming and coalition building;
- developing and implementing management objectives and practices designed for stability, but open to innovation;
- using local epidemiologic and demographic data for evaluation and programming;
- expanding best practices from successful experiences to other communities;
- preparing future leaders for the practice of population medicine.

Each of these principles has been and continues to be pursued by the Mayo Clinic, which continues in its visionary development of community-based and -oriented programs. Mayo offers a model that can be adapted and adopted by other academic health centers. As a validated approach to improving community health, it also warrants consideration as a model for the design of larger health care systems in the United States and elsewhere.

At the opening of the Mayo Medical School in 1972, the Founding Dean, Raymond D. Pruitt, articulated the mission of the new school. He remarked that the mission included dedication "to ... a revolution in academic spirit uniting faculty and students alike [who] cherish an imperative for the humane in an age made rich by technology and service." He called for "the yardstick of the humane" to measure the benefits of science. That imperative is apt for considering what CBHC models bring to the health of individuals and communities.

ACKNOWLEDGMENTS

The authors would like to acknowledge the assistance of Mr. Andrew Lucas of the History of Medicine Library (Mayo Foundation, Rochester), Dr. David R. Sanderson, Emeritus Staff (Mayo Clinic, Scottsdale), and Ms. Sara Howen, Division of Preventive Medicine (Mayo Clinic, Rochester).

RESOURCES

Braasch, William F. 1969. *Early Days in the Mayo Clinic.* Springfield, IL: C.C. Thomas.

Clapesattle, Helen. 1989. *The Doctors Mayo.* 3d ed. Rochester, MN: Mayo Foundation for Medical Education & Research.

Mayo Clinic & Foundation. 2001. Web sites: www.mayoclinic.com and www.mayo.edu.

Nagel, Gunther W. 1966. *The Mayo Legacy.* Springfield, IL: C.C. Thomas.

Nelson, Clark W. 1990. *Mayo Roots: Profiling the Origins of the Mayo Clinic.* Rochester, MN: Mayo Foundation.

Wilder, Lucy. 1941. *The Mayo Clinic.* 4th ed. New York: Harcourt, Brace.

13 Blending Community-Oriented Primary Care and Managed Care to Create Community-Based Health Solutions

Paul Boumbulian, S. Sue Pickens, Samuel Ross, and Ron J. Anderson

Involving community members in decision-making is essential in any successful community-based health care program, but there is too much diversity in any community for residents to speak with a unified voice. Only the stronger, more articulate voices typically influence decisions. Health care institutions must therefore determine how and from whom community input will be sought. It is important to differentiate between community control and community input. Institutions must be honest about whether there will be a real sharing of decision-making or simply an opportunity for communities to air their opinions, especially when the allocation of resources is involved. Sharing decision-making power is appropriate some but not all of the time. Parkland Memorial Hospital appears to have created community partnerships that are advantageous to community members, as evidenced by a significant increase in utilization of services.

—Gail Price

Parkland Memorial Hospital is one of the nation's largest and busiest public hospital and health systems. It has been serving the citizens of Dallas County for over 106 years and evolving to meet changing community needs. Since 1943, the distinguished faculty at the University of Texas Southwestern (UTSW) Medical Center at Dallas has provided house staff supervision and direct patient care at Parkland. Parkland has made significant changes in the delivery of health care over the last 20 years in response to an evolving community and medical marketplace. It now has a regional trauma facility and burn unit, a Level 3 neonatal intensive care unit, and several other highly sophisticated tertiary and quaternary services critical to the broader North Texas community.

Under Texas statute, the Dallas County Hospital District (the parent of the Parkland Health and Hospital System), which was created by local referendum, is mandated "to provide for the establishment of a hospital or hospital system to furnish medical aid and hospital care to the indigent and needy persons residing in the hospital district [Dallas County]." The hospital district can provide or purchase these services. An independent board of managers governs Parkland. However, local elected officials, the county judge, and four commissioners appoint this board. One of the responsibilities of the commissioners is to set property tax rates for the county and Dallas County Hospital District.

In the 1970s, Dallas was in the throes of a major recession brought on by the collapse of the oil and gas industry and the real estate market. The recession had two significant impacts on Parkland. First, it increased the number of individuals who sought care at Parkland. In 1987, Parkland had 41,000 admissions and nearly 15,000 births each year (representing 40% of all babies born in Dallas County). Outpatient visits have now reached nearly 1 million. The second impact of the recession was on the local tax base. Local property values declined steeply with the recession, and new construction was virtually at a standstill. Parkland was facing a dilemma. Its newly renovated and constructed facilities were at capacity the day they were opened and the recession had increased demand beyond what had been projected. Tax dollars were not readily available to support the care of the "new poor" (Anderson and Boumbulian 1995).

Given the problems with capacity and the shift from inpatient to outpatient care, Parkland decided to decentralize by making high-volume, low-cost primary care services more accessible to residents. This allowed the system to concentrate low-volume, high-cost specialty care services on the main campus. Decentralization not only made primary care health services more accessible to patients, it made it easier to promote prevention services and continuity of care. To determine which services to promote and where they should be located, Parkland performed a community assessment. The assessment was designed to identify communities that most needed public health services and basic primary care. Two panels were established to guide the development of this assessment. One was made up primarily of faculty from the medical school, and the other included community institutional providers and citizens.

Using data from the census, vital statistics, patient origin data, and provider availability studies, 64 communities within Dallas County were evaluated, and then clustered according to demographic, socio-economic, and epidemiological variables, and the availability of primary care physicians (Bass, Anderson, and Boumbulian 1987). The eight clusters identified as needing health care services represented the diversity of Dallas County, which was primarily Anglo and African-American with a small Hispanic presence.

COMMUNITY-ORIENTED PRIMARY CARE AS A FRAMEWORK FOR DECENTRALIZATION

The assessment documented not only the need for primary care but also the health status of the residents of the communities in need. The assessment indicated that the residents of these communities had significant issues related to poor health status that could not be addressed by the provision of medical care alone. For a community-based primary care system to be viable and successful, the system had to address the causes of illness. A review of the literature revealed that the community-oriented primary care (COPC) concept addressed many of the concerns found in the communities of need (Anderson and Boumbulian 1995). The COPC concept not only brings primary care to the community but also addresses the issues of ill health. It is a blend of traditional medicine with public health, improving the health of the individual as well as improving the health status of the community.

In 1984, the Institute of Medicine released its report and case studies on COPC in the American context (Nutting and Connor 1984). The four basic components of the COPC concept—assessment, community prioritization of health issues, delivery of services, and evaluation—presented in the study were felt to be appropriate structural elements with which to establish the Parkland initiative.

In 1987, the assessment and a conceptual document were combined in a plan that was accepted and approved for implementation by the Dallas County Commissioners Court. Parkland began its decentralized COPC system with six existing clinics and one new health center. Institutions included four Youth and Family Centers, the East Dallas Health Coalition, and the Oak Cliff Clinic. The group of health care facilities is now known as the Parkland Health & Hospital System.

PARKLAND TODAY

Since the approval of the COPC program in 1987, the Dallas-Fort Worth metropolitan area, with a population of nearly 5 million people, has undergone a major demographic transformation. It has emerged from the depths of a recession to become one of the nation's major transportation and communications hubs (affectionately known as the Silicon Prairie) and has an unemployment level of less than 4%. The demographics of Dallas County have also changed dramatically. The population has grown to nearly 2.1 million in 1999. The county's Hispanic population had grown by 40% to approximately 21% of the population in 1999 (Parkland Health & Hospital System 2000).

Even with a very low unemployment rate, Dallas County has approximately 480,000 residents who live below 150% of the poverty level, which by PHHS policy qualifies them for tax-supported care. Poverty has followed the freeways and spread from the inner city and southern sections of Dallas County to the suburbs, due to the availability of inexpensive housing stock and federal housing support (Parkland Health & Hospital System 1994). In addition, one in four Texans are uninsured and between 25 and 29% of Dallas County residents are uninsured. Although they work and do not qualify for tax-supported care, they routinely depend on the Parkland system's safety net for services. The percentage of uninsured among PHHS patients is therefore twice as high as for the general population (Anderson, Pickens, and Boumbulian 1998, Texas Health and Human Services Commission 1999).

Population growth has put a strain on hospital capacity in Dallas County. Parkland is at functional capacity, and all of its intensive care units are consistently full. In fiscal year 1999, Parkland had 38,177 adult admissions, 14,416 deliveries, over 1,000 neonatal intensive care patients, 798,771 outpatient visits (on campus and in the community clinics), and 136,084 emergency department visits. The hospital's length of stay has been reduced to 4.4 days, and ambulatory surgery has nearly tripled over the last decade. PHHS handles 60% of all major trauma cases in the county and cares for roughly 60% of patients living with HIV/AIDS, at some time during their illness; too often, Parkland takes on these patients after they experience a loss of health insurance (Parkland Health & Hospital System 1999a, Anderson, Pickens, and Boumbulian 1998).

PARKLAND COMMUNITY-ORIENTED PRIMARY CARE

The Parkland COPC program consists of six elements: assessment of community needs and assets, community prioritization of health care issues, collaboration with community organizations, community health care system, evaluation, and financing. These components provide the means of achieving the goals established in the COPC health policy (Anderson and Boumbulian 1995).

Assessment of Community Needs and Assets

Over the last six years, 16 Dallas County hospitals have worked together under the auspices of the Dallas-Fort Worth Hospital Council to develop a comprehensive community health assessment. The assessment includes local data and local criteria. The data include:

- population variables such as age, ethnicity, and income;
- birth and birth-related information;
- death rate variables;
- access to primary care;
- conditions appropriate for outpatient treatment (to prevent future hospitalization);
- utilization;
- population-based survey data on behavioral risk factors and COPC service areas (Parkland Health & Hospital System 1999b).

Data from the assessment are used to inform decisions about what health issues are most important to the community.

The assessment is epidemiologically based and routinely updated. It is used as a management tool to determine the location of community health centers and focus public health outreach activities. The information also provides a basis for measuring health outcomes.

The assessment tool is also used to determine and measure the health care organization's benefit to the community. It demonstrates the organization's leadership role in improving community health status, ensures appropriate resource allocation, prevents duplication of services, and helps justify tax-exempt status and disproportionate share funding (monies given to hospitals that treat a high volume of Medicaid patients, to support the institutional infrastructure).

Community Prioritization of Health Issues

Community prioritization focuses services on the health issues of most concern to the residents of the targeted communities. Within each community, a health care leadership forum is convened. Members are drawn from the elected officials representing the community and include others who have been identified as community opinion leaders. Forums are chaired by community leaders. The assessment of the community's needs and assets is reviewed briefly at the forum. Forum members then establish the community's priorities and develop action plans for the next one to three years. Typically, community priorities are issues that have direct bearing on health status but have little to do with the medical care system. Issues include education, employment, teenage pregnancy and teenage violence, transportation, and safety (Boumbulian and Anderson 1994).

Parkland has learned from the community prioritization process that imposing solutions does not improve the health of the communities. As John McKnight, John Kretzmann, Peter Berger, and John Neuhaus have pointed out, institutions cannot empower people. Experts may have knowledge of a specific subject, but they do not have expertise in another person's life, family, or community (Kretzmann and McKnight 1993, Berger and Neuhaus 1977). To be successful in a community requires identifying the community's capacities, listening to its residents, and working with them. All communities have opinions and ideas about their problems and solutions, and they all have strengths.

Community Collaborations and Partnerships

PHHS is striving to improve the health of the community through partnerships at both the micro and macro levels. Macro-level partnerships include those with other hospitals, the religious community, associations such as the Dallas-Fort Worth Hospital Council, and coalitions of social service agencies. Partnerships at the micro level include those with neighborhood organizations and residents.

The Dallas-Fort Worth Hospital Council has undertaken one such collaborative venture. The 16-hospital partnership determined that by working together, the hospitals would be better able to affect determinants of health. Given the multitude of needs within the community, and to have a demonstrable impact, the hospitals decided to select one pressing issue identified through the assessment process. The Council's needs assessment committee established four criteria to identify which issue the hospitals should address:

- The issue had to be a significant problem in terms of morbidity, mortality, and cost;

- The issue had to be amenable to early intervention and management;
- Assets had to be available to address the problem;
- The issue had to be important to all parts of the community (businesses, schools, health care organization, etc.).

Based on these criteria, diabetes, hypertension, and high cholesterol together were selected as the first issue to be addressed. The Dallas Area Coalition to Reduce Diabetes and Heart Disease was established. This coalition is made up of representatives from all areas of the community: businesses, political organizations, hospitals, managed care facilities, school districts, restaurants, and neighborhood associations. The coalition is focusing on three interventions: an awareness campaign, a continuum of care, and an education program for primary care physicians. This education program is focusing on the needs of the highest-risk populations in the community, African-Americans and Hispanics. The program will enroll COPC physicians and others that serve the population.

Another partnership is the Dallas-Fort Worth Faith Health Partnership. This partnership brings together members of the medical and hospital communities and the representatives of different religious denominations. The primary project of this partnership has been the development and support of parish nursing initiatives. Parkland's parish nursing program is operated as part of its COPC program. Parkland currently serves 15 churches as part of this program.

The Injury Prevention Center of Greater Dallas was established as part of the community's response to a 38% increase in trauma hospitalizations from 1990 to 1991. The Center was established in 1994 and is a collaborative supported by the major hospitals, foundations, and government grants. The Center is located at PHHS and serves the community through the application of the World Health Organization Safe Communities model. This model is very similar to the COPC concept in that Center staff collaborate with the community to develop, design, and implement community-specific interventions. The Center has gained national and international recognition for its work in the Hispanic community. This community has seen appropriate use of infant car seats go from 19% to almost 70% in three years through interventions such as appropriate education, blessings of car seats by priests, strict enforcement programs, and work with faith healers. There is considerable coordination between the staffs of the Injury Prevention Center and the COPC community outreach team.

A public-private partnership with another nonprofit teaching hospital system, the Presbyterian Health System of Dallas, has been created with Parkland to establish a COPC health center in a neighborhood adjacent to Presbyterian's primary campus. This neighborhood has transitioned over the last decade from one of Dallas' "swinging singles" neighborhoods to one made up of low-income families.

Parkland's Community Health Care System

Parkland and its COPC program serve more than 300,000 individuals in Dallas County yearly. Most of the patients served are minorities. Services are provided through a system of health centers and specialty programs. Currently, there are nine COPC health centers, from which care is provided in nontraditional settings at 22 homeless shelters, 15 schools, 15 churches, and three senior citizen centers via multidisciplinary teams that are a rich mix of midlevel practitioners and primary care physicians.

The health centers are staffed by physicians who are employed by Parkland and belong to a group practice, Community Health and Medical Primary and Preventive Services, Inc. (CHAMPPS). The physicians are board eligible or board certified and have clinical faculty status at the University of Texas Southwestern Medical School. Some of the 136 full- and part-time physicians have advanced degrees in public health. Special efforts are made to match physicians ethnically to the communities served by the system; 60% of the physicians are African-American, Hispanic, or Asian, and 54% are women. Roughly half of the physicians are bilingual in Spanish and English.

The COPC health care team includes an array of other health professionals: nurse practitioners, physician assistants, nutritionists, health educators, outreach workers, translators, psychologists, and social workers. All are integral to the health care team and enhance the program's ability to respond to the health needs of the community.

The scope of primary care services includes pediatric, adolescent, adult, and geriatric medicine, as well as women's health services. Preventive outreach programs for cancer and AIDS have also been implemented. The COPC program also cooperates with existing public health programs to address immunizations, sexually transmitted diseases, disease surveillance, health education, maternal and child heath, and health maintenance examinations for public school students. Dental care is provided at five health centers. The City of Dallas Health Department provides women, infants, and children (WIC) services at COPC health centers. Maternal health and family planning services are available at a majority of COPC sites. Of the over 14,000 women who deliver babies at Parkland each year, 94% receive prenatal services through this system. As a consequence, infant mortality rates in this system are among the lowest in the nation's teaching hospitals, which tend to care for sicker patients. The gap between Anglo and African-American infant mortalities has nearly been closed by this effort (Anderson, Pickens, and Boumbulian 1998, Boumbulian and Anderson 1994).

Evaluation

Measurement of health outcomes and data on the cost of health care services are used to evaluate the effectiveness of health policy. Evaluation is based on the assumption that the delivery of preventive health care will positively influence the health status of the community and that improving a community's health status will reduce health care costs. The evaluation process tests the validity of those assumptions as well as a program's performance.

Parkland conducted a multiyear community assessment in conjunction with the University of Texas School of Public Health in Houston to determine changes in utilization and health status in the community attributable to the COPC program. This assessment comprised a telephone survey of 400 randomly selected adults and parents of 250 children within six COPC service areas, and a similar study of COPC users. Studies in 1996 and 1998 were of the randomly selected community residents. A 1997 study of COPC users showed that COPC users had significantly better access to care, significantly better diagnosis of chronic conditions, and better health care-seeking behavior.

Although the results of this assessment did not clearly show an impact on health status of community residents, the assessment demonstrated significant improvement in access for adults. The enhanced access ranged from an initial reporting of between 61% to 73% enhanced access in 1996, to a range of 69% to 74% in 1998 for the six service areas studied (Community Health Status Survey 1996 and 1998). For children, access increased from a range of 83% to 96% in 1986 to a range of 87% to 98% in 1998.

There was also a significant improvement in identification and diagnosis of chronic diseases within the service areas studied. In five of the six communities surveyed, more adults were diagnosed with diabetes between 1996 and 1998. The range of people properly diagnosed in 1996 ranged from 6.1% to 10.7% in the COPC communities. This improved to a range of 6.2% to 15.5% in 1998. Additionally, five of the six communities saw improvement in the number of people properly diagnosed with high blood pressure. In 1996, the percentage of people properly diagnosed with high blood pressure ranged from 16.6% to 30.3% in the COPC communities. This improved to a range of 19.5% to 35.6% in 1998. Between 1996 and 1998, significantly more adults were properly diagnosed in all communities for high blood cholesterol. In 1996, those properly diagnosed with high blood cholesterol ranged from 16.8% to 21.9% in the COPC communities. In 1998, this improved to 21.4% to 27.0%.

In addition to an increase in the number of people properly diagnosed with chronic conditions in the COPC communities, there was significant improvement in seat belt use for adults in five of the six communities between 1996 and 1998. Seat belt use in 1996 ranged from 69.5% to 82.3%. Likewise, there was an improvement in children's seat belt use in five of the six communities.

Three utilization studies were conducted to evaluate the effectiveness of the COPC program for COPC patients. The first study, which considered pediatrics only, was completed in 1995 and covered admissions of COPC patients and the community at large in 1993 and 1994. The results indicate that COPC pediatric patients had shorter stays (3.4 days on average) than non-COPC patients (5.4 days on average). COPC pediatric patients were four times more likely to be admitted electively or by referral than non-COPC patients. Non-COPC patients were two times more likely to be admitted through the emergency room than COPC patients. A higher percentage of COPC patients had Medicaid coverage than non-COPC patients. Non-COPC pediatric patients' total charges ($8,435 on average) were twice those of COPC patients ($4,594 on average). The differences in length of stay, admission type, expected payment source, and total charges remained statistically significant even after adjusting for age, gender, and ethnicity (Schulmeier 1995).

The second utilization study, completed in 2000, covered only adults. Its findings indicated that COPC patients admitted to Parkland had significantly lower charges than non-COPC inpatients. COPC patients admitted to Parkland were charged an average of $10,769, compared to non-COPC inpatients' average charges of $11,431. A logistic regression controlling for age, ethnicity, and sex also showed that COPC patients admitted to Parkland had significantly shorter stays ($p = .05$) (Tietz 2000).

The third utilization study, conducted in 1999, was part of a large undertaking by the Children's Medical Center of Dallas to understand the population that uses their First Care Program—a 24-hour urgent care program. One of the results of this study shows that children who had a "medical home" in a community clinic, such as a COPC center or with a private physician, had significantly fewer emergency room visits for primary care than children without a medical home (Roy 1999).

Organizations under the COPC umbrella have undertaken many specialized programs and individual projects. Most of these have their own evaluation and outcome components. An example is Healthy Start in Dallas County. Healthy Start focuses on reducing infant mortality. The Parkland program targeted two sectors of the City of Dallas, the southeastern and western areas. In 1990, the infant mortality rate in these areas was 11.9 per 1,000 live births. By 1996, the rate had dropped to 6.7 infant deaths per 1,000 live births.

Financing

With the establishment of the COPC program in 1987, the County Commissioners Court voted to fund the initial program at $2.9 million. This money was for the development of a new health center as well as its continuing operation. Furthermore, a portion of these dollars was to be used to contract with existing providers to expand their services in accordance with the COPC concept. The money was added to financial support from various grants (state and federal) used to fund a 25-year-old Children and Youth Project and two community clinics funded through philanthropic resources that were incorporated into the COPC. These community-based programs required local tax support to maintain their long-term viability. Their combined budgets approached $6 million.

The receipt of Medicaid Disproportionate Share Provider funds permitted the expansion of the program. These monies were used to create a source of multiyear funding for the COPC program by buying down Parkland's government-bond debt service, thereby allowing the tax dollars allocated to this debt service to be reallocated to COPC at a steady (nondeclining) $9.5 million level.

Currently, COPC gross patient service revenue is $50.5 million. These dollars come from three primary sources: patients who pay for their own services (13%); unfunded patients subsidized by local tax dollars, Medicare (17%), and Medicaid (18%); and nonpaying (charity) patients (50%). With the advent of Medicaid managed care, the balanced budget amendment, and tremendous growth in the number of uninsured community members, Parkland's ability to cross-subsidize the care of the poor has been sorely stressed.

To preserve its share of the Medicaid market, Parkland has used its experience as a self-insured entity to develop three products to help improve access to care for all Dallas County residents and to help Parkland continue to be financially able to provide services to residents. These products are Parkland HEALTH*plus*, a sliding-scale payment program; Parkland HEALTH*first*, a Medicaid managed care insurance product; and Parkland KIDS*first*, a children's health insurance product (CHIP).

Parkland HEALTH*plus* is a sliding-scale payment program for Parkland self-pay patients. This program is designed to foster increased patient responsibility while providing access and continuity of care. The bottom line of this program for PHHS is the better allocation of health care resources; it allows Parkland to provide more patients with quality care for the same cost.

Parkland HEALTH*plus* also serves as a crossover program for patients no longer eligible for Medicaid. Many residents of Dallas County, while earning too much money to qualify for Medicaid, still cannot afford traditional health care coverage. Rather than let this population go unserved, Parkland HEALTH*plus* allows them access to quality health care at a cost determined on a sliding scale. In 1999, over 50,000 patients were enrolled in Parkland HEALTH*plus*.

Parkland HEALTH*first*, established in 1999, is one of two Medicaid health maintenance organizations (HMOs) in Dallas County. Over 30,000 Medicaid recipients have joined Parkland HEALTH*first*. Parkland KIDS*first* is one of two CHIP managed care plans in Dallas County. Three thousand members had enrolled by the summer of 2000; by 2001, there were nearly 30,000 enrollees. Parkland HEALTH*plus*, HEALTH-*first*, and KIDS*first* allow patients to keep the same doctors, medical records, benefits, and continuity of care as their coverage changes.

Parkland also has a managed care product for its employees. Over 12,000 employees and their dependents are enrolled. As a provider of health care and insurer for health care, Parkland believes in these products for its employees as well. Other public hospitals could use their employees as a beginning point for building a community-based HMO.

Having developed a COPC service delivery platform and three financing vehicles, Parkland believes that the next steps should concern the fusion of the care model and financing mechanisms. This can be accomplished through community-based HMOs.

NEXT STEPS: COMMUNITY SOLUTIONS

The next step in the evolution of COPC in the United States would be to set up community-based HMOs for service delivery. Community-based HMOs would be managed by and responsible to the community and operated on behalf of the patient and the community's health status rather than for shareholder benefit. This type of managed care organization should consider the patients', providers', and community's input into the design, operations, monitoring of costs, quality, and responsiveness of the plan. Such a plan should be dedicated to reinvesting savings from improved care delivery into prevention and enhancing the community's health status. This concept can be tailored to a wide range of settings: urban or rural communities, special populations (such as American Indian reservations), or aggregations of communities, resulting in regionalized programs. Key characteristics of community-based HMOs follow.

Key Characteristics of a Community-Based Plan

A community-based plan can be formulated many ways. It could be a community-incorporated and -owned plan; a joint venture or partnership between the community and a public- or private-sector provider; or a cooperative model. Sponsoring entities must be willing to assume risks and provide funds to capitalize the plan. Because many public hospitals already assume the risks of serving as a safety net for the uninsured, they may be important participants in the formation of such plans and help finance such models for the chance to truly manage care instead of passively accepting the role of "insurer of last resort."

- A community-based plan would deviate from the current paradigm of employer-based insurance to one based on individual or family membership.
- A community-based plan would be owned by institutions that patients rate as meaningful and of high quality, such as associations (cooperatives, small business consortiums), churches within the community, or joint ventures with nonprofit or public-provider-sponsored health plans (or systems).
- A community-based plan would provide an environment that would merge quality-in-fact (peer and professional evaluation) with quality-in-perception (patient satisfaction).
- A community-based plan would develop special programs based on community assessment and dialogue with its members or community residents. Examples include parish nursing programs, diabetes management programs, student mentoring programs, literacy programs, and training in infant stimulation to promote early childhood development.
- A community-based plan would allow participants to take an active role in their own care through a therapeutic partnership with providers. This is a patient-provider partnership that centers on educating the patient about how to be healthy and edu-

cating the provider about the cultural, social, and belief systems of the patient.

- A community-based plan would provide a medical home (a place where the member can always go and know that medical care will be available) for its members.
- A community-based plan would target its educational initiatives to specific problems identified in the assessment, communicate with the community, and provide incentives to members to achieve agreed-upon goals.
- A community-based plan would have the power to improve the health of the community. Because it would be part of the community, it would not be imposing solutions.

Elements of Community-Based Health Maintenance Organizations

Community-based plans are only one option for providing community-based services. Another option is community-based HMOs following an expanded business model, which incorporates community benefits. The elements of this model are ownership, underwriting and capitalization, governance, management, clinical services, community dividend, and accountability.

Ownership. Models of ownership of community-based HMOs can include a "cooperative," in which a membership organization of community residents pools their funds to capitalize and underwrite an insurance product; an organization of member governmental agencies that pool their health benefit funds to underwrite and capitalize a fund; or a membership organization of corporations that pool health benefit dollars to underwrite and capitalize operations. Many types of organizations may own a community-based HMO, including faith-based community services, charitable organizations, or a consortium of small businesses. These entities could establish a joint venture with a public hospital system willing to help capitalize the effort as an extension of its mandate and mission. If these entities prove to be "profitable" (that is, save money through preventive interventions or reduce overhead or expenses), these resources can be reinvested in the plan and the community, in a manner directed by the community.

Underwriting and capitalization. There are multiple means of underwriting and capitalizing a community-based HMO. Possibilities include public-private partnerships, nonprofit trusts or foundations, conversion foundations (foundations created from the sale of non-profit or public hospitals and/or the conversion of nonprofit health plans into for-profit corporations), access assurance plans, regional rural collaborative models, prepaid voucher systems, child health insurance programs (CHIPs), or state tobacco settlements.

- **Public-private partnerships.** Underwriting and capitalization can occur through public-private partnerships in which one large community corporation or a pool of corporations (such as all the telecommunication corporations in a community or all the nonprofit or public hospitals in a community) underwrite and capitalize a community-based HMO. They do this by using existing community assets for the delivery of care to a specific geographic location or specific low-income population. Another type of pooled effort is the creation of an insurance product (managed care organization) by small businesses, social service agencies, businesses in the service industry, or churches.
- **Nonprofit trusts.** Underwriting and capitalization can occur through nonprofit trusts or through the organization of private community or corporate donations.
- **Access assurance plan.** Underwriting and capitalization can occur through an access assurance plan or prepayment plan such as Parkland HEALTH*plus.*
- **Regional collaborative.** Underwriting and capitalization can occur in rural areas through a regional collaborative HMO model. A competitive model does not work well in rural areas due to a lack of providers. Small rural communities could work with each other to establish a 501(c)(3) nonprofit cooperative to provide, purchase, or arrange care locally and regionally at the level of the area's capability and capacity. It would be necessary to overcome state insurance commissions' concerns about undercapitalization for self-insured products, multiple employer welfare arrangements, or other federally created insurance products.

- **Prepaid voucher system.** Underwriting and capitalization can occur through a prepaid voucher system. This type of system provides a defined service with a portion paid by the employer, a portion paid by the employee, and a portion possibly absorbed by the provider using a sliding scale if all employees are covered.
- **Funding from disproportionate share funds.** Underwriting and capitalization can occur through partial funding from disproportionate share funds.
- **State tobacco settlements.** Underwriting and capitalization can occur through state tobacco settlements. They can be administered as block grants to communities to create and sustain community-based managed care.
- **State Child Health Insurance Program.** Underwriting and capitalization can occur in part through the state funding of the State Child Health Insurance Program, Title XXI of the Social Security Act. Title XXI incorporates an entitlement for states that meet the statutory requirements. States can expand Medicaid, buy private coverage, or use some combination of these methods (Budetti 1998).

Governance. Ideally, the governance structure of these organizations would blend the expertise of community residents with the expertise of health system professionals. Functions such as benefit administration could be contracted out to lower overhead costs. The governing body may be established in various ways to be adaptable to community circumstances. For example, the governing body could be formed as a separate governance structure from the sponsoring entities or a subsidiary board of a publicly sponsored entity, or the governing body could be elected from the membership or appointed by a governmental body with the advice and consent of the sponsoring institutions. The governance structure should promote accountability with regard to costs, access, quality, and member satisfaction.

Management. A community-based HMO must be professionally managed. The managed care organization might establish its own management structure or it might be managed through a joint venture with traditional providers such as hospitals, community health centers, or rural health clinics. Science tells us that communities are complex adaptive systems. Dee Hock (1999), in his book *Birth of the Chaordic Age,* summarizes the nature of complex adaptive systems as follows:

> Complex connectivity allows spontaneous order to arise and when it does, characteristics emerge that cannot be explained by knowledge of the parts. Nor does such order seem to obey linear laws of cause and effect. Scientists speculate that all complex, adaptive systems exist on the edge of chaos with just enough self-organization to create the cognitive patterns we refer to as order.

The organic nature of a community-based HMO allows for the application of organic forms of management, such as the evolving science of complex adaptive systems. The study of such systems teaches that there is a tipping factor. The tipping factor refers to small but vital changes (for example, reducing the infant mortality rate in one discrete area of a community). Multiple small changes result in large systemic changes (Zimmerman, Lindberg, and Plsek 1998).

Clinical services. A community-based HMO must have access to the full continuum of services regardless of who provides those services. This continuum may include services that are beyond the traditional medical model, including traditional public health services. Initially, and periodically thereafter, the community should conduct an assessment to determine the scope of services the HMO should provide and the priorities among these services. Periodically, the plan will assess the community to determine the priorities among the services provided. This should facilitate setting deductibles and copayments.

Community dividend. Unique to a community-owned HMO is the allocation of dividends. If the plan has excess revenues, some of the excess may be put into reserves and the remainder could be used to address predetermined community needs and social determinants of disease.

Accountability. Community-based HMOs should maximize trust between providers and members. If decisions that result in access barriers or rationing are made, they should be clearly explained, and the community should be informed of the rationale involved in the decision (Anderson et al. 1998).

Accountability also means being accountable to the community (including health providers) for the results and outcomes of the care delivered. An approach known as Measurably Enhancing the Status of Health (MESH) can be used by an organization to measure accountability. The aims of this approach are to contribute to overall health surveillance efforts of the community, provide indicators of measurable improvement over time, and provide information for targeting and prioritizing future interventions. MESH can also be a vehicle for quality improvement and outcomes within hospitals and health plans. MESH would be the vehicle by which quality-in-fact (peer and professional evaluation) and quality-in-perception (patient satisfaction) could be merged (Young, Laskowski, and Sussman 1998).

CONCLUSION

Being responsive to the community means caring for the health of a population beyond the traditional approach. There are many options to provide community-based managed care. Each of these concepts approaches the financing and provision of care differently, but they have many common elements. These elements distinguish the community-based HMO from other managed care organizations, which are either corporate-owned and responsible to the shareholder (not the community) or responsible only to their own enrolled population. The model or principles are important, but it must be emphasized that these vehicles are adaptable and can be customized to community needs, strengths, and values.

Attention to the values and needs of the community is the touchstone of community-based HMOs. The foundations of the community-based HMO and the COPC concepts are consistent. Assessment and outcomes measures provide the context to develop the scope of services. By integrating quantitative data and cultural distinctions, community-based managed care organizations can deliver services tailored to a particular community. Community-based HMOs can appropriate money or rebate savings into community reinvestment plans. Reinvesting underscores the priority of the community-based health plan: to optimize the health of community residents. It provides an opportunity to continually reinforce a sense of community and acknowledge the spirit, power, and resilience of people working together on a common issue.

REFERENCES

Anderson, Ron J., and Paul J. Boumbulian. 1995. *Comprehensive Community Health Programs: A New Look at an Old Approach.* Washington, DC: Association of Academic Health Centers in a Managed Care Environment, pp. 119–35.

Anderson, Ron J., Sue Pickens, and Paul J. Boumbulian. 1998. "Toward a New Urban Health Model: Moving Beyond the Safety Net to Save the Safety Net—Resetting Priorities for Healthy Communities." *Journal of Urban Health.* 75: 367–78.

Anderson, Ron J., et al. 1998. *Beyond Managed Care: Community Based HMOs.* The James MacGregor Burns Academy of Leadership, University of Maryland, Leadership and Public Policy Series Paper Number 8. Available at www.academy.umd.edu/scholarship/DLS/WorkingPapers/Anderson.pdf.

Bass, P., Ron J. Anderson, and Paul J. Boumbulian. 1987. *Community-Oriented Primary Care: A Plan for Dallas County.* Dallas, TX: Parkland Memorial Hospital.

Berger, Peter L., and Richard J. Neuhaus. 1977. *To Empower People: The Role of Mediating Structures in Public Policy.* Washington, DC: American Enterprise Institute.

Boumbulian, Paul J., and Ron J. Anderson. 1994. "Survival through Community Services: From Sick Care to Health Care." *Health Management Quarterly* 16: 17–23.

Budetti, Peter P. 1998. "Health Insurance for Children: A Model for Incremental Health Reform?" *New England Journal of Medicine* 338: 541–42.

Community Health Status Survey. 1996 and 1998. Professional Research Consultants (Omaha, NE). Dallas, TX: Parkland Health & Hospital System.

Hock, Dee. 1999. *Birth of the Chaordic Age.* San Francisco, CA: Berrett-Koehler, p. 27.

Kretzmann, John P., and John L. McKnight. 1993. *Building Communities from the Inside Out: A Path toward Finding and Mobilizing Community Assets.* Evanston, IL: Northwestern University.

Nutting, P. A., and E. M. Connor. 1984. *Community-Oriented Primary Care: A Practical Assessment.* Washington, DC: National Academy of Science Press.

Parkland Health & Hospital System. 1994. *The Health of Dallas County: A Management Tool.* Dallas, TX: Parkland Health & Hospital System.

———. 1999a. *Annual Report.* Dallas, TX: Parkland Health & Hospital System.

———. 1999b. *1999 Dallas County Health Checkup.* Dallas, TX: Parkland Health & Hospital System. Available at: www.dfwhc.org/dcna.htm

———. 2000. *2000 Dallas County Health Checkup.* Dallas, TX: Parkland Health & Hospital System. Available at www.dfwhc.org/dcna.htm.

Roy, Lonnie. 1999. "Dallas Area Healthcare Use: Study of Insured, Uninsured and Medicaid Enrolled Children." PhD diss., University of North Texas, Dallas.

Schulmeier, Greg. 1995. *An Analysis of Parkland Health and Hospital System's Community-Oriented Primary Care Program.* Dallas, TX: Parkland Health & Hospital System.

Texas Health and Human Services Commission. 1999. "Projected 1999 Texas Estimates of the Texas Population without Insurance in 1999 by County." www.hhsc.state.tx.us.

Tietz, Michelle. 2000. Study and Analysis. Parkland Health & Hospital System, Strategic Planning Department.

Young, Mark J., Robert J. Laskowski, and Elliot J. Sussman. 1998. "How a Community Teaching Hospital Is Changing to Better Serve Its Community." *Academic Medicine* 73: 488–93.

Zimmerman, B., Curt Lindberg, and Paul Plsek. 1998. *Edgeware: Insights from Complexity Science for Health Care Leaders.* Irving, TX: VHA, Inc.

A Case Management Approach to HIV/AIDS Prevention and Care in Boston

Rebecca Marshall, Heidi Louise Behforouz, Ashok Reddy, and Jim Yong Kim

AIDS presents an unprecedented challenge to health systems in poor communities. Community-based care using community members with specialized training is an extremely promising model for confronting that challenge. Lessons about the effectiveness of a community-based approach stretch across socioeconomic, cultural and political boundaries, as Partners in Health has demonstrated from Haiti to Peru, from inner-city Boston to inside Russian prisons.

Every one of us is now living in the time of AIDS. The global pandemic has surpassed the Black Plague in number of deaths and qualifies as the most disastrous epidemic in history. How we, as inhabitants of this planet, respond to this epidemic will, quite simply, define our generation.

—Jon Rohde and Jim Yong Kim

F orty million people in the world are now living with AIDS; 5 million of these were infected this past year. Of the 5 million new infections, more than 95% occurred in developing countries. In parts of sub-Saharan Africa, some villages have lost almost all of their working adult population, leaving only children and senior citizens to perform all the functions necessary for survival.

Among the poorest populations that are being devastated by HIV, the prevention of further infections is clearly the top priority. Yet without access to treatment for AIDS sufferers, sub-Saharan Africa and other regions with explosive epidemics, such as India and China, will soon undergo fundamental demographic shifts that will threaten the stability of villages, nation-states, and perhaps even whole continents.

Partners in Health has effectively used community-based approaches to caring for people living with HIV/AIDS and other illnesses such as multidrug-resistant tuberculosis in rural Haiti, inner-city Boston, Mexico, and the slums of Lima, Peru. Our community-based model of care does not represent a compromise made out of desperation or simple lack of funds. Rather, we have found that efficient, compassionate, and culturally and linguistically appropriate programs that utilize community-based health promoters can yield outcomes that rival and even surpass those seen in more affluent settings. Community-based care for poor people in poor communities does not have to be a compromise. In Haiti, for example, where we run a program in which highly active antiretroviral therapy (HAART) is delivered by community health workers to rural peasants living with HIV, the viral loads of 88% of the first 40 patients tested were undetectable. These results surpass those reported from many clinical trials in the United States.

THE CHALLENGE OF AIDS CARE IN BOSTON

Few cities in the United States better illustrate the inequities in health care between rich and poor than Boston. In a city containing one of the highest concentrations of physicians in the country (Stark and Jahnke 1992, Massachusetts Division of Health Care Finance 2000) and some of the best hospitals in the world, many of Boston's poor have little or no access to basic health services.

The failure of the Boston public health system to effectively and equitably reach the diverse communities throughout the city is particularly evident in the area of HIV/AIDS. As reported in the 2001 "Health of Boston" study commissioned by the Boston Department of Public Health, the HIV rate among Hispanic residents is 46.1% higher than the rate of the Boston population as a whole. Among Black residents, the HIV rate is 43.0% higher than the rate of the population as a whole—and, incredibly, the AIDS mortality rate among this same group is 72.4% higher than the Boston rate (Boston Public Health Commission 2001).

Working with HIV-positive individuals in the city's poorest communities presents particular challenges. The populations most at risk of contracting AIDS tend to be already marginalized: substance users, the mentally ill, men who have sex with men, women who are commercial sex workers. Accordingly, HIV-positive individuals in very poor communities are often the most vulnerable of any individuals in society. In addition, problems that frequently accompany the disease, such as stigmatization and depression, may increase individuals' feelings of isolation and hopelessness and further discourage them from seeking help (Behforouz et al. 2001).

The HIV Prevention and Access to Care and Treatment (PACT) Project in Boston provides an important model of a case-based approach to reaching HIV-positive populations in poor communities. PACT recognizes that the health of HIV-positive individuals depends not only on their medical condition, but on a range of factors related to their economic status, social environment, and emotional well-being. As a result, the project seeks to help clients address critical issues in their lives—ranging from housing instability to substance use to unemployment—which make dealing with their disease additionally difficult. In the process of resolving these problems, individuals learn how to make and sustain connections with the resources they need to stay healthy.

THE PACT PROJECT

Roxbury, the third largest neighborhood in Boston, is also one of the city's poorest neighborhoods and has some of its worst health indicators. Over 50% of its population lives below the poverty line, as compared to 20% in Boston at large. Not surprisingly, the AIDS mortality rate for persons aged 25–64 is almost double the rate of greater Boston (Boston Public Health Commission 1997).

In 1997, Heidi Behforouz, a senior medical resident at the Brigham and Women's Hospital in Boston, began working with a Roxbury-based community organization called Soldiers of Health. Run by community health workers, Soldiers of Health (recently renamed Partners in Health-Roxbury) focuses on health education, prevention, and social services for poor and marginalized populations in the Roxbury area. It is supported by Partners in Health, an internationally acclaimed Boston-based organization that works in poor communities in several countries.

While working with Soldiers and Partners, Behforouz became concerned about the number of clients with HIV. She was further concerned by statistics suggesting that the incidence of AIDS was rising among poor, inner-city young women and that the AIDS mortality rate in African-American women in Roxbury was 3.5 times greater than that of women in Boston as a whole. These growing concerns prompted Behforouz and colleagues at Soldiers and Partners to apply for a grant to test a model of community-based care in the context of HIV/AIDS. They were awarded a three-year grant from the Office of Minority Health, a federal office under the Department of Health and Human Services that has since been disbanded. The resulting project—PACT—was designed to apply a case-based approach to working with HIV/AIDS patients, to assess the potential of this model for scaling up in the future. While Soldiers had applied a community-health worker model to dealing with general health, it was not clear how successfully this model could be applied to HIV/AIDS care, given the complicating social and medical factors surrounding the disease (PACT 1997).

After three years of operation, PACT has shown that a case-based approach to dealing with HIV/AIDS *can* be highly effective. With five full-time case managers, a physician, and a handful of part-time medical students, the project has over 90 clients with a range of different needs relating to their HIV status. Many of the clients who were completely disengaged from the health care system when first beginning to work with PACT are now connected to needed health services, educated about the prevention and treatment of their disease, and engaged in maintaining and improving their own health.

Each client begins a relationship with PACT by meeting with a case manager. At this meeting, the client and case manager together fill out and sign three forms: an intake assessment form, a needs planning form, and a confidentiality form. This confidentiality form, in particular, is an essential feature of the relationship between the case manager and the client due to the still-prevalent stigma surrounding the disease. Once clients have identified their critical needs, case managers work with them using a step-by-step approach that includes clients in making decisions and in navigating medical and social service systems.

Depending on the client's needs, the case manager contacts him or her on a daily, biweekly, or weekly basis. Some clients need a case manager to help arrange social services, such as having meals delivered or finding a treatment program for substance use. Other clients need a case manager to accompany them to medical appointments, interpret medical terminology, or translate into their primary language. Still others need a case manager to help them with adherence to drug regimens, which often involve taking numerous pills at different times of the day or have unpleasant side effects that make compliance difficult.

The effectiveness of the PACT model can be attributed to one critical element: the case manager. The cases PACT encounters often involve multiple layers of problems—racial discrimination, poverty, unemployment, substance use, sexual assault, abuse, and incarceration, in addition to the financial and emotional burden of AIDS. Peeling away these layers—a critical step in helping the client improve his or her health—requires the case manager to spend a tremendous amount of time with the client, to build trust and come to an understanding of the source of many of these problems. Since most of the case workers are from the client's community, they understand the client's problems and the issues involved with being poor and marginalized. Once trained in case management, they are well equipped to help clients identify their problems, encourage harm reduction and education, and help clients obtain the care they need.

In comparison, many conventional HIV/AIDS programs have been based on an adherence support center: a free-standing adherence clinic to which patients come for medication and therapy. Often these clinics employ outreach workers to contact patients who do not appear as scheduled for their medications. Unfortunately, however, many of these workers have little training or experience in case management; they often fail to address the underlying issues leading to nonadherence, and the patients are lost to follow-up and appropriate treatment.

THE FUTURE OF THE PACT PROJECT

In the future, PACT hopes to implement a method of temporary intensive intervention: directly observed therapy, or DOT. Partners in Health pioneered the use of DOT in the delivery of antiretroviral therapy through a collaboration with its sister organization in rural Haiti. The initiative, called DOT-HAART (DOT with highly active antiretroviral therapy), has yielded surprisingly good results despite being carried out in an extremely impoverished setting (Farmer et al. 2001).

Since DOT in industrialized countries is much more expensive, it will be a last-resort option for consistently noncompliant clients. PACT will intake patients identified by providers as having problems, enroll them in regular case management, and work with them to ensure that they attend their scheduled follow-up visits. A client who repeatedly fails to make these visits will then be enrolled in DOT, in which a case worker will visit the client's home several times a day to observe the client taking his or her medication. Once the client's compliance is stabilized, he or she can move back to regular case management. This process is intended to be dynamic and flexible, because a client who is adherent at one time may, for a variety of reasons, become nonadherent in another six months. A client may be served through case management for a year, be transferred to DOT for a set period, and then return to regular case management.

This approach to HIV treatment is potentially extremely cost effective in comparison to either a standard DOT approach or a clinic-based approach. To begin with, it is much less expensive to use a fluid case management/DOT approach than to maintain DOT for all clients at all times. This approach also saves costs by using community health workers rather than nurse practitioners for client visitation. And finally, in assessing costs to the health system as a whole, this presents a highly effective way to reach individuals who might otherwise fall through the cracks, ensuring that they take their medication and preventing, for example, a $100,000 admission for AIDS-induced *pneumocystis carinii* pneumonia (Behforouz et al. 2001).

Despite compelling evidence of the effectiveness of the PACT model and of the potential effectiveness of PACT's adopting a DOT component in its work, the project is in jeopardy due to lack of funding. PACT's three-year grant from the Office of Minority Health ended in December 2001. While the project has enough support from Boston's Brigham and Women's Hospital to sustain it temporarily, it does not have any long-term financial backing.

This highlights a critical problem for community-based programs in the US and other countries. Many service grants from private foundations are for such small sums of money—$3,000 to $15,000—that competing for them barely justifies the time spent writing proposals. In addition, these grants often last for such short periods—often between one to three years—that there may be barely enough time to develop the staff capacity and systems to get the project off the ground before the funding ends. Desperate for funding, organizations are forced to divert precious resources into writing multiple proposals for small, short-lived grants, rather than focusing on their mandated work. PACT, for example, has submitted eight grant proposals over the past three years.

One potential solution to this crisis could be for projects to apply for follow-on funding from the same donor, once a successful initiative has been completed. However, retaining donors' interest in and commitment to a program often requires the kind of dramatic results that may not be possible to achieve in a relatively short period of time. Thus, rather than investing in developing projects over the long term, donors often move on to fund new initiatives, which may appear to have more potential, leaving those whose funding has been cut scrambling to make up the difference or else having to discontinue their operations.

An obvious alternative to applying for foundation grants is vying for large federal grants. Applying for federal grants complicates the relationship between organizations working in the same neighborhood, whose work is complementary and who therefore have to compete for the same pots of money. In addition, for service-based organizations such as PACT, winning grants is particularly difficult because many federal grants that could offer large sums of money expect a research component that includes data collection with intervention and control groups. While collecting data can provide important evidence of a program's effectiveness, having to meet stringent donor research requirements may distract from the program's intended focus and lead to a sacrifice in service delivery. However, PACT recognizes that its access to this avenue of potential funding depends on its ability to collect sufficient data to prove that a community-based model of intensive case management is cost-effective. PACT is currently working to design studies that compare the costs of care for its clients with costs for patients of similar socioeconomic status who are not followed by a community-based case manager.

In addition to applying for grants from various donors, PACT is working to form strategic partnerships that will provide AIDS case management with a community component. The value of such partnerships should not be understated. From the time of its genesis within Soldiers of Health, PACT has benefited tremendously from its ongoing collaboration with Partners in Health; Partners has provided mentoring, financial support, and a steady supply of student volunteers from Harvard Medical School. PACT has also received funding and support from Boston's Brigham and Women's Hospital, including transitional funding through the newly established Division of Social Medicine and Health Inequalities to sustain itself temporarily. How it will sustain itself in the long run remains to be seen.

As the introduction to this book notes, "During the last decade of the 20th century . . . some communities learned to deal with the devastating threat of AIDS through education, local action, and compassion." This is indeed the approach taken by the PACT Project: working with communities to provide education, local action, and compassion, as those communities learn to deal with AIDS. The PACT model appears to be an effective one. For those who developed it, for those who have developed similar community-based models that work, and for those of us who believe in these models, the future challenge will be to find viable ways to fund them and sustain the critical work that they do.

REFERENCES

Behforouz, Heidi, Ashok Reddy, Stephanie Cohen, Mitul Kadakia, et al. 2001. Interviews by Rebecca Marshall with PACT staff members. Tape recording. Boston, MA.

Boston Public Health Commission. 1997. "The Health of Boston 1997." Boston: Office of Research, Health Assessment, and Data Systems.

———. 2001. "The Health of Boston 2001." [Cited Jan. 11, 2002.] Available from www.bphc.org.

Farmer, Paul, et al. 2001. "Community-Based Approaches to HIV Treatment in Resource-Poor Settings." *The Lancet* 358: 404–9.

Massachusetts Division of Health Care Finance and Policy. 2000. "Massachusetts Health Care Trends: 1990–1999." Boston: Massachusetts Division of Health Care Finance and Policy.

PACT (HIV Prevention and Access to Care and Treatment) Project. 1997. "Comprehensive Community-Based HIV Prevention and Treatment in Roxbury, Massachusetts: Implementation of a Program to Improve Health Outcomes." Proposal for funding.

Stark, Marg, and Art Jahnke. 1992. "Diagnosing Doctors." *Boston Magazine* 84: 62–70.

15 The Connections between Academia and the Practice of Community-Oriented Primary Care

C. William Keck

This chapter focuses on the role of local public health departments in responding to the significant failings described in the 1988 Institute of Medicine report, *The Future of Public Health*. Following that report, local health departments were given new responsibilities for assessment, policy development, and quality assurance. Some health departments are meeting these challenges through linkages with academic institutions. Many community health agencies can also increase their capacity to meet their goals through partnerships with colleges and universities.

—Gail Price

Adapted, with permission, from C. William Keck, "Lessons Learned from an Academic Health Department," *Journal of Public Health Management and Practice* 6: 47–52. Copyright 2000 Aspen Publishers.

In 1988, the Institute of Medicine Study Committee that had reviewed the status of the public health system in this country issued a wake-up call to the public health profession. Its report, *The Future of Public Health* (Institute of Medicine 1988), described a "system in disarray" and listed a number of disturbing findings to support that characterization:

- There was no clear, universally accepted mission for public health.
- Public health professionals had been slow to develop strategies that demonstrate the worth of their efforts to legislators and the public.
- Relationships between medicine and public health were, at best, uneasy.
- Inadequate research resources had been targeted at identifying and solving public health problems.
- Public health practice, unlike other health professions, was largely detached from its academic bases.

The response to the report by public health professionals has been substantial. Particularly heartening has been the response of our national and state public health professional organizations and a variety of federal agencies interested in improving public health services. During the past decade, these groups have collaborated in a remarkable effort to respond to the problems identified. These efforts were spurred on by the changes proposed for the US health system by the Clinton administration in the early 1990s, and by the realities of the managed care approach to health care reform. There was (and is) concern that the historically positive impact of public health measures on health status and quality of life will be underappreciated and the potential for future benefits will be overlooked in the scramble to change the mechanisms of health care delivery to cut the cost of illness care.

The result of this concern is that more attention has been paid to the status of local public health services over the past 14 years than probably at any other time in the history of the United States. The 1990s were full of activities intended to increase understanding of and bolster delivery of public health services. Public health professionals from the local, state, and national levels have come together in a variety of settings to discuss and develop consensus on public health's role and the resources required to fulfill that role. The accomplishments resulting from focusing attention on these issues have been substantial. The mission of public health has been clearly defined (Institute of Medicine 1988, US Department of Health and Human Services 1995).

Agreement has largely been reached on the three core functions of local health departments: assessment, policy development, and quality assurance (Institute of Medicine 1988). Out of the core functions has grown a list of the 10 essential services required for communities to reach their maximum potential for health (US Department of Health and Human Services 1995 and 1997):

1. Monitor health status to identify community health problems.
2. Diagnose and investigate health problems and health hazards in the community.
3. Inform, educate, and empower people about health issues.
4. Mobilize community partnerships to identify and solve health problems.
5. Develop policies and plans that support individual and community health efforts.
6. Enforce laws and regulations that protect health and ensure safety.
7. Link people to needed personal health services and ensure the provision of health care when it is otherwise unavailable.
8. Ensure a competent public health and personal health care workforce.

9. Evaluate the effectiveness, accessibility, and quality of personal and population-based health services.
10. Research innovative solutions to health problems.

Performance standards for local communities based on the 10
essential services are under development at the Centers for Disease
Control and Prevention (Halverson 2000). Other accomplishments
include:

- a growing consensus about the competencies health workers
  must have to deliver those services (US Department of Health
  and Human Services 1997, Sorensen and Bialek 1993);
- an initiative to bring the disciplines of medicine and public
  health closer together;
- a clearer focus by schools of public health on linking with
  practice sites (Association of Schools of Public Health 1998,
  Gordon et al. 1999), and expanding practice linkages with
  other kinds of academic institutions (Healton 1999, Blacklow
  et al. 1995, Seifer 1998, Gale 1998);
- initiation of work to develop a community health services
  guide that will identify effective programs and interventions
  (Chaulik and Kazandjian 1998, Public Health Foundation
  1999, Zaza et al. 2000);
- ongoing efforts to define a research agenda for community
  health (Public Health Foundation 1999, 1998).

As exciting as it has been to observe and participate in these activities, it is also increasingly daunting for directors of local and state
health departments to consider the implications of this work for their
agencies. The growing consensus about the role of public health
departments in ensuring conditions in which people can be healthy
and developing new tools for assessing the effectiveness of interventions will create pressures for change in the structure and function of
local health departments. It will also make those departments more
accountable to communities and external funders.

PARTNERSHIPS

Many local health departments are too small and too resource-poor even to attempt to fulfill many of the roles now expected of them, and virtually all health departments will be challenged to redirect resources and acquire needed skills to be successful. Some will need to rethink structure and governance. All will need to pursue new resources, especially by developing partnerships with others who share elements of the public health mission.

Certainly a new driving force to form partnerships will be the community assessments spawned by the new national performance standards. The standards look not only at the capacity of the health department, but also at a community's capacity to deliver the 10 essential services. As proposed, this assessment of community capacity cannot be done without a partnership effort including most, if not all, parties with an interest in improving health. And these services most certainly cannot be delivered with high quality and in adequate quantity without effective working partnerships. I am especially hopeful that the activities associated with the national performance standards will breathe new life into the initiative to bring the separate cultures of medicine and public health closer together.

ACADEMIC CONNECTIONS

Another type of partnership available to many (but probably not all) state and local health agencies is linkages with academic institutions. The Institute of Medicine focused its recommendations on schools of public health, but there are many other academic settings where linkages would be beneficial. These would include master of public health programs offered in institutions other than schools of public health. Schools of medicine, nursing, and dentistry, and programs on health education, environmental health, counseling, and urban studies could also partner with health agencies.

Indeed, many partnerships exist between institutions that train health professionals and local and state health agencies. The nature of these relationships ranges from a casual connection, involving teaching, research, or consultation, to a highly structured and formal affiliation arrangement. There are four key issues that academics and practitioners working together can be particularly helpful in addressing:

1. Health professions students and many staff members of public health departments are not as well prepared as they should be to meet the needs of communities.
2. Community agencies have limited access to the expertise needed to assess community needs and respond to changing demands for services.
3. Community-based research is currently too limited in quantity and quality.
4. The need for continuing education of health agency staff and academic institution faculty is often not addressed.

Linkages between practice sites, such as local health departments, and academic institutions or programs can help address these issues by connecting practitioners with academicians to improve the practitioners' capacity to describe and solve community health problems. Such linkages can improve practitioners' capacity for critical thinking and foster an epidemiologic approach to problem-solving. Linkages can provide opportunities for students to have real-life experiences and for academicians to have access to community-based data and programs for study and evaluation.

An array of linkage arrangements is possible. A service agency may host a student for a practicum or allow him to participate in a research project. A different relationship may be defined by partnership agreements and contracts dealing with teaching, service, and research. The maximal benefits to be gained by a service agency and academic entity might best be realized if there is a formal affiliation between a health professions school and a local public health agency, similar to the more familiar relationships existing between medical schools and their teaching hospitals. Such an affiliation allows both partners to benefit from the educational connection the relationship represents.

A well-functioning public health agency provides a window on the community that can be of great value to an academic institution. The successful public health agency operates in a highly collaborative mode with many community agencies and institutions. It can also act as a conduit for exchange between academics and a variety of community groups so that access to involvement with community health issues is automatically broad. The academic public health agency, therefore, acts to direct resources to the service, teaching, and research needs of its community. In so doing, the gap between medical professionals and public health professionals is narrowed, and the goal of bringing these separate and often combative groups together into an integrated network of health promotion, disease prevention, and illness care services is more likely to be realized.

AN EXAMPLE FROM NORTHEASTERN OHIO

Several health departments in northeastern Ohio have been linked with academic settings for almost 40 years. The first linkages were between colleges of nursing and a few local health departments serving as sites for instruction in community health nursing. The Northeastern Ohio Universities College of Medicine (NEOUCOM) and the Akron Health Department have been closely linked, by design, since 1976. At that time, the college and the health department joined forces to recruit a new director of health who could also serve on the faculty of the college. The purpose was for this individual to draw the two entities together for the benefit of the mission of each by helping the college to identify its proper role in the area of community health and by helping the health department to increase its academic involvement.

Since that time, a vertically integrated curriculum in community health has evolved at the college that places medical students in community settings several times during their medical school experience. To date, seven local health departments in northeastern Ohio (as well as several other community agencies) have been involved in the teaching of medical students. The Akron Health Department has been the most involved; during the past 20 years it has added health education, graduate nutrition, graduate nursing, and public health students from a variety of educational institutions to the ranks of students mentored on a regular basis.

The Akron Health Department is now an official teaching health department for NEOUCOM. In December of 1997 the department signed an association agreement with the College of Medicine that is equivalent to the agreements signed by the College and its teaching hospitals. This agreement represents a formalization of a relationship that has grown steadily stronger over more than 20 years.

The benefits of this working partnership have been significant for both NEOUCOM and the Akron Health Department. There are currently three public health-trained physicians who work in and receive financial support from both settings. Each physician has both academic and practice responsibilities and provides a physician role model for public health practice. In addition, seven other health department staff members have adjunct faculty appointments at the College of Medicine and/or other area universities in colleges of nursing or in departments of health education and nutrition.

At least 1,000 students have rotated through the Akron Health Department over the past 20 years, approximately 120 in 1999 alone. Some students have come to learn public health practice and others to investigate community health problems. The presence of students in the department and the department's predilection for embracing the contributions that academics can make to public health practice have encouraged academics to undertake research projects that benefit from access to health department patients, programs, and data.

The subjects of research projects carried out in the Akron Health Department include teen tobacco use, compliance with hypertension medical regimens, trials of sexually transmitted disease medications, female sexual decision-making related to prevention of HIV transmission, and the impact of incentives for patients to keep appointments. It has been easy for the department to solicit academics for special services over the years, developing contracts for services when reimbursement has been possible. Included in these activities are assistance with the development of an emergency medical system for the City of Akron, development of an evaluation process for a new grant for lead poisoning prevention from the Federal Department of Housing and Urban Development, data development and analysis for Summit County's Assessment Process for Excellence in Public Health, creation of goals and objectives for the community's health plan (entitled "Healthy Summit 2000"), and medical support services for a multi-county control program for breast and cervical cancer.

CONCLUSION

Communities invest heavily in their educational institutions, public health departments, and other community health agencies. The capacity of most of these agencies and institutions to achieve their missions can be enhanced if academics and practitioners can learn to work together when their interests overlap. The "academic health department" is an example of a community agency with enhanced capacity because of its academic linkages. It is a flexible model that can be replicated in part or entirely in many communities. Its potential should be carefully evaluated when the option for beneficial collaboration is present in any community.

REFERENCES AND RESOURCES

Association of Schools of Public Health. 1998. *Strong Schools, Strong Partners.* Washington, DC: Association of Schools of Public Health, for the Bureau of Health Professions, Health Resources and Services Administration, Dept. of Health and Human Services.

Blacklow, R. S., et al. 1995. "A Required Clerkship in Community Medicine." *Academic Medicine* 70: 449–50.

Chaulik, C. P., and V. A. Kazandjian. 1998. "Directly Observed Therapy for Treatment Completion of Pulmonary Tuberculosis: Consensus Statement of the Public Health Tuberculosis Guidelines Panel." *Journal of the American Medical Association* 279: 943–47.

Gale, J. L. 1998. "Combining Academics and Practice or Seven Years Commuting over Snoqualmie Pass." *The Link (Quarterly Bulletin of the Council on Linkages between Academia and Public Health Practice)* 12: 4, 7.

Gordon, A. G., et al. 1999. "Final Report on Public Health Practice Linkages between Schools of Public Health and State Health Agencies: 1992–1996." *Journal of Public Health Management and Practice* 5: 25–34.

Halverson, P. K. 2000. "Performance Measurement and Performance Standards: Old Wine in New Bottles." *Journal of Public Health Management and Practice* 6: vi–x.

Healton, C. G., ed. 1999. "Research Linkages between Academia and Public Health Practice, 1999." *Supplement to American Journal of Preventive Medicine* 16: 1–132.

Institute of Medicine, The Committee for the Study of the Future of Public Health. 1988. *The Future of Public Health.* Washington, DC: National Academy Press.

Lasker, R. 1997. *Medicine and Public Health: The Power of Collaboration.* New York: New York Academy of Medicine.

Public Health Foundation. 1998. Minutes of the November 19, 1998, meeting of the Council on Linkages between Academia and Public Health Practice. Washington, DC.

———. 1999. Minutes of the March 17, 1999, meeting of the Council on Linkages between Academia and Public Health Practice. Washington, DC.

Reiser, S. J. 1996. "Medicine and Public Health: Pursuing a Common Destiny." *Journal of the American Medical Association* 276: 1429–30.

Seifer, S. D. 1998. "Community-Campus Partnerships for Health." *The Link (Quarterly Bulletin of the Council on Linkages between Academia and Public Health Practice)* 12: 3, 7.

Sorensen, A. A., and R. G. Bialek. 1993. *The Public Health Faculty/Agency Forum: Linking Graduate Education and Practice.* Gainesville: Florida University Press.

US Department of Health and Human Services, Public Health Service. 1995. *Public Health in America.* Report of the Public Health Functions Steering Committee. Washington, DC: Dept. of Health and Human Services.

———. 1997. *The Public Health Workforce: An Agenda for the 21st Century.* Report of the Public Health Functions Project. Washington, DC: Dept. of Health and Human Services.

Zaza, S., et al. 2000. "Scope and Organization of the Guide to Community Preventive Services." *Supplement to American Journal of Preventive Medicine* 18: 27–34.

16 Partnerships for Community Health Care in West Virginia

John C. Pearson and Henry G. Taylor

In West Virginia, there is a long tradition of feeling isolated from the rest of the country, requiring a level of self-reliance and, in health, attention to the unique epidemiology of the population. Following the models of community care pioneered earlier this century, a three-way partnership between government, universities, and receptive communities established a network of 120 community-run clinics, supported by a wide range of services developed in the Department of Community Medicine and sustained by state funding and staff. The strong commitment of academic teaching to community exposure and development of innovative adaptations of technologies to meet community needs has ensured a supply of appropriately trained professionals to run the health services and to collaborate in a constantly evolving system of care responding to epidemiologically demonstrated needs.

—Gail Price

Early writings about community-oriented primary care (COPC) emphasize the fundamental nature of effective collaborations between providers and the community. Sidel and Sidel (1984) cite the Peckham experiment in London, with its community board and physical exams on entry to all patients to document the health status of the population, as the first community-based clinic. Pholela's dramatic success in South Africa stemmed from the effective partnership that developed between academic professionals and the various communities they served (Tollman 1994). Sidney Kark and Joseph Abramson also emphasized the pivotal role of the community as they applied their South African experience to Israel. Jack Geiger and John Hatch in Mound Bayou, Mississippi, and Eva Salber and Benjamin Paul at the University of North Carolina, Chapel Hill, introduced the principles of COPC to the United States in the late 1950s and early 1960s. Epidemiological and analytical tools used for community diagnosis became such a powerful part of planning any community health intervention that the central role of the community became overshadowed, if not entirely forgotten.

As Geiger institutionalized his work during Lyndon B. Johnson's War on Poverty, community members held a mandatory majority on the governing boards for neighborhood health centers. They had to approve decisions, but the degree of true empowerment and control was variable. The COPC Toolkit developed by Nutting (1990) included some chapters on community involvement. However, the literature of the time still reflected a bias that external experts and government programs knew best how to implement community change. The teaching of COPC concepts is required for federal funding of primary care residencies; however, there has been minimal community-based training.

Participants in the COPC National Rural Demonstration Project from 1988 to 1991 (Rhyne et al. 1998) were sharply divided over whether "COPC" emphasized the *community orientation* of primary care (COpc), or the way in which *primary care* practices could become more community oriented (coPC). Both points of view were elegantly balanced in the modified conceptual model that the University of New Mexico developed to summarize the project (see Figure 1).

This model clearly places the community in the center of the diagram but surrounds it with Nutting's four steps. Despite the differences, the literature is clear that all five concepts are required for effective COPC practice.

West Virginia is an example of a community-oriented health and health care organization. The partnership in this endeavor includes the governor, the legislature, academia, nonprofit organizations, and members of the public, communicating together and identifying priorities for action to improve health and health care.

A rural mountainous state, West Virginia effectively used the federal effort to support health care in Appalachia. Many health and social service projects of the Appalachian Regional Commission, the Robert

FIGURE I

University of New Mexico COPC Model

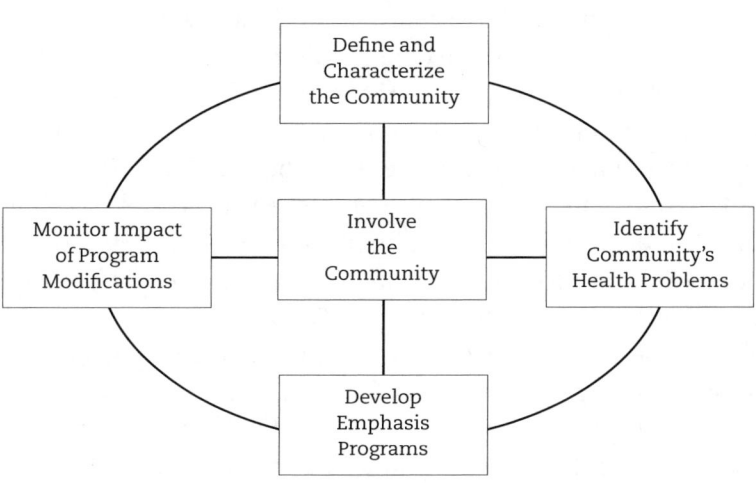

Source: Adapted from Rhyne et al. 1998, 12.

Wood Johnson Foundation, and others addressed critical human needs in this chronically distressed area of the United States. A three-way partnership between communities, universities, and government has sustained successful projects for over 30 years. Six clinics were developed by the United Mine Workers of America in the late 1960s. The New River Family Health Center was then formed as part of the Robert Wood Johnson Rural Practice Project in the early 1970s. Strong community boards worked with the foundation to recruit and sustain community clinics run by teams of local staff, family practice physicians, nurse practitioners, and highly trained administrators. Health services researchers at the University of North Carolina, Chapel Hill (UNC), rapidly translated their research findings into a series of manuals.

Seeing the success of these pilot projects, the state of West Virginia contracted with the newly formed Department of Community Medicine at West Virginia University to extend and support the model in receptive communities throughout the state. The legislature appropriated funds for rural health centers, allowing diversification and modification based on community needs. For more than a dozen years, the University provided technical and management assistance to extend the success of the first two pilot sites to what became a stable network of 63 community-run clinics. Thirty years later, the system has grown to encompass over 120 sites.

Community boards guide and direct operations, while state government provides technical assistance and regulatory oversight for millions of dollars of state and federal funds given as direct grants, cost-based reimbursements, and support for indigent care. Legislative initiatives to improve rural obstetric care, home visitation for first-born infants, enhanced recruitment for the Children's Health Insurance Program, and a network of comprehensive school-based health centers are deployed through a stable administrative structure with tight controls on accountability and cost. Other innovations in rural health education rest on this solid foundation.

The prime example at the present time is the production of the Healthy West Virginia Objectives for 2010 (West Virginia Bureau for Public Health 2001). Three hundred individuals from these constituencies worked together in committees to produce 29 chapters and

190 objectives to be reached by the year 2010. Each of these objectives has measured baseline data and planned outcomes that are realistically reachable. The report includes an innovative chapter on end-of-life care. Money to achieve these objectives has been allocated, with the top priority being to reduce the alarming frequency of smoking during pregnancy.

A very important component in achieving changes is the West Virginia University Health Sciences Center. The University, a public institution with faculty paid from state funds, is the land grant university for the state with responsibility for service to the state, and is also the research university for the state. At West Virginia University when the Department of Community Medicine was established, its responsibility was defined as service to the state through education, research, and collaboration in health planning. Activities of the Department over the years include:

- working with communities in rural areas to help them open primary care clinics, recruit staff for them, and support their management. Sixty-three clinics have been opened in this way, each a little different depending on local circumstances. The Bureau for Public Health has since taken over this role, and 120 rural sites now provide a high proportion of the rural primary care in the state.
- preparing for the development of a chain of small physical rehabilitation hospitals at key points in the state. The Bureau for Public Health supervises the implementation of this plan.
- responding to a request from the Bureau for Public Health; a departmental member was seconded to devise a Medicaid reimbursement system for nursing homes.
- taking over responsibility for the West Virginia census so that it could link demographic data with plans for epidemiological studies. This link enabled the Department to use data on the possession of cars and telephones, for example, to identify pockets of rural deprivation.
- obtaining a Prevention Research Center grant to study not only West Virginia but all of Appalachia.

- establishing a Center on Rural Aging, which conducts educational programs, research, and service activities in the state. It is also sponsored by the United Nations and WHO.
- establishing a Health Policy Center that advises state government through research and consultation.
- offering degree programs in public health (MPH) and community health promotion; an occupational medicine residency program has close research and service relationships with the state's Workers' Compensation department. Community boards supervise all of these programs.
- fostering wellness programs throughout the state at many levels: in communities by writing the first PATCH (Planned Approach to Community Health) grant, by serving on the board of the West Virginia Wellness Council for businesses, and by setting up a wellness center for university faculty, staff, and students. In addition, the State Health Education Council, a forum for health educators in the health professions, was started and for many years staffed by the Department before being taken over by the Bureau for Public Health; this is a very robust organization.
- researching causes of high infant mortality, both neonatal and postneonatal, which has resulted in combined interventions by the state, communities, and the University.
- consulting with community committees of the Bureau for Public Health, which has resulted in improved registries for cancer and infectious diseases.

In addition to participating in such departmental and Bureau for Public Health activities, the Health Sciences Center provides a wide range of services essential to the health of the community:

- The Emergency Medicine Department has a research center (CREM) and not only offers training to emergency personnel statewide but also serves as the state telephone nerve center. This Department is consulted on priorities for expenditures to improve services.

- The MARS telephone service puts community physicians, physician's assistants, and nurse practitioners in quick contact with specialists for advice and consultation. There have been 30,000 calls to date. There is also a Visiting Clinician Program, which enables community physicians to spend days on campus with consultants of their choice.
- The MDTV two-way audiovisual connection between 20 hospitals and clinics statewide offers consultations (more than 3,000 to date) and educational programs (grand rounds and university courses and conferences). The service is currently being extended to the prisons to avoid the transportation of prisoners for clinic visits.
- The Obstetrics Department provides two of the three hubs for high-risk pregnancies, and transports mothers and newborns by ambulance and helicopter. A study has shown that no babies were lost because of a failure of the system during one entire year. This Department also operates the Birth Score Program, which identifies babies at risk for problems in the post-neonatal period and alerts local health departments to initiate follow-up.
- The Poison Control Center for the state responds to calls from both the public and health professionals.
- The Cancer Information Center responds to calls from the public and professionals not only statewide but also in other states.
- Traveling clinics have been operating for many years in the larger cities in the state on a regular monthly or bimonthly basis for patients with tuberculosis and children with congenital heart disease. The latter service has been extended to conducting screening in several rural counties to identify elevated cholesterol levels in schoolchildren (and their parents, if indicated) and to offer advice for its reduction.
- TV and radio programs, led by the Vice-President for Health Sciences, are broadcast weekly on public stations.

In addition to these piecemeal approaches, there are two unique collaborative programs that originated in the department of Community

Medicine but which quickly outstripped the local resources of personnel. They are major statewide efforts that involve large groups of individuals in all walks of life.

The first is the Rural Health Education Program (RHEP). This began with a grant from the Kellogg Foundation, which the then-governor played an important role in obtaining. He persuaded the state legislature to make this an ongoing line item—currently $7.5 million a year—in the budget. Forty-seven of the 55 counties, all rural and underserved medically, participate in 13 training consortiums of health, social, and education agencies. Each consortium is locally governed, with representation from clinics, hospitals, health departments, nursing homes, pharmacies, schools, and welfare agencies. Of the annual budget for the program, $3 million goes to these local consortiums to fund local faculty, staff, and administration, learning resource centers, and the housing of students. The remainder of the money goes to administer the programs at the seven health professions teaching institutions (West Virginia and Marshall University medical and nursing schools, the West Virginia Osteopathic medical school, and West Virginia University's schools of pharmacy and dentistry).

The purpose of this program is to expose health professions students in the state to a combined experience in health care practice in rural areas over a three-month period during the later part of their training, in the hope of demystifying rural practice and encouraging them to work in rural areas. Even if they do not so choose, they will at least have had the chance to understand the problems, difficulties, and pleasures of such practice. The time is spent 80% in appropriate clinical experience, and 20% in combined activities in service, research, or community and school education.

The field faculty number 473 in all available health professions, and each year over 1,000 students participate, spending some 5,500 weeks in the communities, and reaching 150,000 rural citizens. To date, 88 physicians, 55 dentists, 54 nurse practitioners, 14 dental hygienists, and 12 physical therapists from the program have settled in rural practice.

The 18 learning centers have textbooks, audiovisual equipment, and computer workstations with e-mail, Internet access, on-line search databases, and relevant software programs. Ten of the 18 are also connected to MDTV and the universities for consultations, educational programs, and meetings. All 18 have satellite downlinks that provide other educational offerings.

The second innovative program is the Health Services Training Activity (HSTA). This is a program to encourage disadvantaged students in grades 8 through 12 to consider a career in a health profession. Twenty-one counties participate, with 50 schools, 62 teachers, and some 600 students. The teachers spend time in the Health Sciences Center to understand the range of opportunities and then have their students conduct a community or laboratory project during the school year. In the summer, the students spend two weeks at the Health Sciences Center, touring the facilities and attending lectures. The program focuses on rural and disadvantaged students and emphasizes problem solving. The program has appeal in some African countries and will apparently be taken up there. The University initiated the program, but it is run by a board with a majority of community members. Parents, teachers, and students also run local governing boards.

In summary, the level of collaboration to improve health and health care in West Virginia is high. It comes not only from state government and universities but also from practicing health professionals, researchers, teachers, students, business executives, nonprofit organizations, and interested members of the community from none of these backgrounds.

This unique collaborative relationship has succeeded through the perseverance of individuals and organizations too numerous to credit here. Our collective experience suggests that the following principles sustain our long-term efforts:

- The trust and confidence in a common vision allowed us to effectively challenge each other as difficulties arose.
- Our history of shared successes allowed continued communication to overcome barriers.
- Synergies have been fostered by change and information sharing at four levels: (1) individual growth and development, (2) social networks (which can be both supportive and otherwise), (3) organizational capacity and leadership, and (4) community-wide collaboration, ranging from social gatherings to political rallies.

- All participants must focus on analyzing their performance towards mutual goals.
- The emphasis needs to be on achieving *equity of outcomes,* not merely *equality of access.* Equity demands the strategic alignment of limited resources to truly serve those in greatest need.
- Most importantly, we have found that planning has an inherent value. Effective strategic plans are not static documents but collaborative learning activities.
- We have come to an understanding that people and communities change best through groups and group processes.
- In Healthy People 2010, coalitions have been an important tool. To paraphrase Roz Lasker's definition of a coalition (Lasker 1998): it is when a group of people work together towards a common goal, but they all know they cannot get there on their own.
- The first step towards being an effective partner is realizing who we are, what our own agenda is, and trusting others to help us along the way.

In clinical care, the quality of the doctor-patient relationship clearly enhances healing and speeds recovery. When our focus shifts to "treating the community as our patient," caring relationships become even more important. Rarely, an Albert Schweitzer or a beloved country doctor succeeds through sheer charisma. Sometimes, hospitals or other health care organizations earn a level of community trust and respect. Sustaining such relationships, however, presents even the most dedicated with a continuing enormous challenge.

REFERENCES AND RESOURCES

Kark, Sidney L. 1981. *The Practice of Community-Oriented Primary Care.* New York : Appleton-Century-Crofts.

Lasker, Roz D. 1998. *Medicine and Public Health: The Power of Collaboration. With the Committee on Medicine and Public Health.* Chicago: Health Administration Press.

Madison, Donald L. 1980. "Starting out in Rural Practice: The Rural Practice Project—Report of the Director." Dept. of Social and Administrative

Medicine, School of Medicine. Chapel Hill: University of North Carolina.

Nutting, Paul A. 1990. *Community-Oriented Primary Care: From Principle to Practice.* Albuquerque: University of New Mexico Press.

Pearce, I. H., and L. H. Crocker. 1943. *The Peckham Experiment: A Study in the Living Structure of Society.* London: Allen and Unwin.

Rhyne, Robert, et al. 1998. *Community-Oriented Primary Care: Health Care for the 21st Century.* Washington, DC: American Public Health Association.

Sidel, Victor W., and Ruth Sidel, eds. 1984. *Reforming Medicine: Lessons from the Last Quarter Century.* New York: Pantheon Books, chapter 1.

Tollman, S. M. 1994. "The Pholela Health Centre: The Origins of Community-Oriented Primary Health Care (COPC)." *South African Medical Journal* 84: 653–58.

West Virginia Bureau for Public Health. 2001. *West Virginia Healthy People 2010.* www.wvdhhr.org/bph/hp2010/objective/contents.html. [Cited July 3, 2001.]

17 Community Mental Health: The German Experience

Niels Pörksen

The author of this chapter played a significant role in modernizing psychiatric services in Germany, transforming them from an archaic system of institution-based custodial care to the modern day decentralized system of community-based programs. The current emphasis is on preventing as well as treating acute and chronic episodes of mental illness through social support services offered in outpatient settings. This transition holds important lessons for developing countries as well as rich countries; in both, mental health is an increasingly evident need in all communities.

—*Gail Price*

T here is no community-based health care without mental health care. The development of community mental health services in Germany reflects this necessary integration.

My first contact with the Harvard School of Public Health in 1962 was in northern India, at Ludhiana Medical College, where I first encountered the concept of community medicine. As an inexperienced young resident, I had been asked to write a report for the German Protestant Church, which had stopped funding the Medical College. The American president of the college had resigned. He had wanted to establish highest American standards, while the Indian government as well as the staff wanted basic community medicine for the people in India. A research team from the Harvard School of Public Health supported me in writing my report in favor of public health concepts.

The 1960s were also a period of energetic development of the Mental Health Movement (National Institute of Mental Health 1966) in the United States. During my one-year stay at the Laboratory of Community Psychiatry at Harvard Medical School in 1967–68, I was influenced by the concepts of preventive psychiatry and mental health consultation emerging from the work of Erich Lindemann (1963) and Gerald Caplan (1964). Caplan's *Principles of Preventive Psychiatry* became our guide.

After my return to Germany, I got the chance to establish the department of Community Psychiatry and Mental Health Consultation at the Central Institute of Mental Health, which worked under the auspices of the University of Heidelberg. One fine day in 1970, Dr. Joan Altekruse showed up in her old, brightly colored Buick. She became an important member of our multidisciplinary team. The team included members trained in adult and child psychiatry, psychiatric nursing, public health, social work, and psychology. Young professionals and graduate students from education, administration, and medicine rotated through the different fields of the service.

Idealistic notions propagated by the American Mental Health Movement led us to assume that *primary preventive principles,* infused into the health, education, and social service system, would prevent or significantly diminish vulnerability to psychiatric illness in the population. Although that premise was overly optimistic, it had the favorable effect of embedding public health philosophy in our design. It solidified the intent to focus on the community as our client, emphasize prevention, and integrate mental health consultation practice (Caplan 1970) into the general health and social systems of the defined population served.

This ethos carried over into our basic activities. We provided consultations for the staff of the city welfare department, government-subsidized housing projects, and organizations providing shelter for the homeless. We fostered neighborhood initiatives and community programs, particularly in economically disadvantaged and physically rundown areas. We developed and supported social and service clubs for individuals discharged from hospitals and for the chronically mentally ill. In cooperation with a nonprofit student organization, we established a large self-help organization for alcoholics. In sum, we "interfered in community social politics" (Pörksen 1974), encouraging new ways of engaging people in an improved mental health environment.

We were successful in the service delivery aspects of our work. But we became less and less appreciated by local politicians, who were afraid to change classical patterns of psychiatric care. After 1968, they feared our social change initiative even more. The mayor and some heads of the city health and social service departments disliked our interference in their territory. The University of Heidelberg, to which our Institute reported, preferred to dissociate itself from the politics of social change in an attempt to maintain scientific neutrality. My supervisor, the leader of the Central Institute, feared for his own scientific reputation and forced me out. After I left, I wrote a book about the Mannheim model (Pörksen 1974), and the department changed direction.

Apart from our endeavors, German psychiatry 30 years ago was still very traditional. Only 20 years earlier, the Nazi regime had killed more than 100,000 psychiatric and handicapped patients and forcibly sterilized more than 400,000. After World War II, traditional psychiatry was re-established. The major intervention was custodial care in large institutions. Programs for outpatient care did not exist. Psychotherapy was limited. The time had not yet come to put ideas of primary prevention and mental health consultation into practice.

Happily, however, we were not far from an important turning point. In the early 1970s, pressured by a small group of community and social psychiatrists, the German Parliament set up a national commission to study and reorganize psychiatric services in Germany. I became part of that commission. We learned a lot by looking into the changes that had taken place in American and Western European psychiatric service systems. De-institutionalization and decentralization of psychiatric clinical and outpatient services evolved. Community-based services for the chronically mentally ill and for alcoholics had to be established. As a result of the work of this national commission, the government set up a national program to establish community psychiatry in all regions in 1975 ("Bericht zur Lage der Psychiatrie" 1975, Aktion Psychisch Kranke 1988).

Let me give you an example of these changes: In the early 1980s, I became responsible for a large, church-run institution in Bielefeld, a city of some 300,000 inhabitants. I was hired to reform the institution, which hosted more than 1,000 psychiatric patients from all over Germany. To create a community-based, comprehensive psychiatric service, we:

- converted a hospital with more than 250 beds and an average stay of six weeks into a community psychiatric treatment service with an inpatient program and five day-hospitals in the city;
- initiated a large outpatient program for all the groups for which we were responsible: general psychiatric patients, geronto-psychiatric patients, and alcohol- and drug-addicted persons. In Germany, the health insurance system, to which almost everyone belongs, covers all the expenses of treatment for these groups;
- established a large dehospitalization program for more than 700 patients. Some were sent to their hometowns; most were moved to small sheltered housing in Bielefeld. This program was accompanied by a large dehospitalization research project

by the Public Health Faculty of Bielefeld University. This faculty grew out of the Department of Sociology, not Medicine.

- established a community-based, comprehensive psychiatric service program responsible for the care of all chronically ill psychiatric patients in the community. It includes programs for coping with daily life, day care centers, and sheltered working conditions. The community pays for living expenses and professional care, the State for all institutional services, such as day centers or residential care.

- set up, with the community, a 24-hour crisis intervention program, a primary health care program, called Street Med (a minibus with basic medical equipment, a general practitioner, and a nurse), and a comprehensive care program for chronic alcoholics, the homeless, and the drug addicted.

A mental health board and a city steering committee are responsible for comprehensive care in the community. After a full service program for all psychiatric patients in the community was established, it became possible to restart mental health consultation and public health-oriented projects.

What we learned from the Bielefeld experience was: you have to do your own professional job, even the most difficult one, before you go out and advise other social or health service organizations. And we learned another lesson: Until 2000, our basic social service and health care system was functioning and health insurance covered full- or part-time hospitalization. The new health service law in 2000 introduced diagnosis-related group (DRG) systems for hospital payment, but not in psychiatry. In psychiatry, we have a different system for hospital payment for all patient groups: general psychiatry, gerontopsychiatry, and alcohol and drug addiction in six different groups: intensive care, regular treatment, rehabilitative treatment, long-term treatment (one year or more), psychotherapy, and day treatment. The staff decides, within defined periods, how many patients are treated in which groups. A control commission from the insurance company is allowed to examine the data. In other words, the system works so well that the new law has reaffirmed it (Kunze and Kaltenbach 1994 and "Gesetz zur Reform" 2000).

Outpatient treatment is covered by psychiatrists in practice within a managed care system, and hospitals are allowed to establish multiprofessional outpatient treatment services for the expensive care of chronically ill patients. While the communities are responsible for community care programs for chronically ill patients, the State pays for residential care.

I hope that Germany will retain this system of comprehensive treatment and care for all psychiatric patients rather than adopt other managed care systems or health maintenance organizations. Mental health for all, and adequate treatment and care for everyone in need, are still the best way of promoting public health.

Nowadays, communities and their local governments are taking the responsibility for planning, operating, and coordinating the psychiatric service system for chronically ill patients and for crisis intervention. They have recently started to enter into contracts with organizations for the homeless and the psychiatric service systems in order to implement comprehensive services for chronic alcoholics and psychiatric patients in the community. The local governments require contracts with all organizations working with chronically mentally ill patients in the communities to secure comprehensive care. They also compel the small and highly selective programs for young people with problems to participate in comprehensive and integrated services.

The Ministry of Health supports programs to initiate comprehensive care programs in community psychiatry. In addition, in May 2000 the Ministry of Labor and Welfare set up a three-year initiative to organize a program for jobs and sheltered working facilities for all people with mental and alcohol problems in the country. The idea is not to have just a variety of nice little programs, but to establish solutions to the work problems of all people with chronic mental illnesses ("Bestandaufnahme zur Rehabilitation" 2000).

SUMMARY

Now, 25 years after the beginning of the reform process, German psychiatry has been professionalized. Community-based psychiatric services have been established, and most chronically mentally ill patients live in the community. Public health concepts and practices have been integrated into German psychiatric care as part of a professionalization process that emphasized preventive and population-directed psychiatry. At the same time, administrative reorganization mandated and supported these goals through the national health system. Other ministries and local service departments now collaborate in providing a widened range of comprehensive services—social, educational, occupational, and recreational—to meet the needs of defined populations within their own communities. Organizational plans are created and implemented by individuals who represent the interests and priorities of the area's population. While traditional, institutionally based psychiatrists are slow to join these efforts, wide support and active involvement come from community representatives, patients, and family-organized support groups, and from departments and individuals in municipal offices, state agencies, national ministries, and a few progressive academic programs. Those coalitions are nurtured and enhanced by committed multidisciplinary colleagues, who make up a strong advocacy group as members of the German Association for Social and Community Psychiatry.

It is disappointing, however, that the theory and practice of community psychiatry in Germany in the medical field and within the social service system at the community, state, and federal government levels are not part of the scientific world and of the professional psychiatric associations. The Aktion Psychisch Kranke reviewed the development and perspectives of the last 25 years in German psychiatry (1999 and 2001). Its findings were: Germany reached a high standard in community-based psychiatric services, although there is a lack of coordination between services and case management, and problems with supervision and quality.

We have confidence that community mental health programs can provide effective interventions. We are encouraged to proceed with both vigor and vigilance, aware that ongoing assessment of the content, quality, and efficiency of our work will ultimately be validated by measures of improved mental health status of the people and the communities we serve.

REFERENCES

Aktion Psychisch Kranke. 1988. "Empfehlungen der Expertenkommission der Bundesregierung zur Reform der Psychiatrie in der Bundesrepublik." Bonn: Bundesministerium Jugend, Familie, Frauen und Gesundheit.

———. 1999. *Qualität und Steuerung in der Psychiatrischen Versorgung.* Cologne: Rheinland Verlag.

———. 2001. *25 Jahre Psychiatrie-Enquête.* Bonn: Psychiatrie Verlag.

"Bericht zur Lage der Psychiatrie in der Bundesrepublik Deutschland." 1975. Deutscher Bundestag 7/4200.

"Bestandaufnahme zur Rehabilitation Psychisch Kranker in der Bundesrepublik durch die Aktion Psychisch Kranke." 2000. Bonn: Bundesministerium für Arbeit und Sozialordnung.

Caplan, Gerald. 1964. *Principles of Preventive Psychiatry.* New York: Basic Books.

———. 1970. *The Theory and Practice of Mental Health Consultation.* New York: Basic Books.

"Gesetz zur Reform der gesetzlichen Krankenversicherung." 2000. Deutscher Bundestag Drucksache 14/1977.

Kunze, H., and L. Kaltenbach. 1994. *Psychiatrie Personalverordnung.* 2d ed. Stuttgart: Kohlhammer-Verlag.

Lindemann, Erich. 1963. "Mental Health and the Environment." In *The Urban Condition,* ed. L. D. Duhl. New York: Basic Books, pp. 3–10.

National Institute of Mental Health. 1966. *Essential Services of the Community Mental Health Center: Consultation and Education.* Bethesda, MD: NIMH, pp. 4–5.

Pörksen, Niels. 1974. *Kommunale Psychiatrie: Das Mannheimer Modell.* Reinbek: Rowohlt Verlag.

Conclusion: Toward the Next Alma-Ata

Primary health care (PHC) has been called by so many names in an effort to emphasize its different elements that it serves little purpose to attempt to choose the one that is most appropriate. Surely it is more than primary medical care—all agree on the importance of social factors and the primacy of prevention—hence preventive and social medicine. Recognizing the importance of involvement of clients, the term community is often added: community medicine at first, then community-oriented and, more recently, community-based primary care. Whatever term we choose, the elements of prevention, promotion, curative care, rehabilitation, social and behavioral factors, orientation to defined populations, and their involvement in the design and implementation are all agreed components of PHC.

Since Alma-Ata, elements of sustainable human development have also been added, with concerns particularly for the poor to enlarge their choices and opportunities as well as their participation in decisions. James Speth of the United Nations Development Program has described sustainable human development as "development that is pro poor, pro nature, pro jobs, pro democracy, pro women and pro children." Additionally, the concept of equity—not only more equal sharing, but also raising the "bottom" to normative levels of decency in living, even at greater cost—is critical to the distributional concept of PHC. More than simply equality of access, equity embraces distribution of health outcomes, efficiency in the management and allocation of resources, and accountability to the public for their use. Unfortunately, the recent attention of WHO to measures of the burden of illness, to health system performance, and to the cost of health care seem to pay little attention to fundamental elements of PHC based in communities and addressing the many determinants of health outside of medicine.

No doubt health services must deal with the proximate causes of ill health, while intersectoral activities deal more with the distal or indirect causes. There is a real question about how far the health system can go in addressing these indirect causes. Poverty, food insecurity, illiteracy, and social prejudices against various groups, especially women, have an enormous influence on health yet are based on social, cultural, and environmental factors outside the normal purview of health staff. Yet Amartya Sen reminds us that health is the ultimate outcome of inputs aimed at improving or maintaining the quality of life. Thus, it could be said that it is incumbent on health personnel to lead the attack against these more basic problems and advocate for their solution so that health can be achieved.

A central lesson that emerges from the history of PHC is the critical role of leadership, at all levels. Most often attributed to an individual, dedicated leadership seems particularly important given the complexity and social and cultural foundations of PHC. Many projects are directed by doctors, whose initial acceptability in the community may be facilitated through their technical skills. But real leaders are characterized by cultural sensitivity, a vision that is well articulated and widely embraced, a dedication to serving the needs of all—particularly the poorest and most marginalized—commitment to working in a team, and responsiveness to dialogue with the people they are serving. No doubt, leaders must make good technical choices and sound financial decisions to enable sustainability of a project but they must nurture in all participants a sense of belonging, responsibility, motivation and pride. Most of all leaders care, and are seen to care for all. Compassion is central to their success.

These same leaders are often unable to manage large-scale expansion of successful, local PHC projects. More than charisma and caring, expansion requires management and delegation. The leadership of BRAC follows the management principles of large responsible corporations. BRAC is led by an accountant, while leadership in Indonesia's *posyandu* system came from a nationwide family planning organization headed by a social scientist, who successfully developed a team approach extending down to the community. Too often doctors find compromise for the greater good incompatible with their medical ethics. Standard medical models are frequently not affordable or even required. Some doctors find it hard to relinquish control and to respect the capacity of nonmedical personnel, particularly community volunteers, to carry out simple but critical tasks at the community level. Herein lies the strength of Indonesia's posyandu system, where volunteer women weigh and accurately plot the growth of children each month, determine who needs immunization, and administer simple medications for common illness. In Roxbury, only a few kilometers from the symposium site, community volunteers are far more effective than professional social workers in reaching into homes and dealing with the most fundamental cause of ill health: domestic violence. Good leadership requires good tradeoffs.

Leaders need to nurture participation and accept the involvement of people with diverse talents in meeting health needs. Important characteristics of leaders that cannot be measured were highlighted in Jamkhed, where the quality of leadership was more important than the quality of health technology, although the importance of good hospital-based medical care was critical to the success and credibility of the entire PHC system developed by the Aroles. The role of leadership is nowhere more obvious than in large international organizations such as WHO and UNICEF. One need only recall the decline in influence and effectiveness of these global agencies following the departure of Halfdan Mahler and James Grant to see how critical inspired leadership is to an entire system devoted to "health for all."

Like politics, all health is local and leaders need to dialogue, listen, and adapt to local realities. Leadership begins to expand when a critical number of community members extend caring beyond themselves to the entire community and achieve an effective and equitable system. This lesson emerged from years of community preparatory work in

Chakaria, Bangladesh; the Bolivian altiplano; and Tibet. Local leaders are a key to sustainability.

Finally the vision: envisioning a system that works and is responsive seems critical to successful PHC projects. Whether in the United States or poor countries, it is a key role of leaders to articulate, facilitate, and spread that vision. In essence, it is the belief in health for all that must precede its realization. Colin McCord pointed out at the symposium in Boston that vision itself will carry some ideas widely, scaling them up even without a system to do so. When people have a vision of a better life and have been empowered to know that it is possible, some ideas spread even without a formal system.

How then do we create leaders for PHC? Missionary zeal, be it religious or otherwise, is not generally taught or nurtured. But experience in the community, working with a team, and exposure to inspiring mentors do much to encourage those with an innate ability and motivation. Medical curricula all too often support a medical model, leaving the graduate devoid of many required skills for leadership in PHC. The Rockefeller Foundation has attempted to establish comprehensive long-term programs in medical schools to provide students with managerial, team-building, epidemiological, analytical, and presentation skills and experience in a real community that will attract them to PHC programs. Foundation efforts developed useful models in Brazil, Colombia, India, Indonesia, Nigeria, the Philippines, and Thailand, but they were all too often supplanted by clinical medical concerns soon after the Foundation staff departed. Like community-based PHC programs themselves, the training of new leaders requires inspiring leaders as role models. Many of the symposium participants have spent a lifetime doing just that!

The second common finding about successful community-based programs was the importance of objective information and the role of measurement in motivating and sustaining the programs. Starting with the pioneering work of John Gordon in tracking streptococcal infections in Romania, household-based information systems for understanding the dynamics of health in a defined population have been central to effective PHC interventions. This effort was extended with John Wyon in the Khanna Study in India, where monthly household surveillance provided valuable insights not only into fertility determinants and use of contraceptives, but also into risk factors for mortality, especially among the young. These approaches were adapted in the Matlab field surveillance area of Bangladesh by the Cholera Laboratory—now the International Centre for Diarrhoeal Disease Research, Bangladesh (ICDDR,B)—and have provided numerous insights into population dynamics, public health determinants, and service efficacy over the past four decades.

Sound epidemiologic studies are often needed to choose appropriate health technologies in order to adapt and apply these technologies in ways that are both acceptable and sustainable. The tetanus control efforts in Haiti and nutritional Mothercraft centers are models of such informed adaptation. The information needed for planning is often best gathered by the community members themselves, so they can establish their own priorities, make informed choices about system design, and identify all members of the population to be served. Equally important, when communities gather the information, they believe in it and the results that emerge from its use. Moreover, they can then measure progress and see improvement objectively. A system without ongoing monitoring rapidly loses its way. Defining a population, enumerating families, tracking clients, and ensuring that no one is left out provide a sense of community pride and caring. This was repeatedly illustrated during the symposium: from the house-to-house training in oral rehydration therapy of BRAC to the individual records for an entire community pioneered by the Mayo Clinic, from the individual growth cards in Haiti to Indonesian posyandus that measure children and motivate mothers to improve nutrition. Information on each family, aggregated to reflect the health status and risk factors of communities, is central to successful PHC. Information on costs and benefits provides justification both to those who fund services and to those who use them, whether it be a huge campaign such as global polio eradication or local food used to rehabilitate a malnourished child. The information system itself must be affordable in order to be sustainable and continue to provide useful guidance.

The simplest information system was described in the Soldiers for Health intervention in Roxbury, a neighborhood of Boston, where the "cries from behind closed doors" were considered an adequate indicator of the need for direct intervention. The posyandu system in Indonesia collects and publicly posts data on the number of children weighed and those not gaining weight each month, thereby identifying those most in need of intervention at home and stimulating community action to improve child growth. The EPI cluster survey pioneered by WHO and used in most countries throughout the world has proven a critical motivating tool for field workers, as well as ensuring the distributive equity of PHC by showing which communities are fully immunized and which are not. The interesting simplified lot quality assurance sampling method developed in Nepal (chapter 9) is a lovely example of how sophisticated statistical techniques can be used by community members to improve PHC performance and coverage.

Interestingly, the role of research in the design and support of community-based PHC often emerged from the discussion. Research can make key contributions to the success of PHC not only by adapting advances in medical knowledge and technology that can be applied in PHC settings, such as vaccines, oral rehydration, contraceptives, and the newer medicines for tuberculosis, but also by inquiring into how things can work in a given sociocultural setting. Projects in Bangladesh have benefited from close collaboration with the ICDDR,B, which has not only developed important lifesaving technologies like oral rehydration therapy for widespread application, but also has a highly responsive operational research division that pioneered approaches to family planning services in remote villages, affordable nutritional interventions, and adaptations of diagnostic and therapeutic protocols that placed treatment reliably in the hands of illiterate workers. Virtually all effective PHC projects discover new methods and solve problems through well-designed applied research inquiries.

The role of universities and research institutes is therefore highly appropriate in a PHC setting. Such partnerships have contributed to program design and feedback and have supported funding requests and expansion of pilot projects to larger populations. When research institutions take on the responsibility for generating knowledge and refining its practical implementation, their teaching environment contributes to equity and distributive justice as well as to quality of care and efficiency. When institutions accept responsibility for defined populations, such as those of the ICCDR,B, Mayo Clinic, Parkland Hospital, or Hôpital Albert Schweitzer in Haiti, with a denominator comprising all individuals and families captured in an information system, the impact of health services and other determinants of health outcomes can be measured and articulated. BRAC has measured the effect of education and credit schemes on fertility and infant mortality rates, while the Mayo Clinic has determined many subtle risk factors for cardiac and degenerative disorders only through a carefully maintained record system. Simplified information systems used by the community themselves can be designed and validated by more sophisticated epidemiologic techniques. The broad involvement of social scientists and other academicians enhances the relevance of PHC research findings. And the health system develops more comprehensively with a full range of university disciplines brought to community-level inquiry.

The introduction of PHC often requires a careful choice of service mix at the outset, with phasing in of well-chosen technologies thereafter. Most projects, such as the small hospital at Jamkhed, begin with medical care for common or urgent conditions. Another example is the elimination of tetanus by vaccinating all women in Haiti, which solidified the acceptance of the Hôpital Albert Schweitzer by an often skeptical community. BRAC chose a focused approach to a prevalent and widely felt problem—the management of diarrhea in the home—as the first and only thing that a single NGO could afford to do to make a lasting impact on health in the entire nation. This "vertical" approach was at once affordable and time limited, and it established BRAC's bona fides in the health field. BRAC subsequently added layers of services as needs were identified, quantified, and costed. The organization provided immunization in partnership with government and other NGOs, trained local volunteers to support diagnosis and treatment of simple illnesses by algorithms, and developed a successful approach to the complex and demanding therapy of tuberculosis, a major killer of adults. Most of these efforts were funded by BRAC as operational research until a viable cost recovery scheme could be built into their design. Then they went to scale across the entire country.

Some propose getting close to the community for months or even years to enable them to measure and articulate more fundamental needs before ever starting health activities. In Chakaria, Bangladesh, workers exercised "restrained generosity," insisting that the community establish its own committees and discussions and a contractual relationship with government and private providers that they could afford. Carl and Henry Taylor provide examples where community self-surveys identified ecological concerns, access to credit, and agricultural issues as more important than medical interventions. James Grant's choice of the GOBI interventions (growth promotion, oral rehydration, breast-feeding, and immunization) was based on their availability, universality, and affordability. His emphasis on what mothers could do for themselves at home dominated the choice of interventions in all cases except immunization. Indonesian posyandus became viable only when it was realized that children could be weighed using a marketplace beam balance with a basket suspended from it, rather than a costly imported scale. In Jamkhed, age-old caste barriers were broken by siting new water points in the low-caste areas of the villages, with the help of a water diviner who collaborated in locating the "optimal sites" for drilling, invariably amid the low-caste shanties. Successful PHC efforts are replete with wise choices and careful tradeoffs.

But concern for the quality of medical services consistently seems to draw PHC back into larger clinics and buildings and to transfer service delivery to increasingly high levels of professionals. This concern pulls health care away from outreach services delivered in the home and prevents communities from taking responsibility for their own health. Outreach seems to be the first thing to be dropped in a financial crunch. The discontinuance of community health workers in many poor countries undergoing "structural adjustment" guided by international financial institutions is paralleled in the United States by cost-cutting measures in federally funded programs, measures that hit community outreach first and hardest. Cost recovery or containment all too often starts in PHC rather than in the expensive hospitals.

Community orientation, involvement, or actual control of PHC was a subject of debate throughout the symposium. While all agree that the community being served must be defined, understood, listened to, and respected, there is a range of opinions about the extent to which the community should control and own health services delivered under PHC programs. People feel cared for when those caring for them stop to listen, understand, assimilate their values, and consider cultural context. In violence-plagued homes in Roxbury, although government social services are available nearby, it is the intervention of women of the same social and cultural group that makes a real difference. The continuity of volunteer workers in Indonesian posyandus depends on a cultural pattern of community recognition and respect for those who serve community needs. Volunteers are rewarded by this recognition.

BRAC's programs, while highly uniform, consult regularly and continuously with communities to learn what works and how to make things better. Through universal coverage with a careful choice of technologies, BRAC ensures improved health outcomes along with efficiency in resource use, but to suggest that BRAC communities control the design and implementation of PHC is idealistic hyperbole. While quality and acceptability of services are not often measured per se, the outcomes of improved life expectancy, reduced malnutrition, and reduced fertility are the ultimate measures of quality. While there is a dialogue with users of services, there is a form of stewardship held by higher authorities in BRAC and in many other notably successful PHC programs, who figure prominently in the choice and implementation of health interventions.

In the United States, while community participation is readily seen as important, the more difficult question of community control was a matter of debate. Communities rarely control resources, and most decisions about health services require resources to implement. Furthermore, communities rarely speak with one voice; there is perhaps never a consensus. Determining what is true representation in a US community is a challenge. Thus, while the emphasis on community-directed and -controlled care is still the exception, the symposium illustrated universal consultation and responsiveness to community needs and efforts to be sure that community voices could be heard.

The importance of distributive goals in health was universally emphasized. While the richer countries emphasize "HEALTH for all," the emphasis of PHC is more on "health for ALL." Reaching everyone in need seems more important than the quality and responsiveness of services per se. The difference is important, but it is not a mutually exclusive dichotomy.

Alma-Ata urged health systems to address nonmedical factors as critical determinants of health. BRAC has measured the improvement in nutrition, reduction in fertility, and improved life expectancy in controlled trials involving families that participate in the BRAC credit, female literacy, and life skills programs. No doubt poverty remains the key determinant of ill health in poor and rich countries alike. In addressing fundamental poverty, bad housing, illiteracy, violence, and environmental deterioration, programs often remain fractionated among different agencies, with results equally fractionated and ineffective. Should or can health programs take on the job of trying to coordinate? Recognizing the important and powerful role of women's education and its effect on fertility, infant and child mortality, family nutrition, and other health parameters, one might even suggest that a greater health impact could be obtained by diverting health resources into better and more education for women. Such a reallocation of resources has yet to be tried or even costed.

While numerous smaller PHC projects have been successfully implemented around the world, the question of scaling up to cover large populations remains the most critical challenge. Quality suffers as contact with the community is sacrificed and the very elements at the heart of PHC success are often jeopardized in the effort to reach larger and larger populations. In India in the late 1970s, recognition of the success of the Jamkhed experiment in serving more than 200,000 people prompted the national government to adapt parts of this model in a nationwide campaign to train community health workers. What they neglected to recognize was the central role of leadership at several levels in the hospitals and supremely in the villages, and the principles that the Aroles progressively recognized and adopted of the critical linkage to an effective health referral system and the comprehensive approach to community development exemplified by Jamkhed initiatives in water supply, agriculture, small credit, and improved roads and housing. Half a million community health workers were recruited, trained, and sent back to their villages, but their effectiveness was limited and their duration of service brief. The system collapsed within a few years. While the Chinese Barefoot Doctors' system did become nationwide and was sustained for up to two decades, it too collapsed with the disappearance of communal farms and factories. Market forces are generally unkind to PHC! The posyandu system reaches into every village in Indonesia, but the recent financial austerity has placed even the support of a volunteer system in jeopardy.

Carl Taylor has written extensively on the strategy of scaling up successful village-based programs and believes that this can be done through an increasing expansion of demonstration and sharing of successful health projects between villagers and leaders. Of course, where government commitment is strongest, effective programs of community PHC have been enlarged with long-term sustainability guaranteed by tax revenues. The Cuban, Costa Rican, and Sri Lankan health care systems are excellent examples, along with the social health care systems of many European countries. The United States still lags considerably behind, with as many as 40 million people deprived of any regular system to meet even their medical needs, much less the broader scope of PHC.

The financing of PHC is the key element of sustainability in all countries. Chakaria proposes that the community expect nothing from outside and build services that its members can afford and its own resources can support. Ultimately, this may be the most sustainable approach, but it takes time and compromise in terms of health benefits forgone for the sake of self-reliance. Some health programs and institutions, like the Hôpital Albert Schweitzer in Haiti, can count on long-term outside assistance, which makes a quality system affordable, even sustainable, because of outside generosity in recognition of a well-designed, responsive program. All too often, however, outside help is limited in time and extent, and expectations can be raised beyond sustainable levels. Health projects linked to income production activities, as in BRAC, are unusual. More often, local funding from small fee payments or village insurance like Dana Sehat in Indonesia covers the costs of medicines or simple services, but this funding often collapses when the local leadership changes. The entire Barefoot Doctor system of China was funded through communal work points and local purchase of supplies, which collapsed precipitously with the end of communal farms in China in 1980.

In almost all countries, essential public health activities that serve the welfare of the nation or community are considered public goods and remain the responsibility of governments. While fee-for-service policies can raise some funds—typically 5–12% of total costs—the full cost of comprehensive health care for the poor is invariably a responsibility of governments. The challenge is to develop means of cost recovery from those who can afford to pay without excluding or putting aside the needs of the poor. Equity is about meeting the needs of those whose needs are greatest! For richer countries, community demands to mobilize tax support can enable community programs to continue and expand, as found in the examples from the United States and Germany. Again, well-documented proof of efficiency is critical to fiscal viability and continued funding—a role for information systems.

The symposium papers and discussions were surprisingly mute on the issue of HIV/AIDS. The epidemic rages out of control in much of southern Africa, where 30–40% of adults have already contracted the infection, hospitals are overflowing with dying patients, orphans number in the millions, and already weak economies are devastated. With the exception of Haiti, where remarkable efforts have been made to educate the public, change habits, and provide effective interventions for those infected, the meeting did not discuss experiences in nations that have faced the onslaught of AIDS. Yet important lessons have been learned. In Uganda, after nearly a decade of silence and denial, understanding HIV and preventing infection have become a national obsession, with a resulting decline in new infections and a host of community demonstrations of care for those suffering and for those left behind. Thailand, under the tireless leadership of Mechai Viravaidya, has pursued successful nationwide "condomization," with a resulting fall in HIV and other sexually transmitted infections. Brazil, invoking the World Trade Organization emergency provisions to bypass restrictive patent laws, produces and provides full antiretroviral therapy to all its citizens who test positive for HIV, with a resulting decline in new infections. There *are* solutions to HIV. The dramatic fall in HIV infections in the United States gay community was achieved largely through the community members themselves, educating, lobbying, insisting on behavioral change. PHC offers the *only* solution to HIV, but it requires fundamental changes in the economics of the world order and a more comprehensive application of the full range of principles embodied in community-based PHC.

Is it time for a new Alma-Ata? Surely the principles from 1978 still stand. But clarification is needed. As health technologies advance, communities need to know how these can be widely applied and available to all when resource constraints make the private sector an impossible option for many. As WHO increasingly turns its attention to the provision of medical care and the evaluation of those medical services, there is a new opportunity and need to underscore the health needs of the poor and to emphasize equity as a goal in itself. While economic analysis and burden of disease considerations seem to be drawing national health systems increasingly to the provision of curative services for aging populations, the needs of the poor, the very young, and the marginalized can be lost in the welter of statistics. More and more are living to old age and face diseases of degeneration and aging. Meanwhile, the poor, who continue to suffer infections, nutritional disorders, and violence, with high death rates among the young, are relegated to the sidelines as more articulate groups reach the ears of decision-makers. The "epidemiologic transition" is resulting in an "epidemiologic polarization" as resources swing to the aged, leaving the agenda of the poor undone.

Equity—ensuring what is needed for those who need it most—is becoming eclipsed as society's goal in health. The principles embraced by John Grant 80 years ago and rediscovered in PHC programs designed in the decades since are often threatened by the attractiveness of technological solutions to social problems. Perhaps it is again time to remind the health ministers of the world that choices in health must always put the people first and that only by their active involvement in determining the nature of health services will the health of society, of all the people of the world, reach a level that can reasonably be described as health for all. Perhaps it is time for another Alma-Ata!

—Jon Rohde
MSH EQUITY Project
Bisho, South Africa

Glossary

Census-based, impact-oriented (CBIO) approach: An approach to primary health care developed in Bolivia. It emphasizes house-to-house collection of data and repeat home visits depending on conditions found, with regular measurement of program impact.

Community-based health care (CBHC): A system of health care in which community members and health professionals work together to assess and prioritize health problems and to define ways to solve them.

Community-oriented primary care (COPC): First used by Sidney Kark to describe primary health care services that stress the socioeconomic and environmental factors underlying ill health; emphasize preventive medicine and health promotion; and promote community-based approaches to improving health.

Conscientization: Term used by Paulo Freire in *Pedagogy of the Oppressed* to describe the development of critical consciousness that has "the power to transform reality" (Paul V. Taylor, 1993, *The Texts of Paulo Freire*, Philadelphia, PA: Open University Press).

Lot quality assurance sampling (LQAS): A methodology for assessing small samples, which was adapted from industrial quality control methods to enable health workers and supervisors to monitor community-level activities and coverage of key programs.

Population medicine: The provision of health services to a defined population.

Positive deviance: Positive difference from the usual health status or behavior, for example, a well-nourished child in a community where many children are malnourished.

Primary health care (PHC): "Primary health care is essential health care based on practical, scientifically sound and socially acceptable methods and technology made universally accessible to individuals and families in the community through their full participation and at a cost that the community and country can afford to maintain at every stage of their development in the spirit of self-reliance and self-determination.

Primary health care:

1. reflects and evolves from the economic conditions and socio-cultural and political characteristics of the country and its communities and is based on the application of the relevant results of social, biomedical and health services research and public health experience;
2. addresses the main health problems in the community, providing promotive, preventive, curative and rehabilitative services accordingly;
3. includes at least: education concerning prevailing health problems and the methods of preventing and controlling them; promotion of food supply and proper nutrition; an adequate supply of safe water and basic sanitation; maternal and child health care, including family planning; immunization against the major infectious diseases; prevention and control of locally endemic diseases; appropriate treatment of common diseases and injuries; and provision of essential drugs...." "Declaration of Alma-Ata," International Conference on Primary Health Care, Alma-Ata, USSR, Sept. 6–12, 1978.

Primary medical care (PMC): "First-contact treatment of illness . . . with referral to institutional, specialist therapy at secondary, tertiary, and higher levels" (Taylor and Taylor, chapter 6).

Scaling up or going to scale: Expanding a successful development program to reach a larger population and/or a higher administrative level.

Vertical program: A health program that functions independently of the normal health care system, having its own staff, budget, transport, and information system. A vertical program is usually aimed at a single health problem, such as malaria, bilharzia, or family planning. Many focused efforts, such as the Expanded Programme on Immunization (EPI), vitamin A supplements, or tuberculosis treated in the primary health care system, are given direction, extra resources, and emphasis from central authority but are *not* truly vertical.

Selected Bibliography

Abbott, Julie. 2000. "Community Health Report Card for Olmsted County." Rochester, MN: Mayo Clinic, Sept. 7, 2000.

Abed, F. H. 1999. *The BRAC Story: Development and Change in Bangladesh.* Cambridge: Harvard Center for Population and Development Studies.

Arole, Mabelle. 1988. "A Comprehensive Approach to Community Welfare: Growth Monitoring and the Role of Women in Jamkhed." *The Indian Journal of Pediatrics* (Suppl.) 55: S100–105.

Arole, Mabelle, and Rajanikant Arole. 1994. *Jamkhed: A Comprehensive Rural Health Project.* London: Macmillan.

Bhore, Josiah. 1941. "The Bhore Commission Report." New Delhi: Government of India.

Bhuiya, Abbas, and Claude Ribaux. 1997. *Rethinking Community Participation: Prospects of Health Initiatives by Indigenous Self-Help Organizations in Rural Bangladesh.* Special Publication No. 65. Dhaka: International Centre for Diarrhoeal Disease Research, Bangladesh (ICDDR,B).

Bhuiya, Abbas, et al. 1997. *Community Participation in Health, Family Planning and Development Programmes: International Experiences.* Special Publication No. 59. Dhaka: International Centre for Diarrhoeal Disease Research, Bangladesh (ICDDR,B).

Bruce, Thomas, and Steven Uranga McKane. 2000. *Community-Based Public Health: A Partnership Model.* Waldorf, MD: American Public Health Association and the W. K. Kellogg Foundation.

Chavez, Adolfo, and Celia Martinez. 1982. *Growing up in a Developing Country.* San Fernando y Viaducto Tlalpan, Mexico: Instituto Nacional de la Nutrición.

Counts, Alex. 1996. *Give Us Credit: How Small Loans Today Can Shape Our Tomorrow.* New York: Times Books. About the Grameen Bank in Bangladesh.

Cuéllar, Carlos, William Newbrander, and Gail Price. 2000. *Extending Access to Health Care through Public-Private Partnerships.* Stubbs Monograph Series No. 2. Boston: Management Sciences for Health.

Daniels, Norman, Donald Light, and Ronald Caplan. 1996. *Benchmarks of Fairness for Health Care Reform.* New York: Oxford University Press.

Deuschle, Kurt. 1982. "Community Oriented Primary Care: Lessons Learned in Three Decades." *Journal of Community Health* 8: 13–22.

Evans, Timothy, et al. 2001. *Challenging Inequities in Health: From Ethics to Action.* New York: Oxford University Press.

Farmer, Paul. 2001. "Infections and Inequalities: The Microbial Burden of Poverty." Testimony to US Congress. September 26, 2001.

Gladwell, Malcolm. 2001. "The Mosquito Killer: F. Soper's Global Malaria Eradication Programme." *The New Yorker* 77 (July 2, 2001): 42–51.

Gwatkin, Davidson R., Janet R. Wilcox, and Joe D. Wray. 1980. *Can Health and Nutrition Interventions Make a Difference?* Overseas Development Council Monograph No. 13. Washington, DC: Overseas Development Council.

Halstead, Scott B., Julia A. Walsh, and Kenneth S. Warren, eds. 1985. *Good Health at Low Cost: Proceedings of a Conference Held at Bellagio Conference Center.* New York: Rockefeller Foundation.

Institute of Medicine, The Committee for the Study of the Future of Public Health. 1988. *The Future of Public Health.* Washington, DC: National Academy Press.

Kark, Sidney L. 1981. *The Practice of Community-Oriented Primary Health Care.* New York: Appleton-Century-Crofts.

Kark, Sidney L., and Emily Kark. 1999. *Promoting Community Health: From Pholela to Jerusalem.* Johannesburg: Witwatersrand University Press.

Kidder, Tracy. 2000. "The Good Doctor." *The New Yorker,* July 7, 2000, pp. 40–57.

Kielmann, Arnfried A. 1983. *Child and Maternal Services in Rural India: The Narangwal Experiment.* Vol. 1: *Integrated Nutrition and Health Care* and Vol. 2: *Integrated Family Planning and Health Care.* Baltimore, MD: Johns Hopkins University Press.

Knowles, J. H. 1977. "Introduction: Doing Better and Feeling Worse: Health in the United States." *Daedalus* Winter: 1–7.

Kolehmainen-Aitken, Riitta-Liisa, ed. 1999. *Myths and Realities about the Decentralization of Health Systems.* Boston: Management Sciences for Health.

Lewin, Marion Ein, and Stuart Altman, eds. 2000. *America's Health Care Safety Net: Intact but Endangered.* Committee on the Changing Market, Managed Care, and the Future Viability of Safety Net Providers. Washington, DC: Institute of Medicine, National Academy Press.

Lovell, Catherine H. 1992. *Breaking the Cycle of Poverty: The BRAC Strategy.* West Hartford, CT: Kumarian Press.

Mata, Leonardo J. 1978. *The Children of Santa Maria Cauque: A Prospective Study of Health and Growth*. Cambridge: MIT Press.

McGinnis, J. M., and W. H. Foege. 1993. "Actual Causes of Death in the United States." *Journal of the American Medical Association* 270: 2207–12.

Morley, David, Jon E. Rohde, and Glen Williams, eds. 1983. *Practising Health for All*. New York: Oxford University Press.

Mosley, W. Henry, and Lincoln C. Chen, eds. 1983. *Child Survival: Strategies for Research*. Based on a workshop organized by the Rockefeller and Ford Foundations. Bellagio, Italy.

Muñoz, Carlos, and Nevin S. Scrimshaw, eds. 1995. *The Nutrition and Health Transition of Democratic Costa Rica*. Boston: International Foundation for Developing Countries.

Newbrander, William, David Collins, and Lucy Gilson. 2000. *Ensuring Equal Access to Health Services: User Fee Systems and the Poor*. Boston: Management Sciences for Health.

Newell, Kenneth W., ed. 1975. *Health by the People*. Geneva: World Health Organization.

Perry, Henry B. 1999. "Attaining Health for All through Community Partnerships: Principles of the Census-Based, Impact-Oriented (CBIO) Approach to Primary Health Care Developed in Bolivia, South America." *Social Science and Medicine* 48: 1053–67.

———. 2000. *Health for All in Bangladesh: Lessons in Primary Health Care for the Twenty-First Century*. Dhaka: University Press.

Rohde, Jon, Meera Chatterjee, and David Morley, eds. 1993. *Reaching Health for All*. New Delhi: Oxford University Press.

Schauffler, Helen H. 1994. "Health Promotion and Disease Prevention in Health Care Reform." *American Journal of Preventive Medicine* 10: 1–31.

Scrimshaw, Nevin S., ed. 1995. *Community-Based Longitudinal Nutrition and Health Studies: Classical Examples from Guatemala, Haiti and Mexico*. Boston: International Foundation for Developing Countries.

Sen, Amartya. 1981. *Poverty and Famines: An Essay on Entitlement and Deprivation*. Oxford: Clarendon Press.

———. 1999. *Development as Freedom*. New York: Knopf.

Slocum, R., et al., eds. 1995. *Power, Process, and Participation: Tools for Change*. London: Intermediate Technology Publications.

Streefland, Pieter, and Jarl Chabot, eds. 1990. *Implementing Primary Health Care: Experiences since Alma-Ata*. Amsterdam: Royal Tropical Institute.

Taylor-Ide, Daniel, and Carl E. Taylor. 1995. *Community Based Sustainable Human Development: A Proposal for Going to Scale with Self-Reliant Social Development*. New York: UNICEF.

————. 2002. *Just and Lasting Change: When Communities Own Their Futures.* Baltimore, MD: Johns Hopkins University Press, forthcoming.

US Public Health Service. 2000. *Healthy People 2010: Understanding and Improving Health.* 2d ed. Washington, DC: Government Printing Office. Available at www.health.gov/healthypeople/document.

Valadez, Joseph J. 1991. *Assessing Child Survival Programs in Developing Countries: Testing Lot Quality Assurance Sampling.* Cambridge: Harvard University Press.

————. 1998. *A Manual for Training Supervisors of Community Health Workers to Use LQAS: A User's Guide.* Arlington, VA: OMNI Research.

Valadez, Joseph J., and M. Bamberger. 1994. *Monitoring and Evaluating Social Programs in Developing Countries.* Washington, DC: World Bank.

White, Kerr L., ed. 1992. *Health Services Research: An Anthology.* Washington, DC: Pan American Health Organization.

White, Kerr L., and Julia E. Connelly, eds. 1992. *The Medical School's Mission and the Population's Health: Medical Education in Canada, the United Kingdom, the United States, and Australia.* New York: Springer-Verlag.

World Health Organization. 1978. *Primary Health Care: Report of the International Conference on Primary Health Care, Alma-Ata, USSR, 6–12 September 1978.* Geneva: World Health Organization.

Wyon, John B., and John E. Gordon. 1971. *The Khanna Study: Population Problems in the Rural Punjab.* Cambridge: Harvard University Press.

About the Contributors

Anthony I. Adams, MD, MPH, is Professor of Public Health at the National Center for Epidemiology and Population Health at the Australian National University, where he helped establish a public health training program for indigenous students. He earned his medical degree from the University of Adelaide and an MPH in Tropical Public Health at Harvard. After finishing his MPH, Dr. Adams established the International Clerkship Program in the Department of Community Medicine at the University of Kentucky. He then taught public health at the University of Sydney for eight years before becoming Chief Medical Officer of the New South Wales State Health Department in Sydney. Dr. Adams served as Secretary of the International Epidemiological Association from 1977 to 1981. From 1988 to 1997, he was Australia's Chief Medical Officer, leading the Australian delegation to World Health Organization meetings and other international visits.

"While I was always interested in international health, my commitment was strengthened during my MPH year at Harvard, thanks to the influence of Thomas Weller and Carl Taylor. Returning to Australia in the mid-1960s, I found myself helping to change public health services at the national level. This included assisting with the introduction of community health services to meet the public health and health care needs of defined regional communities. Later, I was in charge of handling the AIDS pandemic in the focal city of Sydney. Representing Australia at WHO meetings and serving on regional and global commissions on polio eradication have maintained my involvement in international health."

Joan M. Altekruse, MD, MPH, DrPH, MDS, is the past president of the Harvard School of Public Health Alumni Council and Professor Emerita in Preventive Medicine at the University of South Carolina. She earned her MD degree from Stanford, an MPH from Harvard, a DrPH from UC-Berkeley, and an MDS from Loyola University Institute of Ministry.

"A desire to combine a career in medicine with public service motivated me to enter the US Public Health Service as a medical officer. I became increasingly aware of the need for preventive and restorative health care, which made it clear to me that each person's rightful claims to health care were far from realized. This recognition gave me the personal impetus to extend public health practice to encompass social justice issues.

"I have had the good fortune to be associated with innovative models that bring health and related services to specific communities. The first, in post-World War II Germany, was a comprehensive social rehabilitation experiment responding to the homeless and mentally ill. The second was in Northern Ireland, where I worked with the Irish Peace Institute to assist those suffering from conflict. As Chair of Preventive Medicine and Community Health at the University of California, I worked with students, residents, and faculty to adopt a community-based learning approach. This helped them gain technical proficiency, skills in the application of intellectual content, and sensitivity to the perspectives of different populations— all requisite for medical specialists preparing for service and leadership in public health. Since 'retiring,' I have earned a graduate degree in pastoral ministry and worked as a lay volunteer on a comprehensive approach for the care of populations such as hospital patients and incarcerated women in central Tennessee. I am committed to integrated, community-based care that responds to those in greatest need."

Ron J. Anderson, MD, President and Chief Executive Officer of Parkland Health & Hospital System in Dallas, became CEO of Parkland in 1982. He previously served as Parkland's Medical Director for Ambulatory Care and Emergency Services. Dr. Anderson has remained on the faculty of the Medical School as Professor of Internal Medicine.

Dr. Anderson served on the executive committee of the State Task Force on Indigent Health Care and in 1985 played a major role in the passage of landmark legislation concerning indigent health care in Texas. He was appointed Co-Chair of the Attorney General's Task Force to study not-for-profit hospitals and unsponsored charity care in 1988, and he served as a member of Governor Richards' Health Policy Task Force in 1991–92. Dr. Anderson is past chairman of the Dallas-Fort Worth Hospital Council, the Texas Association of Public and Non-Profit Hospitals, the Texas Board of Health, the National Association of Public Hospitals, the National Public Health and Hospital Institute, and the Texas Hospital Association. Dr. Anderson was also a member of the Kaiser Commission on the Future of Medicaid.

"My interest in community-based primary health care began perhaps because I had the opportunity to run Parkland Memorial Hospital's central clinic and emergency room. It was clear to me that to be effective, we had to create more accessible and accountable delivery systems. We had to move into the community if we were to create healthier communities."

Mabelle Arole (and her husband, Rajanikant Arole) graduated from Christian Medical College in Vellore, determined to serve the poor of India.

They prepared themselves with medical and surgical residencies, respectively, in the United States, and study at Johns Hopkins in public health before returning to central India in 1970 to establish a small hospital among the poorest, remote communities around Jamkhed. In its first 15 years, the Comprehensive Rural Health Project grew to embrace a full range of community development activities that transformed the lives of over 200,000 people. The Aroles' success influenced first the State of Maharashtra to train doctors and health managers at Jamkhed, and later, the Government of India to introduce the Health Guide Scheme in an effort to bring the benefits of community-based primary health care to all of India's 600,000 villages. Mabelle and Raj were articulate spokespersons for primary health care, especially the central role of women in development. She joined UNICEF as the Regional Advisor for Health, turning over the leadership of Jamkhed to her husband and their daughter, Dr. Shobha Arole, who has followed in her footsteps. Dr. Mabelle Arole, who died in 1999, has left a legacy of quiet, persuasive leadership and a model that has influenced thousands of workers across South Asia and the world.

Heidi Louise Behforouz, MD, is an attending physician at the Brigham and Women's Hospital in Boston and a fellow of the Open Society Institute's Medicine as a Profession advocacy program. A graduate of Harvard Medical School, Dr. Behforouz has focused her career on the health issues of the urban indigent. In her work as a primary care doctor at the Women's Health Center at the Brigham and Women's Hospital, Dr. Behforouz treats a large number of HIV-positive individuals. She also serves as the medical director of the Prevention and Access to Care and Treatment (PACT) Project in Roxbury, Massachusetts. Sponsored by Partners in Health, this program uses community health promoters to advocate for the health and well-being of inner-city residents infected with HIV.

Gretchen Glode Berggren, MD, MSc, is a semi-retired international health consultant who specializes in practical approaches to nutrition and women's health. She was trained at the University of Nebraska College of Medicine, the Institute of Tropical Medicine and Hygiene in Antwerp, Belgium, and the Harvard School of Public Health (HSPH). She began her career in 1959 as a medical missionary to the Congo and later concentrated on management of family planning programs and on census-based, community-oriented primary health care programs in developing countries. Dr. Berggren's work to develop methods to reach poor families has been recognized through a 1993 Presidential citation as a Health Hero for Children, the Donald McKay Medal of the American Society of Tropical Medicine, and honorary degrees from universities in the United States and overseas.

As a faculty member of HSPH and the Harvard Center for Population Studies, Dr. Berggren taught in field project sites in Haiti and the Dominican Republic. As a visiting scientist under the direction of Dr. Nevin S. Scrimshaw at MIT, she directed an international research project on home- and village-prepared weaning foods. Her publications include documentation of reduced age-specific and disease-specific mortality rates, age-specific fertility rates, and migration rates in Haiti. She has undertaken training and management assignments for Save the Children in more than 26 developing countries.

"My husband Warren and I met at the University of Nebraska School of Medicine, where both of us were preparing to become medical missionaries. Together we sought opportunities for service and found one when we helped open a clinic for the homeless under the Open Door Mission of South Omaha. Working together in service was a satisfaction that never left us.

"Warren went to the Belgian Congo, and I later joined him. We were assigned to an interdenominational hospital near Kinshasa, where we trained Congolese auxiliary workers in the face of the drastic changes of political independence. We realized that most of the diseases we treated could have been prevented by such workers if given the chance to bring services to the village level. A turning point for us was the arrival of Dr. C. Everett Koop, then a well-known pediatric surgeon, who came to help. He encouraged us to go into preventive medicine. We studied at the Harvard School of Public Health and then became faculty members while commencing community-health field projects in Haiti."

Abbas Bhuiya, PhD, is Head of the Social and Behavioral Sciences Program at the International Centre for Diarrhoeal Disease Research, Bangladesh (ICDDR,B) in Dhaka.

"I am a Bangladeshi who grew up in a village in the central east side of the country bordering India. After receiving a degree in statistics from Chittagong University, I joined ICDDR,B in 1980 and had a chance to work with the Matlab Demographic Surveillance System. Subsequently I earned my MA and PhD in Demography from the Australian National University, Canberra. During the fieldwork for my theses, I was faced with difficulties while weighing children because around 6% of the mothers reported not having had a full meal for a couple of days. I was bothered by this and subsequently convinced ICDDR,B to collaborate with the Bangladesh Rural Advancement Committee (BRAC) to implement BRAC's poverty alleviation programs in Matlab and to study the joint and independent effects of the health and poverty alleviation programs on health and human well-being. This is an ongoing study. While studying many of the poverty alleviation and health programs, I realized that they are not participatory in the real sense of the term. From my own experience in my village of birth, I knew that there exists a lot of social capital in Bangladeshi society that can be fruitfully utilized for the betterment of health of the villagers. This contention of mine encouraged me to take up a project to promote self-help for health in a remote rural area in my country called Chakaria. The project has been ongoing since 1994 and is trying to activate village-based self-help organizations to take health initiatives. I feel privileged to share our experiences from that project."

Paul Boumbulian, DPA, MPH, is an associate professor in the MPH program at the University of Texas in Dallas. Throughout his career, he has been involved in working with communities to develop community-based solutions for the delivery of medical and health services. He earned his MPH from Berkeley and his doctorate in public administration from the University of Georgia. He served for 15 years as the Senior Vice-President for Strategic Planning for the Parkland Health & Hospital System, and he held a similar position at the University of California Davis Medical Center. Preceding his work with health systems, he directed comprehensive community-based health planning initiatives in Utah and in the Appalachian region of Georgia. Dr. Boumbulian has published widely and received numerous awards for his work, including a fellowship from the Fetzer Institute.

"I was humbled early in my career when I learned that professional expertise was not sufficient to create a sustainable improvement in a community's health. Effective change required professionals working within the values, beliefs, and priorities of the community. Luckily, I learned this lesson early. It has served me well."

John H. Bryant, MD, PhD, is former Dean of the Columbia University School of Public Health and former Chair of the Department of Community Health Sciences at the Aga Khan University in Karachi. Dr. Bryant has also worked at Mahidol University in Bangkok, the Office of International Health in the US Department of Health and Human Services, and with the Council of International Organizations for Medical Sciences. While at DHHS, he was responsible for treaty relationships in health between the United States and other countries, including India, China, and Russia. In 1969, Dr. Bryant authored *Health and the Developing World*. With Halfdan Mahler and Carl Taylor, he played a formative role at the Alma-Ata Conference on Primary Health Care in 1978. Presently he is on the Board of Trustees of the Hôpital Albert Schweitzer in Haiti.

"In 1994, I was asked to write an article for *Health Policy and Planning,* entitled "Stepping Stones: Reflections on Careers in Health." In that article, I listed critical events in my professional life and six guiding concepts for working toward health development: (1) *equity:* A concept as old as justice, given new life at Alma-Ata, and the fundamental challenge for health systems development in all countries; (2) *ethics:* There, often unused, like a silent scream, waiting to call attention to violations of human rights and sensibilities. Important for both individual and institutional thinking and action; (3) *values:* Respect the indigenous values, culture, and religion of a society, and beware of importing values uncritically from the developed world; (4) *trust:* I asked Raj and Mabelle Arole in Jamkhed, India, to what they attributed their remarkable success. 'The community trusts us!' they replied. To encourage the vulnerable to enter into a relationship of trust is at the heart of development; (5) *patience:* Personal and institutional patience for the development process to allow the integration and consolidation necessary for sustainability; and (6) *vision:* So you know where you are going, and have the support of clear vision for work on the complexities of the development process."

A. Mushtaque R. Chowdhury, MSc, PhD, is Deputy Executive Director and Director of Research at the Bangladesh Rural Advancement Committee (BRAC) in Dhaka. He earned MSc and PhD degrees at the University of London.

"The War of Liberation in 1971 that led to the creation of Bangladesh was the most important event of my career. This motivated me to think about the country and its people, particularly the poor. Considering the population explosion to be a major problem facing Bangladesh, I decided to study demography in graduate school. But soon I discovered that there were other underlying and probably more important reasons that the people were so poor. This led me to concentrate on public health, primary education, environment, and poverty alleviation.

"Having read statistics as an undergraduate major, I was constantly faced with its limitations in explaining human behavior. Use of ethnography solved some of it. While studying the reasons for low usage of oral rehydration therapy (ORT) in rural Bangladesh, I discovered how the villagers perceived diarrhea and its causes, which was entirely different from what is taught in medical schools. This clearly explained to me why many villagers were not using ORT even when knowing very well how to prepare it with home ingredients. BRAC, which was implementing the ORT program nationwide, quickly incorporated this finding; and the usage rate shot up fast. This confirmed two things for me: first, the value of integrating qualitative and quantitative methods into research; and, second, that BRAC is a unique organization that listens to research findings. The Research and Evaluation Division (RED), developed over the years at BRAC, has derived its existence and excellence from the applied creativity of the BRAC organization. With more than 125 interdisciplinary staff, RED is an important department at BRAC and is playing increasingly important roles nationally and internationally. I have been with BRAC for all 23 years of my professional career, and the joy of seeing one's own research being implemented nationally is certainly an important reason for this continued association."

Hugh S. Fulmer, MD, MPH, is Executive Director of the Center for Community Responsive Care, Inc. (CCRC), a national organization whose board of directors is made up of institutions representing medicine and public health. Dr. Fulmer, who is trained in family practice, internal medicine, and public health, believes that the education of health professionals must focus on integrating community health into undergraduate, graduate, and continuing medical and public health education. While working toward this goal, he has held faculty appointments at Syracuse and Cornell Universities and the Universities of Kentucky and Massachusetts.

As Director of Ambulatory and Community Services at the Carney Hospital in Boston from 1983 to 1988, Dr. Fulmer designed and directed the COPC multidisciplinary fellowship at Carney and a network of community health centers. In 1993, he and colleagues founded, and have continued to direct, the CCRC, which trains multidisciplinary health professionals to merge medicine and public health in caring for communities. As a consultant to the Griffin Hospital (1995–98), a Yale-affiliated community hospital in Derby, Connecticut, he was involved in the design of the now fully accredited four-year combined residency in medicine and preventive medicine. He has been the founder and/or director of five residencies in preventive medicine throughout the country. Most recently, he has become associated with a new medical school, St. Eustasius, which will train 21st-century physicians from the United States and developing countries in the five-step COPC process to improve community health in their countries of origin.

Philip T. Hagen, MD, MPH, has provided community-based primary care to diverse populations at Mayo Clinic for the past 15 years. Dr. Hagen learned the science and art of providing population-based care and individual care through fellowships in internal medicine and preventive medicine at the Mayo Graduate School of Medicine and through public health training at the University of Minnesota School of Public Health. He is currently Vice-Chair of Clinical Preventive Medicine at Mayo Clinic Rochester, Director of the Mayo Preventive Medicine Residency Program, and Medical Director of Mayo Health Management Services.

Dr. Hagen has led the development of a number of innovative projects, including a comprehensive health promotion program for populations. This includes a monthly newsletter, self-care book, Web site (MayoClinic.com), online Health Risk Appraisal, and training in implementation. He has helped develop a computerized structured medical questionnaire, called Patient Provided Information, which has been administered to more than 500,000 people and supports the Rochester Epidemiology Project with data on symptoms and behavior to assess health and disease profiles of the community.

"I feel the guiding hand of many bright people in Mayo's past 100 years, people who by dint of diligence, creativity, and dedication to their community developed a system to care for that community that is simultaneously caring and cutting edge. This care takes both the big picture and the personal perspective into account. I was drawn to it like a kid to a candy shop. I have the privilege daily of moving from looking a patient in the eye, to planning a population health initiative, to teaching residents, to tinkering with an experimental high-tech tool."

C. William Keck, MD, MPH, FACPM, is Director of Health for the City of Akron, Ohio, and Professor and Director of the Division of Community Health Sciences at the Northeastern Ohio Universities College of Medicine. Dr. Keck is past president of the American Public Health Association, the Ohio Public Health Association, the Association of Ohio Health Commissioners, and the Summit County Medical Society. Dr. Keck is board certified in preventive medicine/public health. He is a Fellow of the American College of Preventive Medicine and a member of the Association of Teachers of Preventive Medicine. His career has focused on providing quality public health services, teaching community health sciences to medical and other students in the health professions, and linking public health practice with its academic base.

Jim Yong Kim, MD, PhD, is a physician-anthropologist and trustee of Partners in Health (PIH), a public charity that works to make a "preferential option for the poor" in health care. Dr. Kim and colleagues founded PIH in 1987. Dr. Kim earned his MD degree and a PhD in social anthropology at Harvard University. He completed his residency in internal medicine at the Brigham and Women's Hospital in Boston, where he is now Chief of the new Division on Social Medicine and Health Inequalities. Dr. Kim is also Director of the Program in Infectious Disease and Social Change at Harvard Medical School.

In 1994, Dr. Kim, with PIH and Peruvian colleagues, founded Socios en Salud (SES), a nongovernmental organization based in a poor urban-squatter settlement on the outskirts of Lima, Peru. In addition to providing food and health care for children and building both latrines and more than a dozen community pharmacies, PIH/Socios en Salud has successfully treated patients suffering from multidrug-resistant tuberculosis (MDR-TB). The

World Health Organization had previously recommended to national TB programs that patients suffering from MDR-TB not be treated. After the results of the PIH/SES project were announced, WHO initiated TB control projects that included the treatment of MDR-TB. As a result of PIH's successful MDR-TB treatment project in Peru, the Bill & Melinda Gates Foundation awarded a $45 million grant to the organization for further work on drug-resistant TB in Peru and other countries, including Russia. Dr. Kim is principal investigator of this grant, which is the largest private gift for TB control in history.

Dr. Kim has authored papers in various scholarly journals and served as editor-in-chief of *Dying for Growth: Global Inequality and the Health of the Poor.* This book, which includes case studies from Haiti, Peru, Cuba, Senegal, Mexico, and Russia, explores the relationship between neoliberal economic policies and the health of poor people.

Judith Kurland, BA, has, since 1997, been Regional Director of the US Department of Health and Human Services Region I, comprising the six New England states. From 1988 to 1993, Ms. Kurland served as Commissioner of Health and Hospitals for the City of Boston, the only woman ever appointed to that position. Previously she was Vice-President for Strategic Planning at New England Medical Center and a founding member of the Neighborhood Health Plan (an HMO based in community health centers) and the International Society for Technology Assessment in Health Care. She has been a faculty member at Tufts University Medical School, Boston University Medical School, and Simmons College, and presently teaches at the Harvard School of Public Health.

Ms. Kurland's career has been guided by two fundamental principles: first, communities possess the strength and integrity to create and sustain social change; and second, powerful institutions must be led to act in ways that support and advance that change. Working at the federal, state, and local levels, she has shaped public policy, generated fresh political discourse, and developed innovative health and human service programs, all of which have been directed at harnessing the power of these principles to improve peoples' lives and strengthen their communities.

Ms. Kurland is recognized as the architect of Healthy Boston, a widely hailed and much-copied model of urban social change. It integrates community empowerment, economic development, service delivery, and population-based health and education programs. Her commitment to local empowerment has also taken Ms. Kurland overseas, where she has advised the North and West Belfast Health and Social Services Trust, the Department of Health and Social Services of Northern Ireland, and the Institute of

Public Health in Ireland on the use of public health as a vehicle for community renewal. Since 1998, she has served as the Acting Editor of *Public Health Reports,* the journal of the US Public Health Service.

Joyce C. Lashof, MD, FACP, DMSci (Hon.), is currently Professor Emerita of Public Health at the University of California at Berkeley, where from 1981 to 1991 she was also Dean of the School of Public Health. Dr. Lashof's distinguished career has combined academic medicine with public service. In 1965 she carried out a study of health care needs of populations living in poverty in Chicago, where she was instrumental in establishing, and then directed, the Mile Square Neighborhood Health Center. She served on the Institute of Medicine Committee on Community Oriented Primary Care and has maintained a lifelong interest in the relationship of public health and primary care.

"From academic internist to dean of a school of public health may seem like a strange route but there is some logic to it. I have always had an interest in issues related to the health care system and universal health insurance. With the advent of the War on Poverty, I had the opportunity to develop and run an Office of Economic Opportunity Neighborhood Health Center. This experience served to demonstrate forcefully the importance of social and economic factors in determining health status. So moving to become Illinois State Director of Public Health was a logical step, which led to my further governmental positions. Throughout I worked to integrate public health and medical care. I owe a great deal to Mark Lepper, who served as a mentor throughout, and to Jack Geiger, from whom I learned much about community-oriented primary care."

Rebecca Marshall, MA, is a writer and editor at Management Sciences for Health. She earned her BA in English literature from Smith College and was awarded a two-year fellowship to pursue graduate studies at Clare College, Cambridge University. Since beginning work with MSH in 1998, she has worked with health programs around the world, including programs in Bangladesh, India, Kenya, and Boston.

"I decided to forgo further graduate studies in literature to pursue my interest in health, particularly in relation to issues of poverty and human rights. But even now, working to understand complicated issues related to international health care, I'm drawn most strongly to people's stories, rather than other kinds of evidence. Such compelling truths emerge from the voices and experiences of individuals. In working with domestic and international organizations, most recently the PACT Project through Partners in Health, I've been convinced by the stories I've encountered—from clients, case managers, health care providers, and volunteers—that a community-based approach to care is not only the most ethical, but also the most effective way to increase equity in health care."

William Newbrander, MA, PhD, is the Director of MSH's Center for Health Reform and Financing. He is a health economist and hospital administrator, with master's degrees in hospital administration and economics as well as a PhD in health economics from the University of Michigan.

Dr. Newbrander served with the World Health Organization for eight years in Papua New Guinea, Thailand, and Switzerland. He managed hospitals in the United States and Saudi Arabia prior to his work with WHO. Today, in addition to managing the Center for Health Reform and Financing, he provides technical assistance for MSH in health reform and health policy, social health insurance, issues of equity and the poor, hospital management, and decentralization. Dr. Newbrander teaches health financing at universities and international organizations, and directs international teams of technical experts. He directed the Asian Development Bank's Second Regional Conference on Health Sector Reform: Issues Related to Private Sector Growth.

Dr. Newbrander has published widely on health reform, health financing, decentralization, and issues of equity. His most recent book is *Ensuring Equal Access to Health Services: User Fee Systems and the Poor.*

"My family's involvement in international work came naturally from my childhood, since I was born in Japan of missionary parents and spent my early years in Asia, and my wife was born in Afghanistan and lived there for nearly 20 years. Having people from many countries in our home gave our family a global perspective. I was also influenced to become involved with public health generally, and management and international work specifically, by those I worked with earlier in my career: Dr. Avedis Donabedian not only taught me the importance of quality health care but also helped me bring intellectual rigor to my work. Colonel Richard Hansen of the US Army taught me much about managing people and health institutions. And Dr. Dragan Stern of WHO inculcated in me the importance of public health issues in national health systems."

Robert R. Orford, MD, MS, MPH, a native of Canada, earned his medical degree from McGill University in Montreal, Canada, in 1971. He earned his MS degree from the University of Minnesota and an MPH from the University of Washington, Seattle. He is board certified in internal medicine, general preventive medicine and public health, aerospace medicine, and occupational medicine. He joined Mayo Clinic, Rochester, in 1988, and moved to Mayo Clinic, Scottsdale, Arizona, in 1996, where he is Chair of the Division of Preventive and Occupational Medicine.

Dr. Orford has extensive experience in public health, as a member of the Alberta Board of Public Health from 1979 to 1986 (Chairman 1985–86) and as Deputy Minister of Community and Occupational Health for the Province of Alberta from 1985 to 1987. While in Rochester, he worked closely with the Olmsted County Public Health Department, where he served as a member of the Olmsted County Environment Commission from 1991 to 1996 (Chairman 1993–94). He was the Director of the Mayo Preventive Medicine Residency Program from 1992 to 1996 and plans to develop a preventive medicine residency in Phoenix, with the Maricopa County Department of Public Health.

"As a Canadian, I have lived and worked for many years in a country with a strong public health tradition, and was privileged to work within that system at a senior level. Following my return to Mayo in Rochester in 1988, I was struck by the many similarities between the public health system in Alberta and the system in Olmsted County. The basis for both systems is the love for the community of both county residents and health care professionals. Support from volunteers was strong in both areas. Both systems were relatively well funded and employed superlative staff. Both systems are models for the practice of community-oriented preventive medicine."

John C. Pearson, MA, MD, MPH, is Professor Emeritus of Community Medicine at West Virginia University, where he was Chairman of the Department for 20 years. His original goal was family medicine, but after two years as Medical Officer, he appreciated having a wider role as a physician and pursued an MPH at Yale to add to his pediatrics training. He had a wonderful succession of preceptors and colleagues: John Paul, Ig Falk, and Dick Weinerman at Yale; Bob Logan at Manchester, UK; Kerr White and Osler Peterson; and John Last at Ottawa. His three greatest professional joys have been working in Manchester with the inspirational Bob on multiple regional and cross-national studies, working in West Virginia shepherding the state to a higher level of health and health care, and being able to work and lecture around the world.

Henry B. Perry, MD, is an international public health specialist whose major focus is on community-based primary health care. Dr. Perry worked in Bangladesh from 1994 to 1999 with ICDDR,B, the BASICS Project, and the World Bank. He holds honorary faculty appointments at Emory University and Johns Hopkins.

"I visited the Hôpital Albert Schweitzer in Haiti in 1979, when I learned about its innovative community-based health program that reached out to every household in the population through routine systematic home visits. By this process, a register was maintained of everyone, and the health information system made it possible to determine which persons were in need of basic services. Furthermore, vital events (births, deaths, and migrations) could be recorded on a prospective basis, making it possible to determine mortality and fertility rates in the population. In addition, the most frequent, serious, preventable, or readily treatable conditions could be identified along with those persons at greatest risk; and program activities could be directed to them. I was inspired at that time by this fresh new approach and learned that Warren and Gretchen Berggren had developed it with guidance from their professor at Harvard, John Wyon.

I lived in Bolivia from 1981 until 1984, trying to establish a similar community-based health care program on the rural altiplano with the guidance of John Wyon. Although the start-up proved to be terribly slow and difficult, the seeds sown eventually took root. Today, an organization has arisen from this effort—Andean Rural Health Care—and ARHC has as its central focus what we call the census-based, impact-oriented approach. This approach continues to guide my own professional thinking as well. I believe that it has enormous potential for maximizing the benefits of community-based health care among impoverished and difficult-to-reach populations. My own time in Bangladesh as a technical advisor and researcher has convinced me further of the validity of this approach. My current role as Director General and CEO of the Hôpital Albert Schweitzer in Haiti is giving me further opportunities to develop this methodology and to document its effectiveness."

S. Sue Pickens, MA, Director of Strategic Planning at Parkland Health & Hospital System, has worked in health planning and community needs assessment for the past 25 years. She is a graduate fellow in the Healthy Communities Program sponsored by the Healthcare Forum and serves on many committees assessing the health of populations and working to improve the determinants of health for all populations. She holds a master's degree in education from the University of Texas and is currently a PhD student in sociology at the University of North Texas. Sue has published widely in the area of community health and community health assessment.

"I have discovered that my purpose in life is to create a world of joy and learning. To reach this goal, I see myself working on projects that create a community environment healthy enough to support learning as a natural course of community and individual growth. I am also creating this world by teaching and learning at the University of North Texas, Texas Woman's University, and the University of Texas Southwestern School of Allied Health. I am very fortunate to be able work in an organization such as Parkland Health & Hospital System that is mission driven and allows me to live my values."

Niels Pörksen, MD, now retired, was from 1984 to 1999 the Director of Psychiatric Services at Bethel, in the city of Bielefeld, Germany. Before that he was the director of a psychiatric hospital at Lüneburg in northern Germany.

Dr. Pörksen completed his postgraduate training at the Laboratory of Community Psychiatry at Harvard Medical School. In 1970, he founded the German Society of Social Psychiatry, also serving as a member of the board and the president. He was a member of the Mental Health Commission of the German Federal Government from 1970 to 1975 and from 1980 to 1988. He is a member of the board of the German Psychiatric Association, president of an organization of psychiatric hospital directors, and current President of the German-Polish Association of Mental Health. From 1986 to 1994, he was President of the German-Italian Association of Mental Health. He received the Friendship Prize awarded by both governments in 2000. Dr. Pörksen is a member and past President of the Mental Health Board of Bielefeld.

Gail Price, MS, has spent much of her career identifying ways in which the health care systems in different countries can learn from each other. Ms. Price completed her master's degree at the Harvard School of Public Health in 1986. She joined Management Sciences for Health (MSH) in 1994. At MSH, she has led several projects to improve community-based services in the United States by adapting international models for the domestic environment. Before joining MSH, Ms. Price worked for the Boston Department of Health, where she was instrumental in launching Healthy Boston, a citywide project to improve community-based health and human services. Ms. Price is President of the Harvard School of Public Health Alumni Council. She has written several articles on innovative health and development projects, and she has co-authored an article on transferring the lessons of international health to the United States. Ms. Price has traveled in 23 countries and speaks Spanish fluently.

"My interest in community-based primary health care began when I was working with a team at the Harvard Institute for International Development to evaluate a community development project in Cali, Colombia. Healthy Boston was, in part, based on the Cali model. I later became involved in enhancing the use of lay community health workers (CHWs) in the United States and have educated policymakers about the importance of CHWs. I am currently leading a project to improve community-based services for culturally diverse populations in the United States."

Ashok Reddy, BA, completed his bachelor's degree in anthropology at Emory University in 2000. In 2001, he joined the Boston-based community health project, Prevention and Access to Care and Treatment, of Partners in Health. As a case manager, Mr. Reddy has contributed a unique perspective to the project, having worked as an emergency medical technician and seen the effects on the urban poor of the inability to access proper health care. He intends to attend the University of Washington School of Medicine in the fall of 2002. In his career in medicine, he is committed to calling upon his background in anthropology and social work to help him provide outstanding service and to facilitate long-term follow-up care among the underserved.

Nathan Robison, BA, was born and raised in Bolivia and has spent all of his professional life working in rural development on the high plains of Bolivia. Mr. Robison earned his bachelor's degree in economics from Vanderbilt University in 1974. For 11 years, he worked in assorted rural development efforts, including rural electrification, the organization of cooperatives, and the management of nongovernmental organizations. In 1986, he became field director for Andean Rural Health Care's activities in Bolivia, eventually engineering its transition from a US-based private voluntary organization to a prestigious national nonprofit specializing in community-based primary health care. Mr. Robison has participated on Bolivian Ministry of Health commissions for restructuring the national health information system and for monitoring the EPI program. He is a recognized leader in the national NGO community, particularly among those dedicated to public and community health.

"I became interested in community health as a result of my association with Andean Rural Health Care, which I joined primarily because of the organization's keen interest in measuring the results of its work. Henry Perry and John Wyon, pioneers of ARHC's census-based, impact-oriented approach to community health care, rapidly brought me to the cutting edge of this vital field."

Jon E. Rohde, MD, is the Senior Technical Advisor to the EQUITY Project in South Africa. He graduated from Harvard Medical School and completed a pediatrics residency at Children's Hospital in Boston. Following his medical training, he joined the Rockefeller Foundation as Visiting Professor of Pediatrics in Indonesia. He came to MSH as the Chief of Party for the Rural Health Delivery Project in Haiti and then served as the Chief Technical Advisor for Child Survival for the PRITECH Project, funded by USAID, in India. His subsequent work in India included working as the Special Advisor to the UNICEF Executive Director and serving as the UNICEF Representative.

"When I left Boston for Dhaka in 1968 with the USPHS to do research on cholera, I didn't expect to stay 'out there' for the next 30 plus years; but 'way leads on to way' and the challenges of the poor countries have been exciting and rewarding. The avoidable plight of mothers and children has continued to seem such a solvable problem, and also such a deplorable injustice that can be set right, requiring robust available as well as affordable technology, good management, and some common sense. All too often it is the latter that is in shortest supply! The lessons are all around us, most readily learned not in classrooms but in villages and slums, and applied by people close to the problems. Oh, to immerse all experts and bureaucrats in reality once in a while (as Carl Taylor used to do annually at Narangwal)!

I left Boston for a challenge, to apply the gifts of my good fortune in an education and to get away from the crushing materialism of a system that seemed to be losing its soul. In the cyclone of 1970 and the War of Liberation that freed Bangladesh, I found I could bring science to large numbers of people and have fun in the process. I could raise my family with value systems I believe in and sleep well each night."

Samuel Ross, MD, has put the community-oriented primary care concept into practice in Dallas County through expanded access to primary care and a comprehensive community services program that incorporates health center advisory boards and local coalitions to better define community needs and implement effective interventions.

Since completing his residency in family medicine in 1983 at St. Paul Medical Center in Dallas, Texas, Dr. Ross has completed a 4th-year Chief Residency in Family Medicine, served 2 years on the faculty of the Family Medicine Residency Program of the St. Paul/University of Texas Southwestern Medical School, and spent 5 years in private practice. For the past 11 years, he has worked at Parkland Health & Hospital System in various medical and administrative leadership roles. He is currently the Senior Vice-President for Ambulatory Services.

David S. Shanklin, MS, is the Director of International Programs at Curamericas (formerly Andean Rural Health Care), where he has worked for the past 11 years. He has been active in public health research and programming for the past 22 years, specializing in health program evaluation, and nutrition program policy, planning, and evaluation. He holds two master's of science degrees: one in clinical dietetics from the University of Kentucky (1977) and one in public health from the Harvard School of Public Health (1979).

"My interest in and passion for community-based primary health care have come directly from my experiences in Bolivia, and through my association with such consummate public health practitioners as Henry Perry and John Wyon. I have seen firsthand the enormous effect that simple, effective community-based health services have and now feel compelled to share my experiences with all who are interested and care. At present, I am very interested in the improvement of childhood nutritional status in marginalized populations, as well as the reduction of maternal and neonatal deaths through appropriate, field-based actions."

Carl E. Taylor, MD, DrPH, is Emeritus Professor of International Public Health at the Johns Hopkins School of Public Health, where he chaired his department for 15 years. A graduate of Harvard Medical School, Dr. Taylor directed the celebrated Narangwal Study in the rural Punjab of India until 1973. He played a catalytic role—with John Bryant and Halfdan Mahler—in convening the Alma-Ata Conference on Primary Health Care in 1978 and has been an equally strong influence behind USAID's focus on child survival. After retiring from Johns Hopkins, Dr. Taylor served as UNICEF's Representative in China for 5 years. Throughout his career, he has contributed extensively to the literature on public health and primary care.

"Going back to Narangwal days, I like to define myself as a simple Punjabi villager. Actually, I learned most of what I have tried to implement from my medical missionary parents, who served Terai jungle villages in the United Provinces of India for 54 years. Then I learned from John Gordon, my academic guru. I was privileged to sit at the feet of John B. Grant (the father of primary health care) for a week every year in Puerto Rico with my class of Professors of Community Health while I ran that program at Harvard during the late 1950s. Jimmy Yen, the founder of the Ding Xian Experiment and of IIRR (International Institute of Rural Reconstruction), was a role model through the 1960s. It was a privilege to have the inspiration provided by Jim Grant and Halfdan Mahler through the years. I have been blessed by these associations."

Henry G. Taylor, MD, MPH, was raised in Boston, Baltimore, and the Indian subcontinent, and is now a West Virginian by choice. He received his undergraduate degree from Haverford College, then spent a year on a National Geographic project studying temple monkeys in Nepal. He graduated from Harvard Medical School and did his residency in general internal medicine at the Francis Scott Key/Bayview Medical Center of Johns Hopkins University.

Dr. Taylor and his wife, Nancyellen Brennan, a family nurse practitioner, came to West Virginia in 1982. They helped establish Pendleton County Community Care, 1 of 13 national demonstration sites for community-oriented primary care. Dr. Taylor spent 13 years in Pendleton County as a "modern country doctor," practicing internal medicine without a hospital, and developing community-based programs in workplace wellness and elderly care.

Taylor became involved with the West Virginia Public Health Advisory Council and was instrumental in promoting the establishment of an MPH program "without walls" for West Virginia. In 1995, Taylor left clinical practice to earn his MPH at Johns Hopkins. There, he refined his career-long interest in "helping people in communities identify and address their own unique health issues." Central among his successes is the Public Health Transitions Project, which is helping state and local health departments focus on how to provide and pay for essential public health services for the citizens of West Virginia.

Joseph J. Valadez, PhD, MPH, ScD, is Senior Advisor for Monitoring and Evaluation in the NGO Networks for Health Project funded by USAID. He is also Health Programs Coordinator for PLAN International and a Senior Associate in the Department of International Health at the Johns Hopkins School of Hygiene and Public Health. He has more than 15 years of experience working in 36 countries and has authored or edited eight books and written numerous journal articles and monographs.

"I came to the field of public health through a circuitous route. Following an undergraduate social science degree, I studied for a PhD in International Relations in the UK at the Richardson Institute for Peace and Conflict Research. My postdoctoral studies focused on program monitoring and evaluation, and on computer simulation. In 1980, I realized that I wanted to focus my life's work on public health, and I decided to study for an MPH at the Harvard School of Public Health. During my first hour at Harvard, I met John Wyon, my advisor. When I began studying for a second doctoral degree, this one focused on international health, John Wyon again served as my advisor.

After serving on the faculty of the Harvard Institute for International Development for four years, I became the Director of Projects for the African Medical and Research Foundation, an NGO based in Nairobi, Kenya. For four years I developed and managed community-based projects in Tanzania, Sudan, Ethiopia, Uganda, and Nigeria, as well as Kenya. In 1995, I joined Johns Hopkins School of Hygiene and Public Health and worked in JHPIEGO in clinical contraception. During 1996, I returned to work with NGOs by joining Plan International but retained my affiliation with the Department of International Health at Johns Hopkins. Since that time, I have aided PLAN to apply the community-oriented approach in child survival, safe motherhood, family planning, and HIV/AIDS prevention programs throughout the world. In 1998, I was elected as the first Chairman of the Board of the Child Survival Collaborations and Resources Group, a consortium of 35 leading US private voluntary and nongovernmental organizations working in the health sector in developing countries. The members of CORE work together to improve community-based public health practice by sharing resources and experiences."

John B. Wyon, MB/BCh, MPH, is retired Senior Lecturer at the Harvard School of Public Health, where from 1953 to 1988 he was in the Department of Population Sciences and International Health. He earned his medical degrees from Gonville and Caius College, Cambridge University, and an MPH from the Harvard School of Public Health. Dr. Wyon served as a Medical Officer in Ethiopia during World War II and then as a medical missionary in Uttar Pradesh, India, from 1949 to 1952. In 1953 he became Field Director of the India-Harvard Ludhiana Population Study, better known since as the Khanna Study, which he authored—with John Gordon—in 1971. Dr. Wyon received the Distinguished Alumnus Award from Harvard School of Public Health in 1995 and, also that year, a Lifetime Achievement Award for Excellence in International Health from the American Public Health Association.

"In 1943, I was a conscientious objector to military service, but I was permitted to join a Quaker organization. They sent me to join a group already in Ethiopia. I became the only Western qualified doctor in the Province of Tigre, with a government hospital of 100 beds and six outpatient clinics for about 1 million people. Our team included about 20 fine male "dressers," the only woman nurse in Ethiopia, and two briefly trained British staff. In 1945, waiting for boat passage home, I worked in a flooded area around Calcutta. The medical conditions among the villagers were little better than in Ethiopia. I left these two experiences with the conviction that we had contributed little to these people for a limited time and with no lasting effect. I wondered how might it be possible to practice scientific medicine effectively among a poor illiterate people.

As a medical missionary, I set out with my wife for India in 1949. Our missionary society wanted us to find out how to practice medicine in rural India without a hospital. Hospitals had become too expensive. Within three months I had met Carl Taylor, another medical missionary. Two years later, I was invited to join him as an MPH student to prepare myself to work with Carl's adviser, the epidemiologist John Gordon, to test the possibility of changing the birth rate through application of birth control in some Punjabi villages. Gordon had practiced community-based epidemiology in a small town in Romania, where he had recorded an epidemic of scarlet fever from its first case.

I worked with John Gordon for 7 years in India and for 10 years at Harvard analyzing and reporting the results of the Khanna Study in 11 villages in the Punjab, India. After that, I developed a seminar at the Harvard School of Public Health called the Student Project Design Seminar. Each student had to identify a community and a problem, and report to the seminar on his or her definition and analysis of the community and how to address the selected problem in that community. Several of the students went on to implement their projects.

Since 1970, I have been closely connected with community-based projects as a consultant: in India for 2 years; in Sri Lanka for 6 years, working on malaria control with Oxfam America and the Sarvodaya Shramadana Sangamaya of Sri Lanka; and in Bolivia for 18 years, with Henry Perry and Andean Rural Health Care. Currently I am involved with the Greater Boston Interfaith Organization, which guides faith-based organizations to find common goals among their members and to pursue them. In Boston, 100 religious institutions have selected affordable housing and elementary and high-school education as their present focus. This approach has the potential to contribute to the solution of numerous public health problems."

Index

Surveillance for Equity, 20, 25
Espada, Sara, 161
Evaluation, 66–68, 197, 209, 238, 256–58, 315
Evans, Timothy, 118
Ewbank, Douglas, 136
Expanded Programme on Immunization (EPI), 40, 41, 314

F

Fairness, 22–23, 25
Family planning, 6–7, 9–10
  Bangladesh, 36, 39, 41, 65, 68, 70, 91
  Indonesia, 10
  Narangwal (India) Project, 124–26
  Nepal, 180–82, 190–91
  Tibet, 120
Farmer, Paul, 219, 274
Farmers' Clubs, 51–52
Federal grants, 276
Fees, 208
Female Community Health Volunteers (FCHVs), 123, 176
Fendall, N. R. E., 36
Fertility
  Bangladesh, 40, 77–79
  India, 48
Field area supervisors (FASs), 176, 195–97
Financing, 202–10, 258–60. *See also* Bhishi system; Fees; Funding; Sustainability
Firearms, 227
Foege, W. H., 227
Foundation for Medical Education and Research, 243
Foundations, 206, 275–76
Four Great Rivers Nature Preserve, 120
Foyers d'Apprentissage et de Réhabilitation Nutritionnelle (FARN) program, 140

Foyers de démonstration nutritionnelle (FDNs), 138–40
Framework for Assessing Health System Performance, 19–20, 24
Freire, Paulo, 63
Frenk, Julio, 19, 20
Fulmer, Hugh S., 215, 216, 218, 219
Funding, 43, 319–20
  HIV/AIDS, 275–76
  sustainability, 203–8
  vertical programs, 165
Future of Public Health report, 217, 280–82

G

Gale, J. L., 282
Geiger, H. Jack, 116, 224, 225, 290
Gender bias, 51, 68, 72–73, 79
George, Lloyd, 3
German Association for Social and Community Psychiatry, 307
Germany, 218
  health service law, 305
  psychiatry, 302–7
"Gesetz zur Reform," 305
Gibson, Count, 224
GOBI, 207, 316
Goiter, 80, 241
Gonoshasthaya Kendra, 8, 37, 208
Gordon, A. G., 282
Gordon, John E., 7, 38, 44, 170, 312
"Gossip," 131, 145
Government sector, 205–6, 210, 319–20
Grameen Bank, 37–38
Grant, James, 6, 116, 119, 126, 207, 311, 316, 321
Grant, John B., 3–4, 7, 116
Guatemala, 154

About Management Sciences for Health

Management Sciences for Health (MSH), Inc., is a private, nonprofit organization, dedicated to closing the gap between what is known about public health problems and what is done to solve them. Since 1971, MSH has worked with policymakers, health professionals, and health care consumers around the world to improve the quality, availability, and affordability of health and population services.

MSH has assisted public and private health and population programs in more than 100 countries by providing technical assistance, conducting training, carrying out research, and developing systems for program management. MSH's staff of more than 600 work in its Boston, Massachusetts, headquarters, offices in Arlington, Virginia, and field offices throughout the world.

We provide long- and short-term technical assistance through four centers of excellence: Health Services, Health Reform and Financing, Leadership and Management, and Pharmaceutical Management. Our award-winning publications and electronic products augment our assistance through the centers of excellence.

Current major efforts by MSH to address problems in public health include the following:

- MSH manages two global programs funded by the US Agency for International Development: the Management and Leadership Program and the Rational Pharmaceutical Management Plus Program. The worldwide Strategies for Enhancing Access to Medicines (SEAM) Program is funded by the Bill & Melinda Gates Foundation.
- MSH is the managing partner of the Partnership for Child Health Care, Inc., which implements USAID's principal child survival project, Basic Support for Institutionalizing Child Survival (BASICS II). MSH also manages the consortium that carries out Advance Africa, a major program for integrating

365

and scaling up family planning and reproductive health services in Africa.

- MSH is carrying out several national projects, including three
  in Africa (Guinea, Senegal, and South Africa), two in Latin
  America and the Caribbean (Haiti and Nicaragua), four in
  Asia (Bangladesh, India, and two in the Philippines), and one
  in the Newly Independent States (Georgia).